Optometric Management of Nearpoint Vision Disorders

Optometric Management of Nearpoint Vision Disorders

Martin H. Birnbaum, O.D.
Clinical Professor

State University of New York, State College of Optometry,
New York, New York

Butterworth-Heinemann
Boston London Oxford Singapore Sydney Toronto Wellington

Library of Congress Cataloging-in-Publication Data

Birnbaum, Martin H., 1937–
    Optometric management of nearpoint vision disorders / Martin H.
Birnbaum.
        p.   cm.
    Includes bibliographical references and index.
    ISBN 0-7506-9193-X (hardcover : alk. paper)
    1. Behavioral optometry. 2. Visual training. 3. Myopia. I. Title.
    [DNLM: 1. Eyeglasses. 2. Models, Biological. 3. Myopia—
therapy. 4. Vision Disorders—therapy.   WW 320 B619o]
    RE960.B57 1993
    617.7'55—dc20
    DNLM/DLC
    for Library of Congress   92-16159
                                                                          CIP

British Library Cataloging-in-Publication Data

A catalogue record for this book is available from the British Library.

Butterworth–Heinemann
313 Washington Street
Newton, MA 02158–1626

10 9 8 7 6

Printed in the United States of America

To my wife, Phyllis, my parents, and my daughters Jill, Gail, and Andrea, with thanks for their love and support.

Optometry is the discipline of vision. What its boundaries will be depends upon what the word *vision* means to the profession.

A.M. Skeffington, May 1974

Where there is no vision, the people perish.

Proverbs, 29:18

Contents

Preface

When I entered optometric practice in 1962, I encountered many clinical phenomena that seemed inconsistent with what I had learned in school. I saw patients who developed myopia at age 19 or 20, well past the age at which I had been taught that myopia progression usually ceases. I saw patients with asthenopic symptoms, but no apparent visual problem, and others with severe functional vision disorder, but no symptoms. I saw patients who demonstrated exophoria on cover test, but showed esophoria on the von Graefe phoria measure, esophoric shifts during cheiroscopic tracing, or esophoric fixation disparity. I saw patients with convergence insufficiency who shifted into esophoria and convergence excess as vision therapy proceeded. I saw patients with reading or learning difficulties who wished to determine whether vision disorder might be a cause; although I frequently found no significant vision disorder, I was not confident that my knowledge was sufficient to rule out vision-related factors. As a consequence of these experiences, I felt insecure and inadequate. Since I was resolved to provide the very best care possible, I sought to expand my understanding of vision in order to resolve these uncertainties and be better able to care for patients.

Shortly after entering practice, I joined the staff of the Optometric Center of New York and began to learn vision therapy under the tutelage of Dr. William Ludlam, then chairman of the department. In subsequent years, my horizons expanded through interaction with colleagues at the Optometric Center and its descendent, the State University of New York College of Optometry, particularly Drs. Elliott Forrest, Nathan Flax, Irwin Suchoff, Richard Kavner, Arnold Sherman, and Myron Weinstein.

In my interaction with these individuals, as well as with vision therapy authorities who visited the Optometric Center from time to time, I frequently encountered three concepts that seemed so at odds with my traditional education that I experienced simultaneous confusion, insecurity, and a desire to know and understand more. These concepts were (1) the Skeffington model of nearpoint stress, which holds that a drive for convergence to localize closer than accommodation, intrinsic to the near-work demands of our culture, interferes with nearpoint visual efficiency and leads to the development of a broad variety of vision disorders; (2) the notion that individuals with normal visual acuity and binocular function may nevertheless demonstrate visual-perceptual-motor deficits that interfere with reading and with classroom performance, and that such deficits may result from interference with development; and (3) that visual function may both have an impact on and be influenced by patterns of organismic behavior related to visual information-processing and cognitive-perceptual style, personality, and motor and spatial organization.

These concepts, that vision disorders may arise from nearpoint stress or from interference with development, and that such disorders relate closely to broader aspects of behavior, are fundamental tenets of behavioral optometry and are closely associated with the Optometric Extension Program (OEP). In my quest to expand my understanding of vision and its disorders, I joined an OEP study group, attended OEP Congresses, and began to read the monthly OEP papers. As my understanding of OEP models expanded, I found increasingly that these models explained clinical phenomena that had previously seemed paradoxical. The frequency with which clinical observations were found to be consistent with OEP concepts led to increasing confidence in these models. My confidence in the OEP model increased still further when I discovered, as reported in Chapter 3, that Skeffington's nearpoint stress theory is consistent with and explainable on the basis of general stress physiology. Ultimately, the OEP model became the foundation of my approach to clinical practice, guiding clinical care and providing a framework for predicting the respective outcomes if recommended regimens were or were not followed.

In undertaking this project, my intention was to write a comprehensive textbook on nearpoint stress-induced and developmental vision disorders, their behavioral consequences, and their diagnosis and treatment. My goal was to write a text that would facilitate growth and development in behavioral optometry for the student, recent graduate, and established practitioner seeking to expand knowledge and services in this area. Unfortunately, it proved impossible to cover the subject comprehensively in a single text. Therefore I have largely ignored strabismus, amblyopia, and visual-perceptual-motor deficits in order to focus on the diagnosis and management of nearpoint vision disorders.

Traditional and near-work models of nearpoint stress are discussed in Part I; the clinical case analysis systems that derive from these models are described in Part II. Thus, traditional phoria-vergence demand/reserve theories and more recent fixation disparity/vergence adaptation models are described in Chapter 1; case analysis based on these models is discussed in Chapter 7. The Skeffington nearpoint stress model is presented in Chapters 3 and 4; the OEP system of case analysis, derived from the Skeffington model, is presented in Chapter 8. Various other methods for determining the optimal nearpoint lens prescription are presented in Chapter 9. Harmon's model, emphasizing postural and spacial factors in the ediology of vision disorder, is presented in Chapter 5, and the use-abuse theory is reviewed in Chapter 2. Chapter 10 reviews research on the efficacy of low plus lens prescription for near use. Supplementary tests of ocular motility and binocular and accommodative function are described in Part III, and vision therapy models, principles, regimens, procedures, and sequences, as well as a review of the literature on the efficacy of vision therapy, are presented in Part IV.

The management of nearpoint vision disorders is, for me, the heart of optometric practice, and indeed constitutes much of that which is unique to optometry. Although these disorders are widely prevalent, they are commonly ignored; yet they frequently impose major limitations on human potential and achievement. For me, one of the most satisfying experiences is to successfully treat a child with academic difficulty resulting from functional vision disorder, or one whose visual dysfunction leads to disinterest or avoidance of near work, and to see that child develop into a high-achiever, or begin to enjoy reading. This satisfaction is heightened by the knowledge that in many offices such vision disorders go undetected, or go untreated even if detected. It is my hope that this book will in some measure contribute to the care of such patients. Management of these disorders is, in my view, an essential element of high-quality optometric care, and I hope that this text will serve as a useful resource for doctors seeking to provide such care.

Although my clinical experience has led me to accept the validity of many tenets of the OEP, this book is in no way an OEP text. I have attempted to present each of the major theoretic models of nearpoint vision disorder, to illuminate their commonalities and differences, and to indicate the differences in approach to nearpoint lens prescription and vision therapy that derive from these theoretic differences. It is my belief that knowledge of each of the existing models will best allow clinicians to determine which are most consistent with clinical experience and therefore most useful. I believe that practitioners who know and understand the similarities and differences of the various models will find, as I have, that the OEP model explains and predicts many clinical phenomena that appear inconsistent with traditional models.

In closing, I would like to acknowledge the influence of several individuals who have especially contributed to my growth and development: Dr. A.M. Skeffington, the father of behavioral optometry, with whom I unfortunately had little direct contact, but whose breadth of vision and creative thinking make him one of the greatest innovators in the history of our profession; Dr. Elliott B. Forrest, friend, mentor, and guide, who more than anyone else taught me to look at patient care from a functional perspective; Dr. Alden N. Haffner, President of the State University of New York College of Optometry, whose invitation to join the staff of the Optometric Center of New York in 1962 was to shape my professional career, and whose earliest injunction to me was "Never be afraid to question established ideas!"; Dr. William Ludlam, who tutored me, shared with me, and encouraged me to grow; Drs. Nathan Flax and Robert A. Kraskin, whose lectures and writing profoundly influenced my approach to vision therapy; Dr. Stanley Eisenberg, who through his commitment to professional optometry and his dedication to his patients served as an important role model; and Dr. Irwin B. Suchoff, who has always been a source of strength and support.

I would also like to thank the many individuals whose assistance has been invaluable over the course of this project: the Administration of the State University of New York College of Optometry, which provided resources, encouragement, and support; the College librarians, who assisted in so many ways so many times; Drs. Nathan Flax, Ronald Bateman, Robert Duckman, and Barry Tannen, each of whom was most helpful in critiquing sections of an early draft and making suggestions; Martin Topaz of Professional Press, who initiated this project; my editors at Butterworth–Heinemann, Barbara Murphy and Kathleen Higgins, and production editor, Susan Geraghty, whose assistance has been of inestimable value in guiding the text toward publication; Wayne Grofik, Diane Schiumo, and Steve Goodman of the State University of New York College of Optometry Media Center, and my daughter Andrea Birnbaum, who provided the artwork and photography; Robert Williams, Executive Director of the Optometric Extension Program Foundation, who was exceedingly helpful in supplying various materials; my colleagues on the College faculty and behavioral optometrists throughout the world who encouraged me and indicated their belief in the importance of the project; and the numerous individuals in my office and at the College who provided typing and word-processing services, including Jean Cahill, Jennifer Fulgenzi, Randy L. Schulman, Wendy Thomas, and my wife, Phyllis. Finally, I would like especially to thank my wife, Phyllis, whose support and encouragement have meant so much to me during the periods of frustration, stress, and discouragement that accompany a project of this magnitude.

PART I

Models of Nearpoint Stress

Since its earliest days, optometry has been concerned with nearpoint visual function. Various models and theories have been proposed to determine the cause and remediation of discomfort and inefficiency during near work.

Traditional models attribute discomfort and inefficient performance to anomalies of refraction, vergence, and accommodation, and hold that such disorders result primarily from heredity, random biologic variation, and various anatomic and physiologic influences. These models give rise to care regimens that emphasize correcting significant refractive error and identifying and treating vergence and accommodative disorder.

Early case analysis systems such as those of Sheard (1917) and Percival (1928) (both still in common use) emphasize the relationship between fusional demand and reserves. In recent years, the trend has been toward analysis of findings obtained during binocular function, especially fixation disparity measures at varying levels of vergence demand.

In contrast with these traditional approaches, various models attribute the development of vision disorder and asthenopic symptoms to the extensive nearwork demands imposed by our society. Skeffington's (1928–74) nearpoint stress model holds that asthenopia and a broad variety of refractive, vergence, and accommodative disorders arise because near work creates demands that are inconsistent with our physiology. The use-abuse theory holds that myopia is caused by extensive near work. Harmon (1958) emphasizes the relation between vision, posture, and spatial relations, and theorizes that numerous disorders, especially myopia, anisometropia, astigmatism, and hyperphoria, result from performing near work under conditions that create postural distortion. These near-work models lead to therapeutic regimens that stress prevention, as well as remediation, and which emphasize determination of the optimal lens prescription and environmental conditions to minimize stress on the visual system during near work.

Traditional and near-work theories of nearpoint stress are discussed in Part I. Traditional phoria/vergence, demand/reserve theories, and more recent fixation disparity/vergence adaptation models are described in Chapter 1. The use-abuse theory is presented in Chapter 2, and Skeffington's nearpoint stress model in Chapters 3 and 4. Harmon's theory, and derivative recommendations for minimizing postural stress during near work, is presented in Chapter 5.

REFERENCES

Harmon DB (1958). *Notes on a Dynamic Theory of Vision*. 3rd rev. ed. Austin, TX: author.

Percival A (1928). *The Prescribing of Spectacles*. 3rd ed. York: William Wood.

Sheard C (1917). *Dynamic Ocular Tests*. Columbus, OH: Lawrence Press, pp. 58–85.

Skeffington AM (1928–74). *Optometric Extension Program Continuing Education Courses*. Santa Ana, CA: Optometric Extension Program Foundation.

1

Vergence Stress Models

In traditional models, refractive deviation, high heterophoria, fixation disparity, convergence and divergence dysfunction, and anomalies of accommodation are viewed as potential sources of asthenopia, to be treated when they cause significant symptoms.

Anomalies of binocular and accommodative function are attributed to a variety of anatomic, innervational, and pathologic causes, including heredity, random biologic variation, abnormal accommodative-convergence to accommodation (AC/A) ratio, paralysis, ciliary involvement, toxemia, hypoxia, hypertonicity, muscle weakness, fatigue, and systemic disease (Borish 1970).

The *Duane-White classification* (Duane 1896–97; White 1941) organizes vergence disorders into four categories. This system was originally applied to strabismus, but was extended by Tait (1951) to cover nonstrabismic binocular vision anomalies. The major categories are

1. Convergence insufficiency
   - orthophoria or low exophoria at distance
   - high exophoria at near
2. Convergence excess
   - orthophoria or moderate esophoria at distance
   - marked esophoria at near
3. Divergence insufficiency
   - marked esophoria at distance
   - less esophoria at near
4. Divergence excess
   - marked exophoria at distance
   - equal or less exophoria at near

Maddox (1907) presented the concept that various factors contribute to vergence innervation, and that vergence may be considered as the sum of several components:

- tonic vergence (resulting from tonic innervation to the extraocular muscles);

- accommodative vergence (vergence associated with accommodation);
- proximal vergence (vergence induced by nearness of the target);
- fusional vergence (vergence induced by retinal disparity).

Sheard (1917, 1920) extended Maddox's concepts and applied them clinically, suggesting that heterophoria at near occurs when the sum of tonic, accommodative, and proximal vergence is inadequate or excessive for any particular working distance. The near phoria that results is compensated by the opposing fusional vergence. Inability to compensate for heterophoria with adequate fusional vergence is viewed as a source of discomfort and an indication of need for therapy.

Treatment systems derived from traditional models assume that phorias measured at distance and near reflect fusional demand at those distances, and that prism vergence measures indicate the fusional reserve available to overcome this demand. The Percival (1928) and Sheard (1930) criteria for prescription of prism, as well as graphical approaches to case analysis developed by Neumeuller (1946), Fry (1937, 1939, 1943), and Hofstetter (1945, 1968), are based on this reserve/demand concept. These approaches to case analysis are discussed in Chapter 7.

PRISM ADAPTATION AND VERGENCE STRESS

Current models have moved beyond sole consideration of phoria/vergence relationships to explore more subtle aspects of binocular vision. The mechanisms most prominently considered are those related to prism adaptation, fixation disparity, and interactions between accommodation and convergence.

Substantial changes in the phoria, fixation disparity, and prism vergence findings follow prolonged viewing through base-in or base-out prisms. These measures frequently change so as to reestablish (with the prisms in place) the values originally obtained without prism (Carter 1965).

This phenomenon, known as *prism adaptation* or *vergence adaptation*, is characterized by an adaptive change in tonic vergence, which serves to reduce stress on the fusional vergence system (Schor 1983a). When fixation is changed from one distance to another, a fusional vergence movement is required to achieve ocular realignment and single vision. Schor reports that two separate systems mediate these fusional vergence movements, the fast- and slow-fusional vergence systems.

Fast-fusional vergence acts quickly to reduce disparity, achieving single vision within 1 second. However, once fusion is obtained, there is a tendency toward rapid decay of the fast-fusional vergence innervation. Consequently, the second system, slow-fusional vergence, comes into play to reduce stress on the fast-fusional vergence system and to maintain alignment.

Slow-fusional vergence is slower-acting, requiring at least 30 seconds. Slow-fusional vergence is not generated by retinal disparity; it occurs well after disparity has been nulled by fast-fusional vergence. Rather it appears that slow-fusional vergence is induced by the output, or effort, of the fast-fusional vergence system.

Although slow-fusional vergence is slower-acting, it does not decay rapidly. Its effects are long-lasting, producing changes in tonic vergence that supplant the rapid decay of fast-fusion innervation.

Schor (1983a) indicates that vergence adaptation is mediated by and is in fact synonymous with slow-fusional vergence. When vergence adaptation ability is inadequate, the need to continuously replenish the rapidly decaying fast-fusional vergence innervation creates excessive stress on that system and consequently inefficient binocular function.

Carter (1965) proposed prism adaptation as the basic adaptive mechanism to maintain approximate orthophoria in patients with normal binocular vision, a process known as *orthophorization*. Carter notes that sensory fusion is necessary for such adaptation to take place, and suggests that subjects who are incapable of adaptation may lack normal sensory fusion and be more susceptible to high heterophoria.

The adaptation system is deficient in most patients with abnormal binocular vision and asthenopia. North and Henson (1981) found that subjects with binocular anomalies that result in asthenopic symptoms almost invariably have abnormal adaptation mechanisms.

FIXATION DISPARITY

Many individuals demonstrate *fixation disparity*, a small misalignment from bifoveal fixation that exists under fused conditions. Diplopia does not occur, since Panum's fusional limits are not exceeded.

Fixation disparity has been held to occur when the vergence response lags behind the fusional demand imposed by a high phoria, in the presence of inadequate fusion ability (Mallett 1974). It has also been viewed as a normal phenomenon analogous to lag of accommodation, existing as a so-called lazy vergence lag whereby an individual maintains single vision with minimal vergence effort. It has also been suggested that fixation disparity represents an intermediate step between normal binocular vision and strabismus or microstrabismus (Jampolsky et al. 1957).

In contrast with these notions, which view fixation disparity as resulting from stress on the vergence system, it has been suggested that fixation disparity is a purposeful error that serves to reduce vergence stress (Ogle and Prangen 1953; Schor 1983a). Schor suggests that fixation disparity provides a purposeful steady-state error that relieves vergence stress by providing a stimulus to replenish decaying fusional vergence innervation. Fast-fusional responses are initiated and maintained by retinal disparity. Precise alignment eliminates the stimulus necessary for fast-fusion, which then decays until retinal disparity reaches a magnitude that stimulates additional fusional vergence innervation. This fixation disparity, Schor suggests, is then maintained as a constant stimulus to prevent further decay of fast-fusional vergence innervation.

Vergence adaptation (slow-fusional vergence) and fixation disparity are, in this view, alternative mechanisms for maintaining fusional vergence and single vision. Vergence adaptation alters tonic vergence to reduce demand on the fast-fusion system. When vergence adaptation ability is adequate, a steady-state stimulus such as fixation disparity is therefore unnecessary, and fixation disparity is small or absent. When vergence adaptation ability is inadequate, fixation disparity provides a constant stimulus for fast-fusional vergence innervation (Schor 1983a).

Fixation disparity and vergence adaptation thus exhibit a reciprocal relationship. Fixation disparity tends to be small or absent when vergence adaptation is adequate, and to be greater when vergence adaptation is poor. Forced vergence fixation disparity curves are used to evaluate vergence adaptation. The curves are generated by measuring the fixation disparity induced as prism base-in and base-out and are added to stimulate fusional vergence. Adequate vergence adaptation is generally associated with asymptomatic binocular vision (Schor 1983a).

Evidence that adequate vergence adaptation ability is characteristic of individuals with normal binocular function is found in studies of the effect of sustained close work on the horizontal forced vergence fixation disparity curve. Asymptomatic subjects with normal binocular vision showed no significant changes in fixation disparity or shape of the curve following 25 minutes of continuous reading. Symptomatic subjects with large fixation disparities or steep forced vergence curves developed even more distinctively abnormal fixation disparity curves after sustained reading (Garzia and Dyer 1986).

These findings imply that individuals with normal binocular function have adequate vergence adaptation. Such individuals suffer little adverse effect from near work and are likely to be asymptomatic. Individuals with binocular vision disorders, in contrast, are likely to demonstrate poor vergence adaptation. Such individuals are more likely to exhibit deterioration of function following near work, and are more prone to asthenopic symptoms.

ACCOMMODATIVE-CONVERGENCE/ CONVERGENCE-ACCOMMODATION INTERACTIONS

The demands on accommodation and fusional vergence are increased by mutual interaction between accommodative-convergence (AC) and convergence-accommodation (CA), which takes place under fused conditions. When the relationship between vergence and accommodation is such that accommodation generates more convergence than is appropriate for the task distance, a demand is created for negative fusional vergence. However, this innervation for negative vergence also acts, via convergence-accommodation, to reduce the accommodative response. This reduction of accommodation induces blur, leading to increased innervation for accommodation, which in turn stimulates more accommodative-convergence and results in increased esophoria. Additional negative fusional vergence is required, which again, through activation of convergence-accommodation, reduces accommodative response so that greater innervation is required for positive accommodation to reduce blur, again generating accommodative-convergence and progressive increase in esophoria. This ongoing cross-linked interaction between accommodative-convergence and convergence-accommodation continues until equilibrium is reached, creating progressively greater demand on accommodation and fusional divergence. As a result of this interaction, the demand on fusional vergence under fused conditions is always greater than predicted by the dissociated phoria, and the demand on accommodation is always greater than predicted on the basis of target distance (Semmlow and Heerema 1979; Schor and Narayan 1982; Schor 1983a, 1983b, 1985).

In patients with normal vergence adaptation, the effect of these interactions is transient. Vergence adaptation that alters tonic vergence does not stimulate cross-linked interactions (Schor and Kotulak 1986). Therefore, as adaptive vergence innervation replaces fusional vergence innervation, there is a reduction in convergence-accommodation and hence less interactive effect. However, when vergence adaptation is reduced or absent, these interactive effects increase fusional vergence demand well beyond that measured by the dissociated phoria (Schor 1983a).

When vergence adaptation is weak or lacking, as a consequence, the fast fusional vergence requirement is heightened and the convergence-accommodation to convergence (CA/C) ratio elevated. Similarly, when accommodative adaptation is weak, the AC/A ratio will be high (Schor 1988).

When accommodation and vergence show essentially equal capacity for adaptation, the cross-link interactions described by the AC/A and CA/C ratios will be moderate in value. Abnormally high and abnormally low AC/A and CA/C values, according to Schor (1988), result from an imbalance between the adaptation mechanisms of accommodation and vergence. Frequently the amplitudes of the AC/A and CA/C ratios are inversely related, one being high and the other low as a result of unequal adaptation of the two motor systems (Schor 1986, 1988). When vergence adapts readily but accommodation does not, individuals demonstrate high AC/A and low CA/C ratios. When accommodation is more adaptable than vergence, the CA/C is high and the AC/A low (Schor and Tsuetaki 1987).

Schor (1988) suggests that, in cases of convergence and divergence excess and insufficiency, the fundamental cause may not be the large heterophoria, but rather an underlying disorder of adaptation of vergence or accommodation, particularly an imbalance of adaptation in these systems, which leads to abnormally high or low accommodation/vergence interaction. Thus, for example, a patient who demonstrates excessive adaptability of accommodation and insufficient adaptability of convergence would be expected to have a low AC/A ratio and a high CA/C ratio, and to demonstrate convergence insufficiency (Tsuetaki and Schor 1987).

Wick (1985) indicates that proximal vergence, although often neglected, also plays an important role in the near vergence response, contributing as much or more than accommodative vergence. The patient with high proximal vergence may have greater esophoria under actual near-work conditions, when reading or writing, than is measured clinically under either fused or dissociated conditions. Thus, proximal vergence and AC/CA interactions each contribute to an esophoric tendency under fused conditions that may be greater than indicated by the dissociated near phoria test.

SUMMARY

Optometry has long been concerned with the remediation of nearpoint vision disorders that cause asthenopia. Traditional models attribute vergence and accommodative dysfunction to heredity, random biologic variation, and disease. Sheard viewed heterophoria as a demand on fusional vergence; Sheard's and Percival's criteria for comfort, as well as graphical approaches to case analysis, are based on this concept of fusional demand and compensatory fusional vergence reserves. More recent models of vergence stress are concerned with fixation disparity, vergence adaptation, proximal vergence, and mutual interactions between vergence and accommodation that occur during binocular fused conditions.

SUGGESTED READING

Borish IM (1970). *Clinical Refraction.* 3rd ed. Chicago: Professional Press.
Schor CM (1983). Fixation disparity and vergence adaptation. In: Schor CM, Ciuffreda KJ (eds), *Vergence Eye Movements: Basic and Clinical Aspects.* Boston: Butterworth–Heinemann, pp. 465–516.

REFERENCES

Borish IM (1970). *Clinical Refraction.* 3rd ed. Chicago: Professional Press.
Carter DB (1965). Fixation disparity and heterophoria following prolonged wearing of prisms. *Am J Optom Arch Am Acad Optom* 42:141–152.
Duane A (1896–97). A new classification of the motor anomalies of the eye, based upon physiologic principles. *Ann Ophthalmol Otol* Part I, Oct 1896; Part II, Jan 1897.
Fry GA (1937). An experimental analysis of the accommodation-convergence relation. *Am J Optom* 14(11):402–424.
Fry GA (1939). Further experiments on the accommodation-convergence relation. *Am J Optom* 16(9):325–336.
Fry GA (1943). Fundamental variables in relationship between accommodation and convergence. *Optom Weekly* 34:153, 183.
Garzia RP, Dyer G (1986). Effects of nearpoint stress on the horizontal forced vergence fixation disparity curve. *Am J Optom Physiol Opt* 63(11):901–907.
Hofstetter HW (1945). The zone of clear single binocular vision, *Am J Optom Arch Am Acad Optom* 22(7):301–333; 22(8):361–384.

Hofstetter HW (1968). A revised schematic for graphical analysis of the accommodative convergence relationship. *Can J Optom* 30(2):49–52.

Jampolsky A, Flom B, Fried A (1957). Fixation disparity in relation to heterophoria. *Am J Ophthalmol* 43:97–106.

Maddox EE (1907). *The Ocular Muscles*. 2nd ed. Philadelphia: Keystone, p. 227.

Mallett RFJ (1974). Fixation disparity—Its genesis in relation to asthenopia. *Ophthalmic Optician* 14:1159–1168.

Neumueller JF (1946). The correlation of optometric binocular measurements for refractive diagnosis. *Am J Optom Arch Am Acad Optom* 23(6):235–259.

North R, Henson DB (1981). Adaptation to prism-induced heterophoria in subjects with abnormal binocular vision or asthenopia. *Am J Optom Physiol Opt* 58(9):774–780.

Ogle KN, Prangen A (1953). Observations of vertical divergences and hyperphorias. *Arch Ophthalmol* 49:313–334.

Percival A (1928). *The Prescribing of Spectacles*. 3rd ed. New York: William Wood.

Schor CM (1983a). Fixation disparity and vergence adaptation. In: Schor CM, Cuifreda KJ (eds), *Vergence Eye Movements: Basic and Clinical Aspects*. Boston: Butterworth–Heinemann pp. 465–516.

Schor CM (1983b). Analysis of tonic and accommodative vergence disorders of binocular vision. *Am J Optom Physiol Opt* 60(1):1–14.

Schor CM (1985). Models of mutual interactions between accommodation and convergence. *Am J Optom Physiol Opt* 62:369–374.

Schor CM (1986). The Glenn A. Fry Award Lecture: Adaptive regulation of accommodative vergence and vergence accommodation. *Am J Optom Physiol Opt* 63:587–609.

Schor CM (1988). Imbalanced adaptation of accommodation and vergence produces opposite extremes of the AC/A and CA/C ratios. *Am J Optom Physiol Opt* 65(5):341–348.

Schor CM, Kotulak J (1986). Dynamic interactions between accommodation and convergence are velocity sensitive. *Vision Res* 26:927–942.

Schor CM, Narayan V (1982). Graphical analysis of prism adaptation, convergence accommodation and accommodative convergence. *Am J Optom Physiol Opt* 59:774–784.

Schor CM, Tsuetaki T (1987). Fatigue of accommodation and vergence modifies their mutual interactions. *Invest Ophthalmol Vis Sci* 28:1250–1259.

Semmlow JL, Heerema D (1979). The synkinetic interaction of convergence accommodation and accommodation convergence. *Vision Res* 19:1237–1242.

Sheard C (1917). *Dynamic Ocular Tests*. Columbus, OH: Lawrence Press, pp. 58–85.

Sheard C (1920). Accommodative exophoria or the accommodation associated with the act of convergence. *Am J Physiol Opt* 1:234–249.

Sheard C (1930). Zones of ocular comfort. *Am J Optom* 7(1):9–25.

Tait EF (1951). Accommodative convergence. *Am J Ophthalmol* 34:1093–1107.

Tsuetaki TK, Schor CM (1987). Clinical method for measuring adaptation of tonic accommodation and vergence accommodation. *Am J Optom Physiol Opt* 64(6):437–449.

White JW (1941). The screen test and its modifications. *Am J Ophthalmol* 24:156–160.

Wick B (1985). Clinical factors in proximal vergence. *Am J Optom Physiol Opt* 62(1):1–18.

2

Myopia and the Use-Abuse Theory

In contrast with traditional models that attribute nearpoint dysfunction to disorders of the accommodative and vergence systems, to random biologic variation, and to genetic and pathologic factors, near-work theories emphasize the adverse influence of the extensive near-vision demands imposed by our society. Near-work theories hold that the visual system is biologically unsuited for the sustained near-work demands of our culture, and that repeated exposure to such demands leads to the development of vision disorders.

Two major near-work theories exist: the *use-abuse* theory and *Skeffington's nearpoint stress* theory. The use-abuse theory is specific to myopia, attributing myopia to abuse of the visual system caused by excessive use of the eyes for close work. Skeffington's model, to be discussed in Chapter 3, holds that not only myopia, but also a broad variety of vision disorders occur because the nearpoint tasks imposed by our culture are incompatible with human physiology.

Myopia is a source of considerable concern to both patients and practitioners. Myopia creates greater anxiety than other refractive disorders because of its strong tendency to progress, with reduction in unaided acuity and increasing dependence on glasses. As myopia progresses from year to year, many patients become increasingly fearful that at some point visual correction may no longer be possible, with ultimate visual loss or blindness.

Although myopia is indeed a leading cause of blindness (National Society for the Prevention of Blindness 1966; Kahn and Moorhead 1969–70; National Eye Institute 1976; Curtin 1985, pp. 7–10), fears of visual disability are usually ill-founded, since the greatest incidence of myopia-related ocular disease occurs in high-degree pathologic myopia (Curtin 1985, pp. 7–10, 277–385), which is relatively infrequent (Curtin 1985, pp. 237–238). However, even low degrees of myopia are associated with increased incidence of eye disease, particularly glaucoma and retinal detachment (Perkins 1979, Curtin 1985, pp. 173–174, 179–182); consequently, Curtin emphasizes the importance of careful evaluation of eye health in all myopes, particularly with regard to retinal status and intraocular pressure, regardless of the degree of myopia or the age of the patient.

Patients and clinicians may seek to control progression of myopia to improve unaided visual acuity, to reduce dependence on glasses, to prevent the need

11

for increasingly thick lenses, and to prevent the axial stretching of the globe that is associated with increased risk of ocular disease. Clinicians and researchers have long debated the merit of programs to treat, prevent, or control myopia. Disagreement over the potential for myopia control is rooted in controversy as to the causes of myopia progression. Myopia has been ascribed to heredity, random biological variation, nutritional and metabolic disorders, psychological factors, and near work. Theories of myopia etiology have been reviewed by Baldwin (1967, 1981), Morgan (1967), Borish (1970), Birnbaum (1979), Gottlieb (1982), and Curtin (1985, pp. 61–151). Authorities who attribute myopia to biologic and genetic factors generally minimize the potential for control (Borish 1970; Hirsch 1979; Goss 1982; Grosvenor 1989), while those who emphasize environmental factors often advocate regimens to control these factors in order to prevent or slow myopia progression (Skeffington 1952; Roberts and Banford 1967; Oakley and Young 1975; Birnbaum 1979).

MYOPIA AND NEAR WORK

The use-abuse theory holds that myopia results from excessive use of the eyes for near work. This theory is often attributed to Cohn (1867), who ascribed myopia to repetitive overuse of accommodation. He stressed school work and other intense close work as causative environmental factors. Other variations of this theory emphasize the roles of convergence, gravity, and posture as etiologic agents.

Widespread literacy is a recent development in the history of humankind. The industrial revolution and more recent technological advances have led to an evolved society in which books, magazines, journals, newspapers, and other forms of written communication, as well as computers and video display terminals, play an ever-increasing and important role in daily life. Theories that attribute vision disorders to the near-work demands of our society are based on the premise that the human visual system is biologically unsuited for these demands.

The notion of an association between myopia and near work dates back to the observations of Kepler (1611), Ware (1813), and Donders (1864). Although most authorities would agree with Borish (1970) that the relative influence of biological and environmental factors in the production of myopia is not yet clear, recent years have seen increasing evidence that near work plays a significant role.

It is well established that myopia increases in prevalence and degree throughout the school years (Donders 1864; Cohn 1867; Agnew 1877; Tscherning 1883; Straub 1909; Kempf et al. 1928; Sorsby 1932; Tassman 1932; Brown 1938; Slataper 1950; Hirsch 1952, 1961, 1962, 1964; Baldwin 1957, 1967; Morgan 1967; Goldschmidt 1968; Maliuta 1972). Hallett (1931), Luckeish and Moss (1939), and Kephart and Unger (1953) reported an absence of myopia progression in students during the months of summer vacation. However, Hirsch (1952, 1955) did not find this phenomenon.

Although it has been argued that the development of so-called school myopia during childhood may relate to growth factors rather than to near work, numerous studies document that myopes read more and perform a greater volume of near work than nonmyopes (Ochapovsky 1935; Lundgren 1954; Young et al. 1954; Haines 1955; Morgan 1960; Peckham et al. 1977; Angle and Wissman 1978; Richler and Bear 1980). However, Nadell et al. (1957) found no relation between distribution of refractive state and amount of reading.

Young et al. (1969) examined three generations of Eskimo families. They found little myopia among the parents and grandparents, but found a high incidence, approximately 65%, among the younger generation. They attribute the higher incidence of myopia in the younger generation to increased exposure to near work resulting from the introduction of compulsory education.

Critics of the use-abuse theory offer different interpretations of the association between myopia and close work. Some argue that myopes read more because of their reduced distance visual acuity, that is, that they are better suited for near work by virtue of being myopic (Borish 1970, p. 88). They suggest that individuals do not become myopic because they read more, but rather that they read more because they are myopic. Clinically, however, it is found that among those myopes who are intense readers, the interest in reading typically precedes the onset of myopia. It is rarely noted that an individual who was not an avid reader before becomes one as a result of myopia development.

Peckham et al. (1977) and Curtin (1985, pp. 10–14) suggest that the tendency for myopes to read more than nonmyopes stems from parental influences. Families with history of myopia may encourage close work and influence attitudes toward education.

Academically, myopes tend to achieve at higher levels than nonmyopes. Superior reading ability and scholastic achievement have been reported (Ochapovsky 1935; Schwartz 1940; Dearborn and Leverett 1945; Young 1963; Baldwin 1967, 1981; Goldschmidt 1968; Dunphy et al. 1968; Grosvenor 1971; Karlsson 1973; Peckham et al. 1977).

Some authorities suggest that the superior educational achievement demonstrated by myopes may occur because they are better suited for close work by virtue of being myopic (Morgan 1967; Borish 1970). However, Peckham et al. (1977) found that high academic achievement precedes the onset of myopia in most cases. Curtin (1985, pp. 10–14) suggests that the greater academic achievement demonstrated by myopes results from their personality traits and from greater scholarship reinforcement at home by myopic parents.

Myopes generally score higher than nonmyopes on intelligence tests (Nadell and Hirsch 1958; Hirsch 1959; Young 1963; Grosvenor 1970; Teasdale et al. 1988). Myopes demonstrate better visual perceptual skills than nonmyopes, and are more analytical in spatial judgments (Rosner and Gruber 1985). Myopes also tend to reach higher educational levels than nonmyopes (Teasdale et al. 1988). However, several authors suggest that the higher scores achieved by myopes on intelligence tests do not arise from a true difference in intelligence, but rather that myopes are better suited for near work and demonstrate superior reading ability (Nadell and Hirsch 1958; Hirsch 1959; Baldwin 1967, 1981; Grosvenor 1971).

Indirect evidence that myopia development is associated with near work is found in numerous studies that report reduction in myopia progression with bifocals and cycloplegic agents. These studies are summarized in Chapter 10, and have been reviewed by Greenspan (1981), Goss (1982), and Curtin (1985, pp. 217–225).

Further evidence that use of the eyes influences refractive status is found in studies of refractive change in individuals, primarily those with strabismic amblyopia or unilateral corneal scarring, who use one eye for fixation. These studies demonstrate a tendency for the habitually fixing eye to shift toward myopia, whereas the nonfixing eye shows little or no change in refraction (Falkenberg and Straub 1893; Widmark 1902; Lepard 1975; Hentsch and Frank 1977; Lefferstra, 1977). Women engaged in industrial monocular microscopy show a similar tendency to develop myopia unilaterally in the habitually used eye (Tatevosyan 1968).

A restricted nearpoint visual environment has also been reported to induce myopia development in laboratory animals. Young (1961) reported that monkeys confined in cages with hoods that limited vision to within 20 inches developed greater myopia than those raised in laboratory cages without visual restriction, and that monkeys raised wild developed even less myopia than did those raised in cages. Animals maintained under cycloplegia in a restricted nearpoint environment did not develop myopia, suggesting an accommodative basis (Young 1965). Similarly, cats caged under near vision conditions showed a much greater incidence of myopia than did street cats (Rose et al. 1974; Belkin et al. 1977).

Adult-Onset Myopia

It was once thought that myopia progression typically ceased by age 16 to 18. However, recent research and clinical experience indicate that myopia progression frequently continues into the 20s and beyond in college students, and in those engaged in occupations that require extensive near work. Riffenburgh (1965) reported the occurrence of adult-onset myopia in nine subjects aged 20 and older engaged in intensive near work.

Numerous studies document a greater incidence of myopia and greater tendency toward myopia progression among adults engaged in occupations that require substantial close work, such as writers, typesetters, microscopists, musicians, priests, weavers, hosiery loopers, leather cutters, graduate students, clerks, and those in managerial positions. Comparatively, the incidence and degree of myopia are less pronounced in adults with less education or whose occupations do not require fine near work, such as farmers and agricultural workers, fishermen and seamen, chauffeurs, and unskilled laborers (Tscherning 1883; Duke-Elder 1930; Goldschmidt 1968; Pärssinen 1987; Adams and McBrien 1992; and numerous other studies reviewed by Borish 1970 and by Curtin 1985, pp. 117–129).

Several studies document the development and progression of myopia in college students, graduate students, and students at military academies, at ages well beyond those at which growth and heredity are likely causes. At the U.S. Naval Academy, 18% of students entering with 20/20 acuity became myopic between the ages of 17 and 21, during their 4 years at the Academy (Hynes 1956). During World War II, large numbers of Naval Academy pilot candidates were ineligible for flight duty by graduation because myopia developed while at the Academy (Hayden 1941).

O'Neal and Connon (1987) reported significant myopic progression in 17-to 21-year-olds at the U.S. Air Force Academy, with myopic progression in 47.7%, 41.3%, and 74.0% of initially hyperopic, emmetropic, and myopic eyes, respectively. Progression of myopia in law students has also been reported (Dunphy et al. 1968; Zadnik and Mutti 1987). Informal surveys of optometry students indicate that about one third show myopia development or progression during the professional program.

Occupations that impose a visually restricted environment with no opportunity for long-distance vision are conducive to adult-onset myopia. Development and progression of myopia have been reported in submariners (Schwartz and Sandberg 1954; Kinney et al. 1979, 1980) and in personnel at a Minuteman launch control facility (Greene 1970).

MECHANISMS OF MYOPIA DEVELOPMENT

The observation that myopia is often associated with near work has given rise to theories that attribute myopia development to excessive use of accommodation (Ware 1813; Cohn 1867; Sato 1957; Young 1971) and convergence (Von Graefe 1857; Stilling 1885; Foerster 1886; Jackson 1931; Luedde 1932; Greene 1981).

Tonic Accommodation and Myopia

Evidence that myopia may be induced by accommodation is found in studies of the influence of sustained near work on *tonic accommodation* (TA). TA is the resting position assumed by accommodation in the absence of an adequate visual stimulus, for example, in a darkroom or an empty field.

Ebenholtz (1983) found that sustained near work induces an increase in the level of TA. This effect is relatively long-lasting; accommodation fails to relax completely for several hours after even brief periods of sustained accommodation. Ebenholtz suggests that this hysteresis or aftereffect of accommodation may serve as a precursor for induced myopia. Myopia may occur because accommodation fails to relax completely following sustained near work. Ehrlich (1987) reports a low degree of transient myopia (mean, 0.29 D sphere) following prolonged near work. The increase in TA induced by prolonged near work has been demonstrated to occur following work at a video display terminal, as well as on printed material (Wolf, 1985). Press (1987) notes that the increased shift of TA during near work serves to reduce stress on reflex accommodation, and suggests that it is adaptive in nature.

Variations in TA have been reported in different refractive groups. The magnitude of TA is lower in late-onset myopia than in early-onset myopia, hyperopia, or emmetropia. TA increases following sustained near work and mental effort, and this increase is greatest in those whose initial level of TA is low (Ebenholtz 1985; Bullimore and Gilmartin 1987a, 1987b; Gilmartin and Bullimore 1987; McBrien and Millodot 1987). Noting that this parasympathetic-mediated increase in TA is smallest in individuals whose initial TA level is relatively high, Bullimore and Gilmartin suggest that in such individuals the sympathetic system is activated simultaneously with the parasympathetic in order to reduce accommodative hysteresis. Induced myopia may occur in individuals with low TA because sympathetic inhibitory facility is inadequate, so that such individuals are more likely to develop accommodative hysteresis. Differences among late-onset myopes, early-onset myopes, hyperopes, and emmetropes have also been reported with respect to amplitude of accommodation (McBrien and Millodot 1986a), accommodative response (McBrien and Millodot, 1986b), and AC/A ratio (Rosenfield and Gilmartin, 1987).

Noting differences in TA and other aspects of accommodative function between early-onset and late-onset myopia, several authors have suggested that these conditions differ in etiology, attributing late-onset myopes to near work and early-onset myopia to genetic factors (Goldschmidt 1968; Stevenson 1984; McBrien and Millodot 1987). However, since the subjects in these studies were adults, the reported differences in TA in early- and late-onset myopia may not reflect etiologic differences. Rather, such differences may exist because the early-onset and late-onset myopic subjects are in different stages of myopia progression, the early-onset myopes having already stabilized, while the late-onset myopes have not. Research on younger subjects is necessary to determine whether early- and late-onset myopia represent truly different case types, or if both are induced by near work, with age-related differences in myopia development resulting from differing patterns of near-work demand. Consistent with the concept that the mechanism is similar whether myopia is of early or late onset, Grosvenor and Scott (1991) found that differences in the refractive components of eyes of early- and late-onset myopes result from differences in the degree of myopia (early-onset myopes tend to be considerably more myopic), rather than the age of onset.

Accommodation and Axial Length

Accommodative theories of myopia etiology generally ascribe the development of myopia to (1) changes in ciliary tone resulting in increased curvature of the crystalline lens, and/or (2) increased axial length of the eye resulting from weakening and stretching of the coats of the globe secondary to accommodative effort.

Sato (1957) suggests that school myopia is primarily produced by an increase in crystalline lens power caused by excessive accommodation. He found that many myopic eyes show a significant shift toward hyperopia and emmetropia under cycloplegia. However, the research of Stenstrom (1948) and Sorsby et al. (1961) suggests that axial length, rather than lens power, is the most significant component in the determination of refractive state. These authors report that most cases of myopia cannot be explained by increased ciliary tonus, since the power of the lens is less than average in myopes. Eyes with greater than average axial length tend to have corneas and lenses of lower power, suggesting the presence of an emmetropization mechanism that fails when axial length grows too great.

Young (1971, 1975, 1977, 1981) claims that myopia develops in two stages. In the first stage, excessive accommodation during prolonged near work leads to ciliary spasm and inability to relax accommodation at far. This stage of functional myopia or pseudomyopia is easily reversed. However, with time, increased vitreous chamber pressure associated with accommodation (Young 1981) leads to axial elongation of the eyeball, producing a structural myopia that is more difficult to reverse.

Several mechanisms have been proposed to explain how increase in axial length might result from excessive accommodation. Iwanoff (1869) and Newman (1929) postulated that strong accommodation causes stretching of the choroid, which decreases ocular nutrition and leads to chorioretinal degeneration and posterior staphyloma.

More recently, Adel (1966) and Enoch (1975) each reported retinal changes at the posterior pole during accommodation, suggesting that accommodation exerts a force on the choroid, which is transmitted to the back of the eye. Van Alphen (1961) also demonstrated that accommodation increases choroidal tension. However, he suggests that increased choroidal tension acts to reduce stress on the sclera, so that accommodation actually serves as an antimyopic force.

Young (1975, 1981) reported an increase in vitreous chamber pressure during ciliary muscle stimulation in primates. His findings are consistent with Coleman's (1970) theory of accommodation, which suggests that ciliary contraction causes a forward movement of the ora serrata, drawing the anterior vitreous forward against the lens. This produces a relative pressure gradient during accommodation with increased pressure in the vitreous and decreased pressure in the aqueous chambers. Coleman et al. (1969) demonstrated changes in axial diameter of the human eye with changes in accommodation. Young (1975, 1981) and Bell (1980) suggest that increased vitreous pressure resulting from sustained accommodation during prolonged near vision plays an important role in axial elongation and myopia development.

Noting that environmentally induced increases in vitreous pressure have been reported to play an important role in the development of myopia, Kelly (1981) indicates that myopia and chronic glaucoma are each caused by an increase in intraocular pressure. In myopia, the increase in vitreous pressure produces expansion of the young eye. In chronic glaucoma, the eye is too mature to expand and the impact of the increased pressure on the internal blood supply causes pathology. Kelly advocates use of the term *expansion glaucoma* in preference to myopia, to underscore both the mechanism and the significance of the disorder. Curtin (1985, pp. 173–174, 179–182) noted an increased prevalence of myopia in individuals with glaucoma.

Research on plasticity of refraction in the chick eye provides additional evidence that axial length and refraction are modified by ocular use. Chicks raised with various power lenses in front of their eyes, within the range that could be compensated by accommodation, demonstrated changes in axial length and noncyclopegic refraction to compensate the lens-induced defocus. Chicks treated with minus lenses demonstrated greater myopia and increased axial length as compared with chicks treated with plus lenses. Refractive compensation was apparently achieved through alteration in the pattern of ocular growth, since most of the difference in refraction was explained by difference in axial length. The finding that axial length is adjusted to tune the retinal plane to the image plane suggests that ocular accommodation plays a key mediating role in the regulation of ocular growth (Schaeffel et al. 1988).

Greene (1978, 1980) reported that mechanical stress on the posterior sclera is important in the etiology of axial myopia. He evaluated scleral stress-strain behavior, and suggests that scleral stress during alternating cycles of accommodative stimulation and relaxation could cause posterior staphyloma as a result of scleral weakening (Greene 1978). In a later study, Greene (1980) examined the mechanical stress on the posterior sclera induced by accommodation, convergence, vitreous pressure, and the extraocular muscles. He concluded that convergence and extraocular muscle tension, particularly that induced by the oblique muscles, are mechanically more important than accommodation, because they cause a more sizable increase in vitreous pressure.

In adult myopia progression, corneal steepening was the major ocular component change found by Goss et al. (1985). In contrast, Adams (1987) reported one well-documented case in which axial elongation was the most likely basis for adult onset and progression of myopia. Grosvenor and Scott (1991) found that differences in refractive components between early- and late-onset myopes stem from differences in degree of myopia, rather than age of onset.

Form Deprivation, Axial Myopia, and Accommodation

Additional evidence that accommodation plays a role in the development of axial myopia is found in studies that demonstrate the occurrence of axial elongation and high myopia in humans and experimental animals deprived of adequate patterned visual stimuli in infancy. Several studies suggest that the axial elongation that results from such deprivation is caused by the excessive accommodation put into play as the deprived organism actively attempts to obtain a well-defined visual image.

Surgically suturing the eyelids of monkeys before eye growth is completed leads to development of high-axial myopia (Hubel et al. 1975; Wiesel and Raviola 1977). Raviola and Wiesel (1978) found that this myopia does not develop when lid-sutured animals are reared in the dark. They believe that the fused, thin eyelids act as translucent occluders, and that deprivation of patterned vision induces an active visual search that is absent in the dark. They hypothesize that excessive accommodation in the attempt to achieve pattern perception may be the triggering factor in the production of this experimental myopia, and report that atropine did, as predicted, block the development of myopia in one species of monkey, but not in another (Raviola and Wiesel 1980). Axial elongation and myopia were also obtained in monkeys deprived of patterned vision by experimentally induced corneal opacification (Wiesel and Raviola 1979).

Experimental lid-suturing induces axial myopia in other species as well, including the tree shrew (Sherman et al. 1977; McKanna and Casagrande 1978), cat (Wilson and Sherman 1977), and chick (Wallman et al. 1978; Yinon et al. 1980; Shapiro 1981; Hodos and Kuenzel 1984). High-axial myopia also occurs in chicks when translucent occluders are used instead of lid-suturing, or with lateral occluders, which restrict vision to the frontal field (Wallman et al. 1978).

Troilo et al. (1987) found that axial myopia induced by form deprivation in the chick eye occurs even after the eye is disconnected from the central nervous system by cutting the optic nerve. This suggests the presence of an internal mechanism in the eye, related to retinal imagery, which regulates growth.

The axial myopia induced in chicks by restriction to the frontal visual field was markedly reduced by cutting the ciliary nerves (Wallman et al. 1981). Myopia induced in the tree shrew by lid-suturing was markedly reduced with atropine (McKanna and Casagrande, 1981). These findings implicate accommodation as the probable mechanism for this experimentally induced axial myopia.

An increased incidence of myopia has also been reported in human eyes that have been partially or totally deprived of patterned form vision as a result of ptosis (O'Leary and Millodot 1979); hemangiomas of the eyelids and orbits in infancy (Robb 1977; Schultz 1982); neonatal lid closure (Hoyt et al. 1981); and corneal scarring (Widmark 1902; Wilson 1912; Rumpelhardt 1952).

OTHER THEORIES OF MYOPIA DEVELOPMENT

Although considerable evidence suggests that near work and accommodation play a significant role, the etiology of myopia is still controversial. Numerous theories exist, with no consensus among clinicians or researchers. Various authorities attribute myopia to genetic influence, random biologic variation, nutritional and endocrine factors, psychologic factors, and personality. It may well be that there is no single cause, but that a variety of factors, including near work and accommodation, each play a contributing role.

Genetic and Random Biologic Variation

Steiger (1913) suggested that refractive status is a product of random biologic variation, resulting from the free interaction of the various components of refraction. Baldwin (1967) reviewed the literature on refractive status distribution and points out that there is a greater incidence of myopia than would occur if refractive status were normally distributed. Advocates of near-work theories argue that the theory of myopia as a normal biological variation fails to explain the increased incidence of myopia through the school years, or its association with close work in students and young adults. Opponents hold that increased incidence among students results from growth, rather than from environmental factors. Myopia tends to occur earlier in girls than in boys, evidently associated with the earlier onset of puberty (Smith and Woodruff 1951; Pendse and Bhave 1954).

Studies on uniovular twins provide evidence of an inherited element in the etiology of myopia (Sorsby et al. 1962; Karlsson 1974). Baldwin (1981) reviewed numerous studies of refractive state in identical twins, fraternal twins, siblings, and unrelated individuals, undertaken to establish the influence of heredity on refractive status. Baldwin concluded that the incidence of myopia is probably influenced by, but not solely attributable to heredity. Hirsch and Ditmars (1969) found that patients with higher degrees of myopia show hereditary influences, while those with lower degrees show little or no hereditary influence.

Nutritional and Endocrine Factors

Myopia has been attributed to nutritional deficit, endocrine disorder, and systemic disease. Baldwin (1965, 1967, 1981), Borish (1970), and Curtin (1985, pp. 61–151), have reviewed this literature. Most authorities agree that nutrition, endocrine function, and infectious systemic disease may be factors in the etiology of myopia, but do not consider them to be primary factors in the majority of cases.

General malnutrition is associated with a higher incidence of myopia. Increased myopia has been reported among prisoners of war fed markedly deficient diets (Livingston 1946; Reed 1947; Smith and Woodruff 1951) and among malnourished children (Halasa and McLaren 1964).

Most authors who attribute myopia to nutritional deficit postulate that myopia development results from interference with scleral metabolism caused by deficient intake of vitamins, minerals, and protein, as a consequence of which scleral resistance to the intraocular pressure decreases and scleral distensibility increases. Knapp (1939) advocated derangement of vitamin D, calcium, and phosphorus metabolism as a cause of scleral weakness and progressive myopia. Feldman (1950) and Wood (1927) found that myopes have lower blood calcium levels than nonmyopes.

Studies to evaluate differences in dietary intake between myopes and nonmyopes have produced conflicting results. Gardiner (1956, 1958, 1960) found that children with progressive myopia have lower protein intake (especially animal protein) than normal children, and that the addition of protein supplements to the diet leads to a reduction in myopic progression. However, Miller (1940) found no significant difference in protein intake between myopes and hyperopes, and Lane (1981) reported that individuals with increasing myopia consume excessive denatured protein, as well as excessive sugar and refined carbohydrate and inadequate dietary fiber. Lane also found that myopes have abnormally low concentrations of chromium and abnormally high concentrations of calcium in hair tissue.

Inadequate nutrition can contribute to the development of myopia both by interfering with efficient accommodation and by increasing scleral distensibility (Lane 1981, 1985). Lane reports that daily, sustained close-work accommodation causes elevation in intraocular pressure and increase in axial length, especially in individuals with deficient accommodation, apparently as a mechanism for reducing accommodative demand. He found that chromium potentiates ciliary muscle function. Chromium depletion causes inadequate accommodation, which in turn generates elevated intraocular pressure and increasing myopia. These effects are heightened when vitamin C ingestion is low, since vitamin C enhances chromium uptake.

Vitamin C and calcium each play an important role in the formation of collagen and the maintenance of scleral strength and elasticity. Axial length increase may be facilitated when deficient vitamin C or calcium metabolism or intake permits increased scleral distensibility (Bell 1978, 1980; Lane 1985).

Lane (1985) considers that the most common form of myopia is triggered by sustained accommodation, and that the myopiagenic effect of sustained accommodation is exacerbated by inadequate nutrition. He advises that myopia prevention and control programs include adequate ingestion and absorption of nutrients to aid in the maintenance of normal intraocular pressure levels and build scleral strength.

Myopia has also been reported to be associated with higher incidence of hypothyroid function (Bothman 1931; Costello 1936; Morrison 1947), although Andrews and Andrews (1966) found no difference in thyroid function between myopes and controls. Wiener (1927, 1931) and Borrello (1951) implicated adrenal function as a factor in myopia. Wiener emphasized the importance of exercise in increasing adrenal secretion. Topical administration of epinephrine has been reported to arrest progressive myopia (Wiener 1927, 1931; Macdiarmid and Hamilton 1964).

Infectious systemic diseases, particularly measles, are associated with increased incidence of myopia (Sonder 1920; Hirsch 1957). Children of mothers who suffered infectious diseases during pregnancy also showed a high incidence of myopia after age 8 (Gardiner and Griffith 1960).

Psychologic Factors

The relationship between myopia and personality has long been a subject of controversy. Several studies (cited later in this section) report an association between myopia and personality. Others (Schultz 1960; Grosvenor 1981; Brown et al. 1987) do not. In those studies that report a positive relationship, correlations are generally small in magnitude. Findings are frequently inconsistent from one study to another.

Myopia has been reported to be associated with introversion (Mull 1948; van Alphen 1952; Beedle and Young 1976); emotional inhibition, disinterest in motor activity, and inclination toward social leadership (Schapero and Hirsch 1952); a tendency to sharply differentiate memories and to make precise judgments on tests of leveling-sharpening (Stevens and Wolff 1965); achievement, introspection, abasement, heterosexuality, and aggression needs (Young 1967); increased covert anxiety, greater passivity toward stress, a tendency to be cautious and to exhibit excessive control, and decreased motor activity (Rosanes 1967); a deep-seated anxiety pattern, and a unique pattern of abstract thinking (van Alphen 1961).

In reviewing this literature, Lanyon and Giddings (1974), Baldwin (1981), and Curtin (1985, pp. 10–14) each conclude that distinguishing personality characteristics, especially introversion, accompany myopia. In addition to introversion, Lanyon and Giddings list shyness, social awkwardness, need for achievement, and handling anxiety by passively enduring it; Curtin cites anxiety and guilt feelings; and Baldwin notes self-confidence and reflectiveness as personality characteristics common to myopes.

While some authors (Schapero and Hirsch 1952; Curtin 1985, pp. 10–14) believe that the personality traits attributed to myopes result from emotional factors arising from the early use of glasses, or to heightened interest in near work as distance visual acuity reduces, others hypothesize that myopia is caused by psychological factors. Lanyon and Giddings (1974) note that correlations between personality characteristics and myopia have been demonstrated, but that theories suggesting psychologic causes for myopia offer little substantiating evidence.

Palmer (1966) views myopia as a response to psychological difficulties, to reduce stimulus input so as to avoid being overwhelmed, and to aid in reducing contact with the external environment. Kelly (1958, 1962) hypothesizes that myopia occurs as a conditioned response to anxiety, while Freud (1924) viewed the visual loss in myopia as a castration symbol.

Bates (1920) postulated that refractive errors are caused by anxiety, stress, emotional attitudes, effort, and strain. Gottlieb (1982) theorizes, based on Bates' model and on Pribram and McGuinness's (1975) research on the control of attention, that axial elongation and myopia result from chronic isometric contraction of the extraocular muscles, occurring as part of a generalized muscular activity associated with attention, mental processing, and problem solving.

Van Alphen (1961) proposes that stress, emotion, or extreme autonomic activity may interfere with the emmetropization mechanism. He suggests that sustained near-vision tasks related to studying and learning create different psychologic effects than nearpoint tasks of a more leisurely nature. Learning situations involve substantial levels of stress and anxiety, and are more likely to trigger myopic change.

Forrest (1988) views myopia as one of several adaptive outcomes triggered by near work, and suggests that psychologic status is the primary factor influencing both the visual stress response and the adaptive path taken by a particular individual. He suggests that refractive status mirrors one's mental state, attitudes and beliefs. Some individuals react to feelings of being vulnerable and out of control by challenging and attacking the world; such individuals tend to project attitudes outward and are more prone to develop hyperopia. Those who react by assuming the attitude that the world is against them tend to project inward, are easily depressed, feel inadequate, and are more prone to develop myopia. Forrest views myopia as a perceptual and psychologic barrier created by the individual to protect himself from the world.

Gawron (1981) performed several physiologic tests to obtain an index of autonomic activity and reported heightened sympathetic activity in myopes as compared with hyperopes. These physiologic findings may be correlates of psychologic differences between myopes and hyperopes, since patterns of autonomic nervous system activity have been related to personality (Wenger 1947; Eysenck 1953) and emotion (Cannon 1929).

SUMMARY

The use-abuse theory holds that myopia is caused by excessive use of the eyes for near work. Evidence suggests that myopia increases in prevalence and degree throughout the school years; that myopes read more, perform more near work, and achieve educationally at higher levels than nonmyopes; and that adults engaged in college studies and in occupations requiring extensive close work demonstrate greater incidence and progression of myopia than those who perform less close work. Myopia that results from near work has been attributed to increase in tonic accommodation, accommodative spasm, and accommodation-induced increase in axial length. Evidence that use of the eyes influences refraction is also found in reports that, in individuals who habitually use one eye for fixation due to strabismic amblyopia or corneal scarring, the fixing eye shifts toward myopia to a greater degree than the fellow eye, as well as in reports that individuals and laboratory animals subject to form deprivation or to restricted near-visual environment are more likely to demonstrate myopic increase. Other theories of myopia development emphasize heredity and random biologic variation; nutritional, endocrine and psychological factors; and systemic disease. Myopia progression is a source of considerable concern both because patients are disturbed by increasing dependence on glasses and the need for increasingly thick lenses, and because the incidence of serious ocular disease, particularly retinal detachment and glaucoma, increases as the degree of myopia increases.

SUGGESTED READING

Baldwin WR (1965). Some relationships between ocular, anthropometric, and refractive variables in myopia. Thesis, Indiana University, Ann Arbor, MI: University Microfilms.

Birnbaum MH (1979). Management of the low myopia pediatric patient. *J Am Optom Assoc* 50(11):1281–1289.

Borish IM (1970). *Clinical Refraction.* 3rd ed. Chicago: Professional Press.

Curtin BJ (1985). *The Myopias. Basic Science and Clinical Management.* Philadelphia: Harper & Row.

Press LJ (1987). Myopia. *J Optom Vis Dev* 18(1):1–17.

REFERENCES

Adams AJ (1987). Axial length elongation, not corneal curvature, as a basis of adult onset myopia. *Am J Optom Physiol Opt* 64(2):150–151.

Adams DW, McBrien NA (1992). Prevalence of myopia and myopic progression in a population of clinical microscopists. *Optom Vis Sci* 69(6):467–473.

Adel N (1966). Electomyographic and entoptic studies suggesting a theory of action of the ciliary muscle in accommodation for near work and its influence on the development of myopia. *Am J Optom Arch Am Acad Optom* 43(1):27–38.

Agnew CR (1877). Nearsightedness in the public schools. *New York Med Record* 12:34–36.

Andrews EJ, Andrews EJ Jr. (1966). Investigation of hypothyroidism as a possible cause of progressive myopia. *J Pediatr Ophthalmol* 3:14–18.

Angle J, Wissman DA (1978). Age, reading, and myopia. *Am J Optom Physiol Opt* 55:302–308.

Baldwin W (1957). A serial study of refractive status in youth. *Am J Optom* 34(9):486–490.

Baldwin W (1967). Clinical research and procedures in refraction. In: Hirsch MJ (ed), *Synopsis of the Refractive State of the Eye: A Symposium.* Minneapolis: Burgess, pp. 39–59.

Baldwin WR (1965). Some relationships between ocular, anthropometric, and refractive variables in myopia. Thesis, Indiana University, Ann Arbor, MI: University Microfilms.

Baldwin WR (1981). A review of statistical studies of relations between myopia and ethnic, behavioral and psychological characteristics. *Am J Optom* 58(7):516–527.

Bates W (1920). *The Cure of Imperfect Sight by Treatment Without Glasses.* New York: Central Fixation Publ.

Beedle SL, Young FA (1976). Values, personality, physical characteristics, and refractive error. *Am J Optom Physiol Opt* 53(11):735–739.

Belkin M, Yinin N, Rose L, et al. (1977). Effect of visual environment on refractive error of cats. *Doc Ophthalmol* 42:433–437.

Bell GR (1978). A review of the sclera and its role in myopia. *J Am Optom Assoc* 49(12):1399–1403.

Bell GR (1980). The Coleman theory of accommodation and its relevance to myopia. *J Am Optom Assoc* 51(6):582–588.

Birnbaum MH (1979). Management of the low myopia pediatric patient. *J Am Optom Assoc* 50(11):1281–1289.

Borish IM (1970). *Clinical Refraction.* 3rd ed. Chicago: Professional Press.

Borello G (1951). Rilievi sulla choroidite miopica. *Rass Ital Ottalmol* 20:320–322.

Bothman L (1931). The relation of the basal metabolism rate to progressive axial myopia. *Am J Ophthalmol* 14:918–924.

Brown B, Stewart J, Moo G, et al. (1987). Are myopic children more anxious than their non-myopic peers? *Clin Exp Optom* 70(2):46–52.

Brown E (1938). Net average yearly changes in refraction of atropinized eyes from birth to beyond middle life. *Arch Ophthalmol* 19(5):719–734.

Bullimore MA, Gilmartin B (1987a). Tonic accommodation, cognitive demand, and ciliary muscle innervation. *Am J Optom Physiol Opt* 64(1):45–50.

Bullimore MA, Gilmartin B (1987b). Aspects of tonic accommodation in late-onset myopia. *Am J Optom Physiol Opt* 64(7):499–503.

Cannon WB (1929). *Bodily Changes in Pain, Hunger, Fear and Rage: An Account of Recent Researches into the Function of Emotional Excitement.* New York: Appleton.

Cohn HL (1867). *Untesuchen der augen von 10060 schulkendern nebst vorschlagen zur verbesserung der den nachtheiligen schuleinrichtungen. Eine atiologische studies.* Leipzig: F. Fleischer.

Coleman DJ (1970). Unified model for accommodation. *Am J Ophthalmol* 69(6):1063–1079.

Coleman DJ, Wuchinch MS, Carlin B (1969). Accommodative changes in the axial dimension of the human eye. In: Glitter KA, Keeney AH, Sarin LK, et al. (eds), *Ophthalmic Ultrasound.* St. Louis: Mosby, p. 134.

Costello J (1936). Obesity and ocular symptoms in mentally alert children due to hypothyroidism. *Endocrinology* 20:105–106.

Curtin BJ (1985). *The Myopias. Basic Science and Clinical Management.* Philadelphia: Harper & Row.

Dearborn W, Leverett H (1945). Visual defects and reading. *J Educ* 13:111–124.

Donders FC (1864). *On the Anomalies of Accommodation and Refraction of the Eye: With a Preliminary Essay on Physiological Dioptrics.* London: New Syndenham Society. Reprinted 1952, London: Hatton Press.

Duke-Elder WS (1930). An investigation of the effect upon the eyes of occupations involving close work. *Br J Ophthalmol* 14:609–620.

Dunphy EB, Stoll MR, King SH (1968). Myopia among American male graduate students. *Am J Ophthalmol* 65:518–521.

Ebenholtz SM (1983). Accommodative hysteresis: A precursor to induced myopia? *Invest Ophthalmol Vis Sci* 24:513–515.

Ebenholtz SM (1985). Accommodative hysteresis: Relation to resting focus. *Am J Optom Physiol Opt* 62(11):755-762.

Ehrlich DL (1987). Near vision stress: Vergence adaptation and accommodative fatigue. *Ophthalmol Physiol Opt* 7(4):353–357.

Enoch J (1975). Marked accommodation, retinal stretch, monocular space perception and retinal receptor orientation. *Am J Optom Physiol Opt* 52(6):376–392.

Eysenck HJ (1953). *The Structure of Human Personality.* London: Metheum.

Falkenburg J, Straub M (1893). Uever die normale refraction des auges and die hypermetropie bei angeborener amblyopie. *Arch Augenheilkd* 26:336.

Feldman J (1950). Myopia, vitamin A, and calcium. *Am J Ophthalmol* 33:777–785.

Foerster R (1886). On the influence of concave glasses and convergence of the ocular axes in the increase of myopia. *Arch Ophthalmol* 15:399–435. (Translated by J.A. Spaulding.)

Forrest EB (1988). *Stress and Vision.* Santa Ana, CA: Optometric Extension Program Foundation.

Freud S (1924). Psychogenic visual disturbances according to psychoanalytical conception. In: *Collected Papers II.* London: Hogarth Press, 1948. (Originally published 1924.)

Gardiner P, Griffith J (1960). Association between maternal disease during pregnancy and myopia in the child. *Br J Opththalmol* 44:172–180.

Gardiner PA (1956). Observations on the food habits of myopic children. *Br Med J* 2:699.

Gardiner PA (1958). Dietary treatment of myopia in children. *Lancet* 1:1152–1155.

Gardiner PA (1960). Protein and myopia. *Proc Nutr Soc London* 19:96–100.

Gawron VJ (1981). Differences among myopes, emmetropes and hyperopes. *Am J Optom Physiol Opt* 58(9):753–760.

Gilmartin B, Bullimore MA (1987). Sustained near-vision augments inhibitory sympathetic innervation of the ciliary muscle. *Clin Vis Sci* 1(3):197–208.

Goldschmidt E (1968). On the etiology of myopia. *Acta Ophthalmol Suppl* 98:1–171.

Goss DA (1982). Attempts to reduce the rate of increase of myopia in young people—A critical literature review. *Am J Optom Physiol Optics* 59(10):828–841.

Goss DA, Erickson P, Cox VD (1985). Prevalence and pattern of adult myopia progression in a general optometric practice population. *Am J Optom Physiol Opt* 62(7):470–477.

Gottleib RL (1982). Neuropsychology of myopia. *J Optom Vis Dev* 13(1):3–27.

Greene MR (1970). Submarine myopia in the Minuteman launch control facility. *J Am Optom Assoc* 41:1012–1016.

Greene P (1978). Mechanical aspects of myopia. Unpublished doctoral thesis, Cambridge, MA: Harvard University, p. 1.

Greene P (1981). Myopia and the extraocular muscles. *Doc Ophthalmol Proc Ser* 28:163–169.

Greene PR (1980). Mechanical considerations in myopia: Relative effects of accommodation, convergence, intraocular pressure and the extraocular muscles. *Am J Optom Physiol Opt* 57(12):902–914.

Greenspan S (1981). Research studies of bifocals for myopia. *Am J Optom Physiol Opt* 58(7):536–540.

Grosvenor T (1970). Refractive state, intelligence test scores and academic ability. *Am J Optom* 47:355–361.

Grosvenor T (1971). The neglected hyperope. *Am J Optom* 48(5): 376–382.

Grosvenor T (1981). The relationship between refractive error and scores on the Minnesota Multiphasic Personality Inventory. *Doc Ophthalmol Proc Series* 28:157–162.

Grosvenor T (1989). Myopia: What can we do about it clinically? *Optom Vis Sci* 66(7):415–419.

Grosvenor T, Scott R (1991). Comparison of refractive components in youth-onset and early adult-onset myopia. *Optom Vis Sci* 68(3):204–209.

Haines HF (1955). An evaluation of the visual status and academic achievement of a selected group of elementary school children over a period of seven years. *Am J Optom* 32:279–288.

Halasa SH, McLaren DS (1964). The refractive state of malnourished children. *Arch Ophthalmol* 71:827–831.

Hallett DW (1931). The prevention of myopia. *Am J Ophthalmol* 14:143–146.

Hayden R (1941). Development and prevention of myopia at the United States Naval Academy. *Arch Ophthalmol* 25(4):539–547.

Hentsch R, Frank E (1977). Entwicklung der refraktion und sehscharfe bei schielenden kindern. *Klin Monatsbl Augenheilkd* 170:80–83.

Hirsch MJ (1959). Refractive state and intelligence scores. *Am J Optom* 36:12–21.

Hirsch M (1961). A longitudinal study of refractive state of children during the first six years of school—A preliminary report of the Ojai study. *Am J Optom* 38(10):564–571.

Hirsch M (1962). Relationship between refraction on entering school and rate of change during the first six years of school—An interim report from the Ojai longitudinal study. *Am J Optom* 39(2):51–59.

Hirsch M (1964). The longitudinal study in refraction. *Am J Optom* 41(3):137–141.

Hirsch MJ (1952). The changes in refraction between the ages of 5 and 14—Theoretical and practical considerations. *Am J Optom Arch Am Acad Optom* 29(9):445–459.

Hirsch MJ (1955). The relationship of school achievement and visual anomalies. *Am J Optom* 32:262–270.

Hirsch M (1957). The relationship between measles and myopia. *Am J Optom* 34:289–297.

Hirsch MJ (1979). Prentice memorial lecture. *Am J Optom Physiol Opt* 56(3):177–183.

Hirsch M, Ditmars D (1969). Refraction of young myopes and their parents—A reanalysis. *Am J Optom* 46(1):30–32.

Hodos W, Kuenzel WJ (1984). Retinal image degradation produces ocular enlargement in chicks. *Invest Ophthalmol Vis Sci* 25:652–659.

Hoyt CS, Stone RD, Fromer C, et al. (1981). Monocular axial myopia associated with neonatal eyelid closure in human infants. *Am J Ophthalmol* 91:197.

Hubel DH, Wiesel TN, LeVay S (1975). Functional architecture of area 17 in normal and monocularly deprived macaque monkeys. Cold Spring Harb Symp Quant Biol 40:581–589.

Hynes EA (1956). Refractive changes in normal young men. *Arch Ophthalmol* 56:761–767.

Iwanoff A (1869). Beitrage zur anotomie des ciliarmuskels. *Graefes Arch Ophthalmol* 15(3):284–298.

Jackson E (1931). Norms of refraction. *Trans Sec Ophthalmol Am Med Assoc*, pp. 174–190.

Kahn HA, Moorhead HB (1969–70). *Statistics on Blindness in the Model Reporting Area*. Washington, DC: Department of Health, Education and Welfare, Publication No. (NIM) 73–427, US Government Printing Office.

Karlsson JL (1973). Genetic relationship between giftedness and myopia. *Hereditas* 73:85–88.

Karlsson JL (1974). Concordance rates for myopia in twins. *Clin Genet* 6:142–146.

Kelley C (1958). Psychological factors in myopia. Doctoral dissertation, New York: New School for Social Research.

Kelley C (1962). Psychological factors in myopia. *J Am Optom Assoc* 33(11):833–837.

Kelly TSB (1981). Myopia or expansion glaucoma. *Doc Ophthalmol Proc Series* 28:109–116.

Kempf G, Collins S, Jarman B (1928). *Refractive Errors in the Eyes of Children as Determined by Retinoscopic Examination with a Cycloplegic.* Public Health Bulletin No. 182, Washington, DC: Government Printing Office.

Kephart N Unger RM (1953). An investigation of visual performance among selected groups of school children. *Am J Optom* 30:635–643.

Kepler J (1611). Dioptrice: Seu demonstratio eorum quae visui et visibilibus propter conspicilla non ita pridem inventa accidunt. Augsburg.

Kinney JAS, Luria SM, McKay CL, et al. (1979). Vision of submariners. *Undersea Biomed Res* 6(suppl):163.

Kinney JAS, Luria SM, Ryan AP, et al. (1980). The vision of submariners and national guardsmen. *Am J Optom Physiol Opt* 57:469–478.

Knapp AA (1939). Vitamin D complex in progressive myopia: Etiology, pathology and treatment. *Am J Ophthalmol* 22: 1329–1337.

Lane BC (1981). Elevation in intraocular pressure with daily sustained close work stimulus to accommodation, lowered tissue chromium, and dietary deficiency of ascorbic acid (vitamin C). *Doc Ophthalmol* 28:149–155.

Lane BC (1985). Nutrition and vision. In: Jeffrey Bland (ed), *1984–85 Yearbook of Nutritional Medicine*. New Caanan, CT: Keats Publ, pp. 239–281.

Lanyon RI, Giddings JW (1974). Psychological approaches to myopia: A review. *Am J Optom Physiol Opt* 51(4):271–281.

Leffertstra LJ (1977). Vergleichende untersuchungen auf unterscheidliche refraktionsanderungen beider augen bei patienten mit strabismus convergens. *Klin Monatsbl Augenheilkd* 170:74–79.

Lepard CW (1975). Comparative changes in the error of refraction between fixing and amblyopic eyes during growth and development. *Am J Ophthalmol* 80:485–490.

Livingston PC (1946). Ocular disturbances associated with malnutrition. *Trans Ophthalmol Soc UK* 66:19–71.

Luckeish M, Moss FK (1939). Ocular changes in school children during the fifth and sixth grades. *Am J Optom* 16:443–450.

Luedde WH (1932). Monocular cycloplegia for the control of myopia. *Am J Ophthalmol* 15:603–609.

Lundgren P (1954). Myopie in den hoheren lehranstalt schwedens. *Klin Monatsbl Augenheilkd* 124:110.

Macdiarmid DC, Hamilton N (1964). The treatment of myopia. *NZ Med J* 16(suppl):66.

Maliuta GD (1972). Myopia in relation to close up visual work. Vestn Oftalmol 5:58–59.

McBrien NA, Millodot M (1986a). Amplitude of accommodation and refractive error. *Invest Ophthalmol Vis Sci* 27:1187–1190.

McBrien NA, Millodot M (1986b). The effect of refractive error on the accommodative response gradient. *Ophthalmol Physiol Opt* 6(2): 145–149.

McBrien NA, Millodot M (1987). The relationship between tonic accommodation and refractive error. *Invest Ophthalmol Vis Sci* 28:997–1004.

McKanna JA, Casagrande VA (1978). Reduced lens development in lid suture myopia. *Exp Eye Res* 26:715–723.

McKanna JA, Casagrande VA (1981). Atropine affects lid-suture myopia development. *Doc Ophthalmol Proc Ser* 28:187–192.

Miller H (1940). Is myopia a deficiency disease? *Am J Ophthalmol* 23:296.

Morgan MW (1960). Relationship of refractive error to bookishness and androgyny. *Am J Optom* 37:171–185.

Morgan MW (1967). A review of the major theories of the genesis of refractive state. In: Hirsch MJ (ed), *Synopsis of the Refractive State of the Eye: A Symposium*. Minneapolis: Burgess Publ, pp. 8–12.

Morrison FM (1947). Myopia and hypothyroidism. *Trans Am Ophthalmol Soc* 45:527–536.

Mull HK (1948). Myopia and introversion. *Am J Psychol* 61:575–576.

Nadell MC, Hirsch MJ (1958). The relationship between intelligence and the refractive state in a selected high school sample. *Am J Optom* 35:321–326.

Nadell MC, Weymouth FW, Hirsch MJ (1957). The relationship of frequency of use of the eye in close work to the distribution of the refractive error in a selected sample. *Am J Optom* 34:523–537.

National Eye Institute (1976). *Support for Vision Research*. Washington, DC: Department of Health, Education and Welfare, Publication No. (NIM) 76–1098.

National Society for the Prevention of Blindness (1966). *Estimated Statistics on Blindness and Vision Problems*, New York: Author.

Newman FA (1929). Acquired axial myopia. *Am J Ophthalmol* 12:714–719.

Oakley KH, Young FA (1975). Bifocal control of myopia. *Am J Optom Physiol Opt* 52:758–764.

Ochapovsky S (1935). Genesis of the refraction of the human eye. *Arch Ophthalmol* 14:412–420.

O'Leary DJ, Millodot M (1979). Eyelid closure causes myopia in humans. *Experientia* 35:1478–1479.

O'Neal MR, Connon TR (1987). Refractive error changes at the United States Air Force Academy—Class of 1985. *Am J Optom Physiol Opt* 64(5):344–354.

Palmer R (1966). Visual acuity and excitement. *Psychosom Med* 28(4, part. 1):364–374.

Pärssinen TO (1987). Relation between refraction, education, occupation and age among 26- and 46-year-old Finns. *Am J Optom Physiol Opt* 64(2):136–143.

Peckham CS, Gardiner PA, Goldstein H (1977). Acquired myopia in eleven year old children. *Br Med J* 1:542–544.

Pendse G, Bhave B (1954). Refraction in relation to age and sex. *India Med Res Memoirs* 52:404–412.

Perkins ES (1979). Morbidity from myopia. *Sight Sav Rev* 49:11–19.

Press LJ (1987). Myopia. *J Optom Vis Dev* 18(1):1–17.

Pribram K, McGuinness D (1975). Arousal, activation and effort in the control of attention. *Psychol Rev* 82(2):116–149.

Raviola E, Wiesel TN (1978). Effect of dark rearing on experimental myopia in monkeys. *Invest Ophthalmol Vis Sci* 17:485–488.

Raviola E, Wiesel TN (1980). Effects of atropine on experimental myopia in macaque monkeys. Annual meeting, Orlando, FL, May 4–9, 1980. *ARVO Abstracts* pp. 170–171.

Reed JG (1947). Ocular symptoms in prisoners of war in Sumatra. *Trans R Soc Trop Med Hyg* 40:411–420.

Richler A, Bear JC (1980). Refraction, near work and education: A population study in Newfoundland. *Acta Ophthalmol* 58:468–477.

Riffenburgh RS (1965). Onset of myopia in the adult. *Am J Ophthalmol* 59:925–926.

Robb RM (1977). Refractive errors associated with hemangiomas of the eyelids and orbit in infancy. *Am J Ophthalmol* 83:52–58.

Roberts W, Banford R (1967). Evaluation of bifocal correction techniques in juvenile myopia. *Optom Weekly* 58(38):25–31, Sept. 21; 58(39):21–30, Sept. 28; 58(40):23–28, Oct. 5; 58(41):27–34, Oct. 12; 58(423):19–26, Oct. 26.

Rosanes MB (1967). Psychological correlates to myopia compared to hyperopia and emmetropia. *J Proj Techn* 315:31–35.

Rose L, Yinon U, Belkin M (1974). Myopia induced in cats deprived of distance vision during development. *Vision Res* 14:1029–1032.

Rosenfield M, Gilmartin B (1987). Effect of a near-vision task on the response AC/A of a myopic population. *Ophthalmol Physiol Opt* 7(3):225–233.

Rosner J, Gruber J (1985). Differences in the perceptual skills development of young myopes and hyperopes. *Am J Optom Physiol Opt* 62(8):501–504.

Rumpelhardt K (1952). Untersuchungern über die beziehungen myopie und hornhautnarhen. *Klin Monatsbl Augenheilkd* 120:397–403.

Sato T (1957). *The Causes and Prevention of Acquired Myopia*. Tokyo: Kanehara Shuppan.

Schaeffel F, Glasser A, Howland HC (1988). Accommodation, refractive error and eye growth in chickens. *Vision Res* 28(5):639–657.

Schapero M, Hirsch ML (1952). The relationship of refractive error and Guildford-Martin Temperament Test scores. *Am J Optom* 29:32–36.

Schultz LB (1960). Personality and physical variables as related to refractive errors. *Am J Optom Arch Am Acad Optom* 37(11):551–571.

Schulz E (1982). Deprivationsamblyopie und refractionsanomalie bei fruhkindlichen lidhamgiomen. *Klin Monatsbl Augenheilkd* 181:192–194.

Schwartz FO (1940). Ocular factors in poor readers in the St. Louis public school. *Am J Ophthalmol* 23:535–538.

Schwartz I, Sandberg NE (1954). *The Effect of Time in Submarine Service on Vision.* Medical Research Laboratory Report No. 253. New London, CT: U.S. Navy Bureau of Medicine and Surgery.

Shapiro A (1981). Experimental visual deprivation and myopia. *Doc Ophthalmol Proc Ser* 28:193–195.

Sherman SM, Norton TT, Casagrande VA (1977). Myopia in the lid-suture tree shrew. *Brain Res* 124:154–157.

Skeffington AM (1952). The myope. In: *Practical Applied Optometry.* Optometric Extension Program Continuing Education Courses. Santa Ana, CA: Optometric Extension Program Foundation. 24(12):109–120.

Slataper F (1950). Age norms of refraction and vision. *Arch Ophthalmol* 43(3):466–481.

Smith DA, Woodruff MFA (1951). *Deficiency Diseases in Japanese Prison Camps.* Medical Resource Council, Special Report Series No. 274, London: Her Majesty's Stationery Office.

Sonder T (1920). Influence of disease in children on progressive myopia. *Arch Ophthalmol (France)* 37:290–298.

Sorsby A (1932). School myopia. *Br J Ophthalmol* 16(4):217–224.

Sorsby A, Benjamin B, Sheridan M (1961). *Refraction and Its Components During the Growth of the Eye from the Age of Three.* Medical Research Council, Special Report Series No. 301, London: Her Majesty's Stationery Office.

Sorsby A, Sheridan M, Leary GA (1962). *Refraction and Its Components in Twins.* Medical Research Council, Special Report Series No. 303, London: Her Majesty's Stationery Office.

Steiger A (1913). *Die entsehung der spha rischen refraktion des menschlichen auges.* Berlin: Karger.

Stenstrom S (1948). Investigation of the variation and the correlation of the optical elements of human eyes. Translated by Daniel Woolf. *Am J Optom Arch Am Acad Optom* 25:218–232; 286–299; 340–350; 388–397; 438–449; 496–504.

Stevens VA, Wolff HH (1965). The relationship of myopia to performance on a test of leveling-sharpening. *Percept Motor Skills* 21:399–403.

Stevenson RWW (1984). The development of myopia and its relationship with intra-ocular pressure. In: Charman WN (ed), *Transactions of the First International Congress, "The Frontiers of Optometry."* vol. 2. London: British College of Ophthalmic Opticians, pp. 43–50.

Stilling J (1885). Eine studie zur kurzsichtigkeit frage. *Arch Augenheilkd* 15:133.

Straub M (1909). Uber die aetiologie der brechungsanom alien des auges und den ursprung der emmetropie. *Graefes Arch Ophthalmol* 70:130–199.

Tassman I (1932). Frequency of various kinds of refractive errors. *Am J Ophthalmol* 15:1044–1053.

Tatevosyan AA (1968). On the development of unilateral occupational myopia. *Vestn Oftalmol* 81(2):63–64.

Teasdale TW, Fuchs J, Goldschmidt E (1988). Degree of myopia in relation to intelligence and educational level. Lancet 8624:1351–1354.

Troilo D, Gottlieb MD, Wallman J (1987). Visual deprivation causes myopia in chicks with optic nerve section. *Curr Eye Res* 6:993–999.

Tscherning M (1883). Studien uber die aetilogy der myopie. *Graefes Arch Ophthalmol* 29:201–272.

Van Alphen GW (1952). A comparative psychological investigation in myopes and emmetropes. *Proc Koninklijke Nederlandse Academie von Wedenschappen* 55:689.

Van Alphen GWHM (1961). On emmetropia and ametropia. *Ophthalmologica* 142 (suppl):1–92.

Von Graefe A (1857). Beitrage zur physiologie and pathologie der scheifen augenmuskein. *Graefes Arch Ophthalmol* 3:277.

Wallman J, Rosenthal D, Adams JI, et al. (1981). Role of accommodation and developmental aspects of experimental myopia in chicks. *Doc Ophthalmol Proc Ser* 28:197–206.

Wallman J, Turkel J, Trachtman J (1978). Extreme myopia produced by modest change in early visual experience. *Science* 201:1249–1251.

Ware J (1813). Observations relative to the near and distant sight of different persons. *Philos Trans R Soc Lond (Bio Sci)* 103(1):31–50.

Wenger MA (1947). Preliminary study of the significance of measures of autonomic balance. *Psychosom Med* 9:301–309.

Widmark JE (1902). Contribution to the etiology of myopia. *Br Med J* 2:1435.

Wiener M (1927). Epinephrine in progressive myopia. *JAMA* 89:594.

Wiener M (1931). The use of epinephrine in progressive myopia: Further report. *Am J Ophthalmol* 14:520–522.

Wiesel TN, Raviola E (1977). Myopia and eye enlargement after neonatal lid fusion in monkeys. *Nature* 266:66–68.

Wiesel TN, Raviola E (1979). Increase in axial length of the macaque monkey eye after corneal opacification. *Invest Ophthalmol Vis Sci* 18:1232–1236.

Wilson JA (1912). Keratitis as a cause of myopia. *Glasg Med J* 77:241.

Wilson SR, Sherman SM (1977). Differential effects of early monocular deprivation on the binocular and monocular segments of cat striate cortex. *J Neurophysiol* 40:891–903.

Wolf K (1985). *The Role of Accommodation and Binocular Vergence in Visual Fatigue Induced by Near Work at a Video Display Terminal or Hard Copy.* Research Reports and Special Articles, Optometric Extension Program Continuing Education Courses, Santa Ana, CA: Optometric Extension Program Foundation, pp. 61–76.

Wood DJ (1927). Calcium deficiency in blood with reference to spr. cararrh and myopia. *Br J Ophthalmol* 11:394–401.

Yinon U, Rose L, Shapiro A (1980). Myopia in the eye of developing chicks following monocular and binocular lid closure. *Vision Res* 20:137–141.

Young F (1961). The development and retention of myopia by monkeys. *Am J Optom* 38(10):545–555.

Young F (1965). The effect of atropine on the development of myopia in monkeys. *Am J Optom* 42(8):439–449.

Young FA (1963). Reading measures of intelligence and refractive errors. *Am J Optom* 47:257–264.

Young FA (1967). Myopia and personality. *Am J Optom Physiol Opt* 44(3):192–201.

Young FA (1971). The development of myopia. *Contacto* 15:36–42.

Young FA (1975). The development and control of myopia in human and subhuman primates. *Contacto* 19:16–31.

Young FA (1977). The nature and control of myopia. *J Am Optom Assoc* 48(4):451–457.

Young FA (1981). Intraocular pressure dynamics associated with accommodation. *Doc Ophthalmol Proc Ser* 28:171–176.

Young FA, Beattie R, Newby FJ, et al. (1954). The Pullman study: A visual survey of Pullman school children. *Am J Optom* 31(3, Part 1):111–121; 31(4, Part 2): 192–203.

Young FA, Leary GA, Baldwin WR, et al. (1969). The transmission of refractive errors within Eskimo families. *Am J Optom* 46:676–685.

Zadnik K, Mutti DO (1987). Refractive error changes in law students. *Am J Optom Physiol Opt* 64(7):558–561.

3

The Skeffington Nearpoint Stress Model

Skeffington (1928–74) postulated that the near-work demands imposed by our culture are incompatible with our physiology and provoke a stress response characterized by a drive for convergence to localize closer than accommodation. The resulting mismatch between vergence and accommodation interferes with visual efficiency and information-processing, and may lead to adaptive changes within the visual system.

DISTINCTIONS BETWEEN MODELS

The Skeffington model differs in several important respects from traditional models and from the use-abuse theory. Traditional models view refractive, binocular, and accommodative anomalies as causes of nearpoint difficulty, and attribute such disorders to genetic influence, innervational disturbance, and random biologic variation. Skeffington, in contrast, held that these anomalies occur as adaptations to resolve an effector system mismatch intrinsic to the nearpoint task demands of our culture, and are hence products, rather than sources, of nearpoint stress. The primary source of nearpoint stress, in this view, is the task-induced drive for convergence to localize closer than accommodation.

Both the use-abuse theory and the Skeffington model hold that the visual system is biologically unsuited for the sustained near-vision demands imposed by our culture. However, while the use-abuse theory deals primarily with myopia, Skeffington postulates that a broad variety of refractive, binocular, and accommodative disorders arise from nearpoint stress.

The use-abuse theory attributes myopia to mechanical effects arising from excessive accommodation and convergence. The Skeffington model, in contrast, views myopia as an adaptive change to resolve the mismatch between vergence and accommodation, which is held to be intrinsic to the near-vision tasks imposed by our culture.

THE FOUR CIRCLES

To appreciate the Skeffington model, one must be familiar with Skeffington's concept of vision as an organismic process inextricably associated with spatial, motor, and intellectual functions. Skeffington portrayed vision as a product of the interaction of four component subprocesses: antigravity, centering, identification, and speech-auditory. These subprocesses were depicted as four overlapping, intertwined circles, with vision emerging as a product of their interaction (Figure 3.1) (see Hendrickson 1969).

The antigravity system, concerned with balance and position in space, provides a basic frame of reference for orientation and spatial localization.

Centering is an attentional and orienting process that involves selecting an area of space for attention and directing the body, head, and eyes toward the area selected for information-processing. Centering is intimately involved with spatial localization. Convergence is the overt oculomotor component of the centering process (Skeffington 1964).

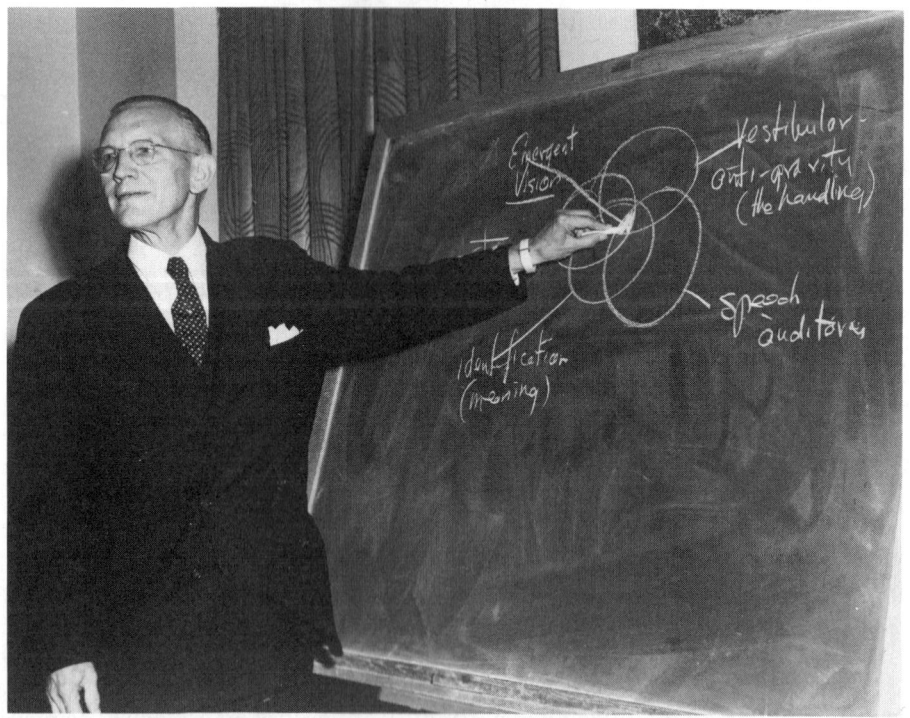

Figure 3.1 Dr. A.M. Skeffington and the four circles. (Photo courtesy Optometric Extension Program Foundation.)

Identification is the process of deriving meaning from those areas of space selected for attention. It involves resolution, discrimination, differentiation, and the determination of relationships between details. Accommodation is the overt oculomotor component of the identification process (Skeffington 1964).

The *speech-auditory process*, Skeffington's fourth circle, is closely entwined with vision. The speech-auditory process is involved with analysis and communication of that which is seen.

OVERVIEW OF THE SKEFFINGTON NEARPOINT STRESS MODEL

Skeffington (1928–74) believed that we are biologically unsuited for the near-vision tasks imposed by society. The demands for sustained concentration, immobilization, and mental effort provoke a stress response characterized by a drive for the centering process to localize closer to the individual than identification, and for the effector mechanism of convergence to localize closer than accommodation.

Efficient reading requires that vergence and accommodation localize at the plane of regard. Without a means of compensation, the drive for vergence to localize closer than accommodation leads to blurred vision or diplopia. Skeffington viewed reading as a biologically unacceptable task, because it triggers a mismatch between vergence and accommodation, yet requires precise matching of these systems for efficient performance.

To avoid blur or diplopia in the presence of a nearpoint stress–induced drive for convergence to localize closer, individuals make a series of characteristic changes in the pattern of relationships between vergence and accommodation (see Chapter 4). Effort directed toward resolution of the effector system mismatch diminishes information-processing capacity, impairs comprehension, and decreases efficiency of task performance. Inefficient visual function causes asthenopia and inability to sustain. Consequently, many individuals avoid close work, demonstrating patterns of disinterest and withdrawal. Others adapt within the visual system, developing myopia or skews in vergence and accommodative function, as means of resolving the drive for convergence to localize closer (Skeffington 1928–74).

The prescription of low-plus lenses for near use is a key element of the Skeffington model. Low-plus lens prescription aids in the resolution of the drive for convergence to localize nearer than accommodation, improves visual efficiency, minimizes interference with cognitive function, and eliminates the need for adaptation (Skeffington 1928–74).

The physiologic basis for a nearpoint stress–induced drive for convergence to localize closer than accommodation, and the clinical signs and manifestations of this drive, are discussed in this chapter. Adaptations to resolve the effector system mismatch are discussed in Chapter 4, and OEP case analysis to determine the optimal nearpoint lens prescription is covered in Chapter 8.

PHYSIOLOGY OF OVERCONVERGENCE

The core element of Skeffington's nearpoint stress model is the statement that a drive for convergence to localize closer than accommodation is intrinsic to the nearpoint visual demands of our culture. Several questions arise with regard to this core element: Why does nearpoint visual activity provoke a stress response? Does the hypothesized drive for convergence to localize closer than accommodation really exist? And if so, why does convergence localize closer? What physiologic mechanisms are involved?

Skeffington held that the nearpoint tasks of our society are biologically unacceptable, and hence provoke a physiological stress response. The stress response is caused not by the near working distance or by the demand on accommodation, but rather by the nature of the task demands imposed.

The nearpoint task demands imposed by society are biologically unacceptable, according to Skeffington, because (1) they require sustained immobilization or containment, while the human organism is designed to move about; (2) they impose unique, intense demands for intellectual application and information-processing through abstract symbols; and (3) in contrast with the three-dimensionality of biologic space, the nearpoint tasks of our culture are performed in an artificial two-dimensional setting.

The visual system evolved in relation to biologic needs, rather than the nearpoint demands of our culture. Reading and other culturally imposed nearpoint tasks present demands that do not occur in a natural setting. The physiological mechanisms used are not shaped by evolutionary pressure, but rather reflect the use of already existing mechanisms for new purposes. While the capacity to do this exists, Skeffington felt that the process by which it is accomplished is inherently stress-producing (Flax 1985).

According to Skeffington, hyperopic and exophoric buffers operate to protect the mechanisms of accommodation and convergence from surges in dominance of the autonomic and skeletal nervous systems. Demands for sustained concentration and immobilization during near work generate a stress response characterized by a pattern of visceral dominance in which accommodation is activated to a greater degree than convergence. Increased innervation to accommodation is accompanied by an associated increase in convergence innervation, which leads to absorption of exophoria. If the degree of stress is greater than can be resolved by the absorption of exophoria, the increased activation of accommodation results in a tendency to converge nearer than the plane of regard.

Skeffington alluded to other reasons why convergence may localize closer than accommodation during near-vision tasks. He noted that convergence, mediated by skeletal musculature innervated by the central nervous system, is a faster-acting system than accommodation, mediated by the autonomic nervous system. Convergence has shorter latency and faster response time than accommodation. Skeffington also suggested that accommodation is a primitive mechanism that evolved to permit resolution of objects at nearpoint, but which is inadequate for efficient performance on culturally imposed tasks requiring sustained inspection of minute, detailed target material. Both factors imply rationales whereby accommodation may lag behind convergence.

Howell (1990) cites ciliary muscle fatigue as a factor that causes accommodation to lag beyond convergence. He suggests that the ciliary muscle fatigues faster than the extraocular muscles, because during sustained near-vision tasks the ciliary muscle must maintain steady contraction without being able to relax to distance, while the extraocular muscles cycle through stimulation and relaxation as the eyes move from side to side.

A SYMPATHETIC ACTIVATION MODEL

Birnbaum (1984) views nearpoint stress in the context of general stress physiology. He suggests that the drive for convergence to localize closer than accommodation arises from the activation of neuroendocrine mechanisms that Cannon (1929) and Selye (1956) reported to underlie general stress. Birnbaum suggests that sympathetic nervous system activation resulting from attention and mental effort while reading, as well as from general stress pervasive in our society, causes a shift of accommodation toward far, so that increased accommodative effort is required to sustain accurate accommodation at near. This heightened innervational effort for accommodation generates overconvergence.

The fight-or-flight response (Cannon 1929) is an all-at-once emergency reaction to prepare the individual for immediate action in response to major stressors. The sympathetic nervous system activates those structures required for immediate action in response to a threatening situation and reduces activity of organs not involved in the emergency reaction. Sympathetic activation generates increased heart rate, increased blood pressure, increased blood flow to muscles and heart, and bronchial dilation to increase oxygen intake. Increased secretion of adrenalin liberates sugar from the liver for immediate use in energy production. Sympathetic activation also quiets the digestive tract and reduces blood flow to the skin (Mountcastle 1974).

Attention and mental effort are intrinsic to the near-work demands of our culture. These are not passive processes, but rather require physiological effort to maintain a state of readiness. This state, known as *physiological arousal,* is one of sympathetic activation similar in nature to the emergency fight-or-flight response described by Cannon (1929), though lesser in degree. The pattern of autonomic activity is similar for conditions of stress, strong emotion, attention, and mental effort, differing primarily in terms of magnitude (Malmo et al. 1950; Kahneman 1973; Pribram and McGuinness 1975).

Heightened *sympathetic arousal* has been demonstrated during visual attention (Kahneman 1973; Libby, et al. 1973; Pribram and McGuinness 1975) and cognitive processing (Hess and Polt, 1964; Beatty and Wagoner 1978). During pleasure reading, sympathetic activation similar in magnitude to that generated by cognitive processing occurs (Nell 1988).

In contrast to the central and parasympathetic nervous systems, which are organized to activate discrete units, the sympathetic nervous system is an all-at-once system that responds with activation of all innervated structures to facilitate action (Mountcastle 1974). The iris and ciliary muscle are among these sympathetically innervated structures.

Sympathetically mediated pupillary dilation is an integral part of the fight-or-flight response, serving perhaps to increase retinal luminance. Pupillary dilation is one of the most commonly used indices of autonomic arousal and attention (Kahneman 1973; Libby et al. 1973; Hess and Polt 1964; Nunnally et al. 1967). Pupillary dilation associated with mental effort increases with task demand and difficulty (Hess and Polt 1964; Beatty and Wagoner 1978), suggesting increased sympathetic activation.

Although the role of the sympathetic nervous system in accommodation was formerly controversial, recent anatomic, physiologic, and pharmacologic studies (reviewed by Toates 1972; Gilmartin 1986) establish the existence of sympathetic innervation to the human ciliary muscle. Evidence suggests that the role of sympathetic innervation in accommodation is to attenuate accommodative hysteresis (retention of accommodative tone) following near-vision tasks (Gilmartin and Hogan 1985; Gilmartin 1986; Gilmartin and Bullimore 1987; Bullimore and Gilmartin 1987). This notion is consistent with the general role of the sympathetic nervous system in triggering an emergency response to stress, in that it facilitates a rapid shift of accommodation from near to far to aid in the fight-or-flight response to environmental stressors.

Randle et al. (1980) and Malstrom et al. (1980) report that mental activity is accompanied by a shift of accommodation toward far, apparently resulting from activation of the sympathetic nervous system. Commercial pilots required to make task-related decisions while viewing a display during a night-landing simulation showed a small (approximately 0.1 D) persistent accommodative shift toward far. This accommodative shift was cumulative with each flight decision, and was influenced by the increasing importance of each decision (Randle et al. 1980).

Malstrom et al. (1980) found that subjects viewing a nearpoint target showed an accommodative shift toward far of 0.25 to 0.75 D following the introduction of a concurrent mental task. This shift was consistent, progressive, and cumulative, increasing as the mental task continued. The authors suggest that concentrated reading involves conflict between an ongoing accommodative shift toward far, associated with concurrent mental activity and increasing with its duration, and a need to readjust accommodation to maintain accurate near focus. They suggest that this conflict may underly asthenopic symptoms accompanying extended tasks such as reading.

Kruger (1975, 1977a, 1977b, 1980), in contrast, found an increase in accommodation when the task demand was changed from reading numbers to adding them, with no change in stimulus to accommodation. This increase was usually small (mean increase, 0.28 D), but was greater than 0.50 D in 20% of the sample, and as high as 2.63 D in one subject. Kruger indicated that the increase in accommodation appeared to reflect a reduction in lag.

These conflicting findings probably reflect differences in experimental design. Studies that report a shift of accommodation toward far with concurrent mental activity used large targets, and mental activity was unrelated to the fixation target. Kruger (1975, 1977a, 1977b, 1980), who found an increase in accommodation with mental effort, used fine print and introduced information-processing demands that were directly centered on the fixation material. Forrest (1988) suggests that accommodation postures beyond the plane of regard when demand is less intense and when cognitive state is less related to the task at hand. With more intense demand, the effort to problem-solve becomes greater. When cognitive aspects are increasingly related to the visual task, and when the periphery is increasingly excluded in attending to the task, the tendency is toward increased accommodation (Kruger 1977a, 1977b, 1980).

The nearpoint visual tasks imposed by society present demands similar to those created during Kruger's experiments. Print is generally small and information-processing demand is centered on the visual task. Under such conditions, Birnbaum (1984) suggests that a parasympathetic-induced increase in innervation to accommodation occurs to override the shift of accommodation toward far, demonstrated by Randle et al. (1980) and Malstrom et al. (1980) to accompany mental effort. Increased parasympathetic innervation to achieve conjugate focus generates increased convergence. Hence, convergence tends to localize closer than accommodation.

Consistent with the notion that the function of sympathetic innervation is to reduce accommodative hysteresis and facilitate the shift to far, Bullimore and Gilmartin (1987) indicate that both parasympathetic and sympathetic excitation may accompany strong attentional demands. Sympathetic innervation to accommodation is greatest during sustained visual tasks that require high levels of accommodative effort (Gilmartin and Bullimore 1987). However, during performance of the near-work task, these authors indicate that the effect of sympathetic involvement is to modify the synkinetic link between accommodation and convergence, with resultant increase in the AC/A ratio. Such an effect, similar to that hypothesized by Birnbaum (1984), is consistent with reports of a shift toward increased nearpoint esophoria (or reduced exophoria) with sustained near work (Forrest, 1960a, 1988; Ehrlich 1987).

In conflict with findings of increased sympathetic activation during stress and cognitive demand, some studies report an increase in TA with stress (Miller and LeBeau 1982) and strong cognitive demand (Bullimore and Gilmartin 1987). This increase in TA is primarily parasympathetic-mediated, and is subject to large differences in intersubject susceptibility.

PSYCHOLOGIC FACTORS IN NEARPOINT STRESS

Lazarus (1969) raises the issue as to whether the physiologic stress response is intrinsic to the stimulus, or is rather a product of one's appraisal of and attitude toward the stimulus. Grunberg (1986) raises a similar question with regard to nearpoint stress: Is stress intrinsic to the nearpoint task demands, or is it generated by the individual's attitude toward the task?

While Skeffington (1928–74) attributed nearpoint stress to task-related factors intrinsic to reading, Forrest (1980, 1987, 1988) and Birnbaum (1984, 1985a) suggest that psychologic factors that increase sympathetic activation may influence and exacerbate the nearpoint stress response.

Although the stress common to modern society usually involves psychologic and emotional factors, rather than physically threatening stimuli, the body's stress response is essentially the same regardless of the nature of the specific stressor (Selye 1956). Whether confronted with demands for sustained concentration and mental effort, threatening stimuli, or psychologic stressors, the body responds with a coordinated neuroendocrine response, the fight-or-flight response, comprising endocrine changes and sympathetic nervous system activation.

Psychologic stress that generates sympathetic activation induces a shift of accommodation toward far. Miller and Takahama (1987) found a decrease in dark focus of accommodation following exposure to emotionally stressful stimuli.

Forrest (1980, 1987, 1988) suggests that the primary factors that influence the visual stress response are attitude and psychologic status. He believes that nearpoint visual activity is the triggering mechanism for functional vision disorders, but that psychologic status, because of its influence on the physiologic stress response, is the primary and most important underlying factor. Forrest cites attentional intensity, central-peripheral organization, and attitude toward the task (and toward life itself) as psychologic factors that influence the stress response.

The intensity with which a task is performed influences the visual stress response (Forrest, 1988). Individuals who engage diligently on a task with maximum concentration and strong drive for achievement, striving to get the work done in as short a time as possible, invest greater attentional energy and generate greater stress activation.

Forrest (1988) cites *central-peripheral organization* as another major factor influencing the visual stress response. Individuals who are highly focal (central) generally exhibit a greater stress response. Such individuals tend to concentrate on figure. They inhibit periphery to minimize distraction. Their attentional intensity in performing the task is often quite high. While attention always requires some degree of energy and effort, focal individuals expend greater attentional energy to tune out the periphery, and consequently tend to exhibit a greater stress response.

Individuals who are highly logical and analytical in their thinking tend to be more highly focal. Reasoning, intellectualizing, and internally verbalizing during the task involve detuning much of the environment. As a consequence, such individuals invest greater attentional energy and exhibit a more severe stress response (Forrest, 1988).

According to Forrest (1988), an individual's fundamental belief systems and attitudes toward life may increase stress activation. Those who resist life as it is, who feel vulnerable and experience feelings of self-doubt and lowered self-esteem, who feel helpless and unable to control the events in their lives, who perceive themselves as being against the world rather than simply in harmony with life's flow, are more likely to experience stress.

Further, according to Forrest, one's attitude toward a particular task, and the intensity or resistance that an individual puts into a particular endeavor, is often a reflection of how life itself is approached, whether one copes with major life events by flowing with them or by resisting. One's attitude toward the task significantly influences the degree of physiological stress activation. Resenting a visual task increases the stress response. Psychological acceptance makes the task less stressful, and enjoying the task makes it less stressful still (Forrest 1988).

Effect of General Stress

Birnbaum (1984) hypothesizes that sympathetic activation generated by psychologic stress exacerbates the tendency toward overconvergence induced by attention, mental effort, immobilization, and intensity of nearpoint application. In modern society, psychologic stress is pervasive and extreme. We live in a highly competitive society, with a social and economic structure and sense of time urgency that subject us to greater stress than has been experienced in the past. Following frequent exposure to psychologic stress, the body may become habituated to high levels of stress activation. Many individuals, exposed to stress repeatedly or for prolonged periods, function at high levels of sympathetic activation, which become the norm during daily life (Pelletier 1977).

Nearpoint activity thus takes place in a milieu of conditioned sympathetic activation arising from psychologic stress (Birnbaum 1984). Further, individuals frequently engage in near work under stressful conditions. Adults study or read when tired or under time pressure; they read material that generates emotional stress or is related to business pressures and decision making; and they read for relaxation when emotionally stressed. Children experience pressure to achieve from parents, teachers, and peers, as well as from within. They may feel threatened during reading instruction, especially when required to read aloud, when reading demands are too difficult or too long, or when they are criticized or feel embarrassed as a result of reading errors. Difficulty or failure in reading adds to negative feelings of self-worth (Allington 1980; Wilson 1981; Deci et al. 1982; Gentile and McMillan 1987). Each of these factors serves to exacerbate the stress response and heighten sympathetic activation when reading.

Thus, the mismatch between convergence and accommodation postulated by Skeffington may arise from two sources: (1) task-related factors intrinsic to reading, which require immobilization and present demands for attention and mental effort which activate the sympathetic nervous system; (2) the psychologic status of the individual, whose personality, cognitive-perceptual style, attitude, intensity, emotional status, exposure to psychologic stress, and stress reactivity may lead him or her to function at high levels of sympathetic activation.

Birnbaum (1984) suggests that, since sympathetic activation induces a shift of accommodation toward far, increased parasympathetic innervation to accommodation is required to achieve conjugacy. This increased accommodative innervation generates a drive toward overconvergence.

CLINICAL EVIDENCE OF OVERCONVERGENCE

According to Skeffington (1928–74), the core element of nearpoint stress is a tendency for convergence to localize closer than accommodation during nearpoint visual tasks. This tendency is not always demonstrable as a measured esophoria at near, since many individuals adapt by creating an exophoric buffer. Nevertheless, test probes that impose heightened demand for sustained attention and concentration, like the nearpoint tasks common to our society, can be used to demonstrate overconvergence clinically, even in patients who show exophoria on the von Graefe test at near.

Forrest (1960a, 1988) reported an esophoric shift when the near-phoria test is taken before and after a brief period of reading. Ehrlich (1987) reported a similar esophoric shift following prolonged near work. He attributes this shift to vergence adaptation and to accommodative fatigue, which results in an increase in accommodative innervation required to maintain focus, and hence an increase in accommodative convergence.

Similar trends toward increased esophoria with sustained attention have been noted by Stenhouse-Stewart (1945), who reported an increase in nearpoint esophoria in subjects who spent one-half hour viewing stereograms, and by Vaegan (1979), who reported an increase in esophoria between first glance and 15 seconds later as a well-known clinical consequence of continued inspection of the Maddox wing.

During cheiroscopic tracing, a task that requires sustained attention and concentration, many patients exhibit a progressive esophoric shift as the tracing proceeds (Figure 3.2). This shift is commonly found in exophores, as well as in esophores. Progressive exophoric shift is rarely observed, except in divergent strabismus (Birnbaum 1985a).

Birnbaum (1985b) reported an esophoric shift of 5 prism diopters (Δ) or more in 18 of 100 subjects when von Graefe phoria measures were obtained in rapid succession. Shifts as great as 16^Δ were obtained. Christenson et al. (1990) reported a similar esophoric shift in 22% of a sample of 50 optometry students, noting that the esophoric shift is more likely to be associated with a type II, III, or IV than with a type I fixation disparity curve.

Birnbaum (1985b) attributes the esophoric shift obtained during repeated phoria testing to autonomic arousal associated with sustained attention and concentration. He suggests that sympathetic activation causes a shift of accommodation toward far, with consequent increase in the accommodative effort required to maintain conjugate focus at the plane of regard, and hence to overconvergence.

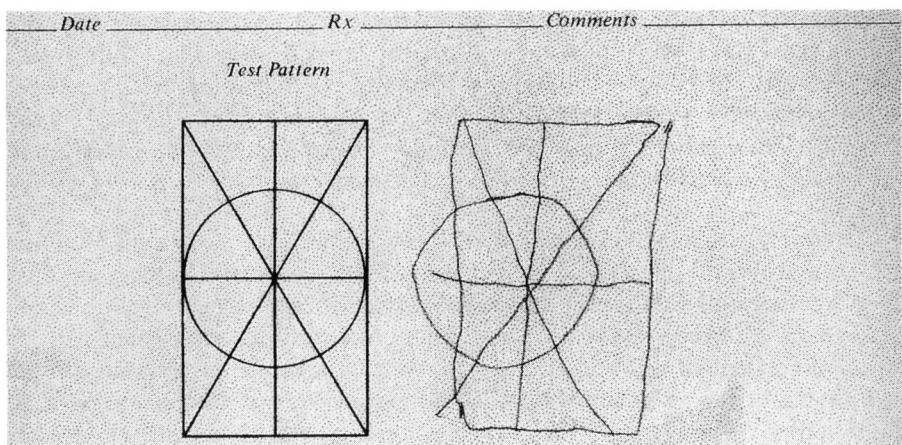

Figure 3.2 Esophoric shift during cheiroscopic tracing. The patient first traced the rectangle, beginning in the upper right corner; then the diagonal, vertical, and horizontal lines; and finally the circle. Increasing esophoric posture is evident as the tracing proceeds.

The associated phoria frequently measures less exophoria or more esophoria than the dissociated phoria, and many patients who show exophoria at near under dissociated conditions nevertheless demonstrate eso-fixation disparity (Ogle et al. 1967). Such findings are consistent with the existence of a drive toward overconvergence under fused binocular conditions.

In the Skeffington model, exophoria present under dissociated conditions is viewed as a measure of the innervational pattern between accommodation and convergence, which has been adopted to reduce overconvergence during fused conditions. Exophoria is viewed not as a fusional demand, but rather as an adaptive response to buffer overconvergence. The presence of exophoria in a particular patient does not rule out the presence of a drive for convergence to localize closer than accommodation, since the exophoria may be an adaptive response to overconvergence. Further, individuals who demonstrate exophoria under dissociated conditions, when attentional demands are minimal, may nevertheless demonstrate overconvergence during habitual fused conditions, especially during sustained concentration.

Accommodative-Convergence/ Convergence-Accommodation Interactions

Schor and Narayan (1982) indicate that the increased esophoria found under associated (fused) conditions results from the interaction between accommodative-convergence and convergence-accommodation (see Chapter 1). The effect of this mutual interaction is such that the demands on fusional vergence and accommodation under fused conditions are always greater than indicated by the dissociated phoria measure and the target distance, respectively.

In individuals who demonstrate esophoria at near on the dissociated phoria test, as well as those who show orthophoria or low exophoria but shift toward esophoria with heightened attentional demand or mental effort, the over-convergence tendency generated by sympathetic activation may be exacerbated by AC/CA interaction so that the tendency toward overconvergence under fused conditions is markedly greater than that measured by the dissociated near phoria.

The evidence that individuals often show greater esophoria under habitual fused conditions and during tasks that require sustained attention supports Skef-fington's premise of a tendency for convergence to localize nearer than accommodation during nearpoint visual tasks. These findings are inconsistent with the traditional concept of dissociated near phoria as a measure of fusional demand under habitual near-work conditions. The overconvergence tendency present under habitual near-work conditions may be much greater than that indicated by the dissociated near-phoria test.

In contrast with these findings, Yekta et al. (1987) report a shift toward increased exophoria at the end of a day's work. They found an increase in dissociated heterophoria, associated heterophoria, and fixation disparity at the end of a working day that included several hours of close work.

EXOPHORIA AS A BUFFER

Skeffington (1947, 1950) notes that the ocular mechanisms of convergence and accommodation are elements of the systemic skeletal and visceral (auto-nomic) systems, respectively, and suggests that systemic changes in neural activity may influence these ocular mechanisms. Skeffington postulates that exophoria and hyperopia serve to protect convergence and accommodation from systemic influences. In the absence of such buffers, changes in systemic innervation would interfere with the maintenance of clear, single vision. Low hyperopia and exophoria are thus viewed as desirable attributes, not as defects or errors.

Skeffington (1953) postulated that approximately 6^Δ of exophoria is ordinarily expected at near, and approximately 0.5^Δ at far, in individuals whose visual function is unimpaired. Studies document that exophoria at near is an expected, normal finding. Haines (1941) reported a mean near phoria of 5^Δ exophoria in a sample of 500 asymptomatic, visually efficient individuals. Shepard (1941) and Morgan (1948) did not eliminate symptomatic or visually inefficient individuals, and found mean near-phoria measures of 5^Δ and 3^Δ exophoria, respectively.

Hyperopic and exophoric buffers designed to protect the mechanisms of accommodation and convergence during momentary shifts in dominance between the systemic visceral and skeletal systems are not sufficient to protect against extreme demands on the visual system itself. When an individual is forced to maintain concentration at near for prolonged periods, the magnitude of these buffers gradually decreases, resulting in emmetropia and orthophoria. Absorption of these buffers is undesirable, since the individual losses protection against increased stimulation (Skeffington 1947, 1950; Manas 1965).

If increased systemic stimulation or intense nearpoint visual activity is prolonged, increased stimulation of the convergence mechanism will cause diplopia unless an active inhibition of convergence innervation is established. This excess convergence innervation is measured, by means of dissociating prism, as an esophoria. Esophoria is viewed as an emergency state in which excess convergence innervation is inhibited to maintain single vision (Skeffington 1947, 1950; Manas 1965).

Since orthophoria and esophoria are inefficient states, it is desirable for the individual to reestablish an exophoric buffer to eliminate them. However, continued dominance of the systemic skeletal system or sustained near-work demand may make it impossible to restore exophoria (Skeffington 1947; Manas 1965).

Orthophoria therefore is not simply a passive, static condition, but is rather a state of dynamic equilibrium. Depending on where the individual is in the esophoria-exophoria cycle, the presence of orthophoria may indicate either that the original exophoria has been completely absorbed as a result of stress on the visual system, or that the individual has eliminated an existing esophoria and is rebuilding an exophoric buffer (Manas 1965).

In some cases, individuals exposed to prolonged visual stress may develop degrees of exophoria so great as to lead to suppression or intermittent exotropia. In such cases, the exophoria itself becomes a source of visual inefficiency (Forrest 1960b; Manas 1965).

Mechanisms for Creating an Exophoric Buffer

The concept of exophoria as a desirable attribute, serving to provide a buffer in the convergence mechanism, is unique to the Skeffington model, but is consistent with the notion of vision as a pliable, adaptive system that is modified as a result of environmental interaction. Mechanisms that can be used to create an exophoric buffer include (1) vergence adaptation (prism adaptation), and (2) modification of the relationship between accommodation and convergence.

Vergence adaptation is a process in which alteration in tonic vergence occurs to reduce stress on the binocular system (Schor 1983a). McCormack (1985) found that exophores whose nearpoint phoria was neutralized with a base-in prism during a 20-minute near-reading task adapted from their prismatically created orthophoria toward their habitual exophoria. By the end of the reading period, the exophoria measured with the prism in place approached that present before prism application. This demonstration that vergence adaptation maintains exophoria, rather than prism-created orthophoria, in normal subjects performing a nearpoint task, suggests that nearpoint exophoria is not a defect, but rather a valuable attribute.

Similar adaptation to experimentally induced heterophoria has been reported by Schor (1979) and by North and Henson (1985). Binocular application of minus lenses stimulates accommodation and accommodative-convergence, with a consequent shift toward esophoria. Under binocular viewing conditions, the phoria is corrected by fusional divergence. When the minus lenses are removed and one eye covered, adaptation results in exophoria. These results are consistent with Skeffington's assertion that exophoria may develop as an adaptive response to buffer or compensate overconvergence during nearpoint visual activity.

Modification of the relationship between accommodation and convergence is a possible alternative mechanism by which one might create an exophoric buffer. Although the AC/A ratio is often described as fixed and resistant to change (Alpern 1969), considerable evidence suggests that the relationship between vergence and accommodation is not static or fixed (Schor 1986).

Adaptive changes in AC/A do occur when such change is required for efficient function, and when the stimulus for change is sufficiently great. The AC/A ratio remains fairly stable during the pre-presbyopic years (Breinin and Chin, 1973), despite increasing rigidity of the crystalline lens. The demand for increasing accommodative effort would be expected to lead to an increase in the AC/A ratio; that this does not occur suggests that an adaptive process is at work (Schor 1983b). Esotropes sometimes maintain a reduced AC/A ratio following discontinuation of miotic therapy, which also suggests that adaptation has taken place (Birnbaum 1963). Changes in AC/A are often found in undercorrected myopes during adaptation to full refractive correction (Flom and Takahashi 1962). The accommodation/convergence relationship develops early in life, yet must be sufficiently flexible to allow modification in response to growth-induced increases in interpupillary distance (Schor 1983c). Adaptive change in AC/A has been demonstrated when demands on accommodative vergence are altered by optically changing the effective interocular separation (Judge and Miles 1981).

Further indication that adaptation influences the relationship between accommodation and convergence is found in reports that adaptation disorders of either vergence or accommodation result in abnormality of accommodative vergence. The AC/A ratio varies directly with adaptability of vergence and inversely with adaptability of accommodation; the CA/C ratio varies directly with adaptability of accommodation and inversely with adaptability of vergence (Schor 1986, 1988; Schor and Tsuetaki 1987).

Transient changes in the AC/A ratio have been reported as a result of orthoptics (Manas 1958; Flom 1960), even though the training performed was not designed to induce such changes. There are reports of cases that demonstrate significant variation in AC/A over a period of several years as a result of refractive status change, lens application, and/or orthoptics (Ogle et al. 1967).

These findings suggest that the relationship between vergence and accommodation is not as rigid and inflexible as was once thought. The demonstration of vergence adaptation to maintain preexisting exophoria, and of plasticity in the relationship between convergence and accommodation, suggests potential mechanisms for the organism to build or rebuild an exophoric buffer as suggested by Skeffington.

CLINICAL SIGNS OF NEARPOINT STRESS

Patients who demonstrate a tendency toward overconvergence are at high risk for development of nearpoint stress—induced vision disorder. Such patients typically experience inefficiency and discomfort during near work, develop adaptations such as myopia, or withdraw and avoid close work as much as possible. It is important that treatment be initiated at the earliest sign of difficulty to prevent these adverse effects.

Signs of nearpoint stress include the following:

- skews and constrictions in the phoria, vergence, and accommodative findings;
- esophoria, orthophoria, or less than the desirable exophoria at near;
- exophoria at near greater than normal;
- shifts toward overconvergence during sustained nearpoint activity;
- absorption of the desirable low hyperopic buffer, with shifts toward emmetropia, myopia, or adverse high hyperopia;
- low positive relative accommodation (PRA) finding;
- asthenopia during near-vision tasks;
- avoidance of near work;
- maintenance of an exceptionally close near-working distance.

A tendency for convergence to localize closer than accommodation interferes with efficient binocular function. Patients frequently demonstrate intermittent suppression and lowered prism vergence findings.

Asthenopic symptoms frequently accompany lowered visual efficiency. However, many patients avoid reading as a consequence of binocular disorder, and hence report little symptomatology.

Absorption of the hyperopic and exophoric buffers is an early sign of nearpoint stress–induced vision disorder. In this context, emmetropia and orthophoria are viewed not as perfect or desirable, but as signs of problems. If the difficulty persists and preventive care is not initiated, reduced visual efficiency and/or adverse adaptation are likely to result (Skeffington 1947, 1950).

Esophoria at near may be an early sign of nearpoint stress–induced overconvergence, or may reflect a conditioned response to long-standing stress on the visual system. High exophoria at near may indicate that the individual has adapted to buffer nearpoint stress–induced overconvergence.

A tendency toward overconvergence is, in this author's experience, the earliest clinical sign of a nearpoint visual problem. The near-phoria measure is an extremely sensitive, bellwether finding. Clinical experience indicates that exophoria of 4 to 6$^\Delta$ is desirable, and that even small deviations from this expected level signal difficulty. Measurement of esophoria, orthophoria, or even a few prism diopters less than the expected 4- to 6$^\Delta$ exophoria are early signs of overconvergence. Failure to recognize these early signs and to apply preventive measures is frequently followed by adverse adaptive change, often myopia (Birnbaum 1985a).

The near-phoria test measures oculomotor balance at a given instant in time, under conditions of relatively minimal demand. Tasks that impose greater attentional and information-processing demand may generate increased overconvergence. Even patients manifesting orthophoria or low exophoria on a dissociated near-phoria test may show overconvergence during sustained near work. The significance of a dissociated near phoria less than the expected 4- to 6$^\Delta$ exophoria lies not in the fusional demand imposed by the phoria, but rather that it signals the lack of an adequate exophoric buffer (Birnbaum 1985a).

Since tasks that require sustained concentration are more likely to provoke overconvergence, the clinician should challenge the patient by either measuring the near phoria before and after a few minutes of sustained reading (Forrest 1960a); measuring the near phoria repetitively as the patient sustains fixation (Birnbaum 1985b); or performing a cheiroscopic tracing test to determine the existence of an esophoric shift (Figure 3.2). Shifts toward esophoria under such conditions are early signs of nearpoint stress. Failure to initiate care often precedes development of nearpoint stress–induced vision disorder. Goss (1991) found that children who develop myopia are likely to demonstrate more esophoria and lower PRA, preceding the development of myopia, than children who remain emmetropic.

A low PRA finding is another important early clinical sign of nearpoint vision disorder. The PRA does not probe accommodative function per se, but rather the flexibility between accommodation and convergence. An individual who has a nearpoint stress–induced tendency for convergence to localize closer than accommodation will have difficulty shifting accommodation closer than convergence. A low PRA is thus an early sign of nearpoint stress–induced overconvergence. A low PRA is characteristic not only of accommodative disorder, but of incipient and progressing myopia and of many cases of vergence dysfunction as well (Birnbaum 1985a).

Working at excessively close distances while reading and writing is common in cases of functional vision disorder. Although individuals with accommodative or convergence disorder might be expected to hold nearpoint material farther away, as does the presbyope, an excessively close near-work distance is common. Since a tendency for convergence to localize closer than accommodation appears to underlie functional vision disorders, an excessively close working distance may reflect a "pulling in" to neutralize this overconvergence, near-work distance moving progressively closer as esophoria increases during sustained nearpoint application.

Close working distances may also result from intensity of application. Highly intense individuals often read and write at close working distances, pulling material in close to block out periphery and facilitate concentration. Such individuals, who invest a great deal of concentration and attentional energy in their near work, may be those most likely to manifest overconvergence as a result of sympathetic nervous system activation.

SUMMARY

Skeffington postulated that the nearpoint visual tasks of our culture provoke a stress response characterized by a drive for convergence to localize closer than accommodation. The resulting mismatch between vergence and accommodation during near work interferes with visual efficiency, impairs information-processing capacity, and leads to asthenopia, avoidance, and adaptations within the visual system. Birnbaum attributes the drive for convergence to localize closer both to sympathetic activation associated with attention and mental effort during near work, and to psychological stress. Forrest suggests that the primary factors that trigger the nearpoint stress response are psychological, particularly attentional intensity, attitude, and central-peripheral organization.

Several reports document a tendency toward increased esophoria (or decreased exophoria) during sustained near work. Early clinical signs of nearpoint stress include esophoria, orthophoria, or too little exophoria at near; a shift toward overconvergence during sustained visual activity; and low PRA.

Exophoria, according to Skeffington, is an innervational pattern that serves to protect the visual system against overconvergence and consequent diplopia. When overconvergence is induced by sustained visual activity, the individual may adapt by creating a greater exophoric buffer.

SUGGESTED READING

Birnbaum MH (1984). Nearpoint visual stress: A physiological model. *J Am Optom Assoc* 55(11):825–835.

Birnbaum MH (1985). Nearpoint visual stress: Clinical implications. *J Am Optom Assoc* 56(6):480–490.

Manas L (1965). *Visual Analysis,* 3rd ed. Chicago: Professional Press.

Skeffington AM (1928–74). Optometric Extension Program Continuing Education Courses. Santa Ana, CA: Optometric Extension Program Foundation.

REFERENCES

Allington RL (1980). Poor readers don't get to read much in reading groups. *Language Arts* 57(8):872–876.

Alpern M (1969). Types of Movement, In: Davson H (ed), *The Eye, vol. 3: Muscular Mechanisms,* 2nd ed. New York: Academic, pp. 137–141.

Beatty J, Wagoner BL (1978). Pupillometric signs of brain activation vary with level of cognitive processing. *Science* 199 (4334):1216–1218.

Birnbaum MH (1963). The use of miotics in the treatment of esotropia. *Opt J Rev Optom* 100(19):29–37.

Birnbaum MH (1984). Nearpoint visual stress: A physiological model. *J Am Optom Assoc* 55(11):825–835.

Birnbaum MH (1985a). Nearpoint visual stress: Clinical implications. *J Am Optom Assoc* 56(6):480–490.

Birnbaum MH (1985b). An esophoric shift associated with sustained fixation. *Am J Optom Physiol Opt* 62(11):732–735.

Breinin GN, Chin NB (1973). Accommodation, convergence and aging. *Doc Ophthalmol* 34: 109–121.

Bullimore MA, Gilmartin B (1987). Tonic accommodation, cognitive demand, and ciliary muscle innervation. *Am J Optom Physiol Opt* 64(1):45–50.

Cannon WB (1929). *Bodily Changes in Pain, Hunger, Fear and Rage: An Account of Recent Researches into the Function of Emotional Excitement.* New York: Appleton.

Christenson GN, Korth CJ, Marcolivio M (1990). An investigation of the "eso-phoric shift" and its relationship to parameters of the fixation disparity curve. *J Behav Optom* 1(7):179–182.

Deci EL, Spiegel NH, Ryan NM, et al. (1982). Effects of performance standards on teaching styles: Behavior of controlling teachers. *J Educ Psychol* 74(6):852–859.

Ehrlich DL (1987). Near vision stress: Vergence adaptation and accommodative fatigue. *Opthalmic Physiol Opt* 7(4):353–357.

Flax N (1985). Functional case analysis: An interpretation of the Skeffington model. *Am J Optom Physiol Opt* 62(6):365–368.

Flom MC (1960). On the relationship between accommodation and accommodative convergence. Part III. Effects of orthoptics. *Am J Optom Arch Am Acad Optom* 37(12):619–632.

Flom MC, Takahashi E (1962). The AC/A ratio and undercorrected myopia. *Am J Optom Arch Am Acad Optom* 39(6):305–312.

Forrest EB (1960a). A modern philosophy of vision. IV. The story of stress. *Optom Weekly*, 51:332–334; 635–636.

Forrest EB (1960b). A modern philosophy of vision. III. The motor components of the visual process. *Optom Weekly*, 51:17–20.

Forrest EB (1980). Stress: A redefinition. *J Am Optom Assoc* 51(6):600–604.

Forrest EB (1987). Going beyond the behavioral model: A challenge for the future. *J Optom Vis Dev* 18(2):3–5.

Forrest EB (1988). *Stress and Vision*. Santa Ana, CA: Optometric Extension Program Foundation.

Gentile LM, McMillan MM (1987). *Stress and Reading Difficulties. Research, Assessment, Intervention*. Newark, DE: International Reading Association.

Gilmartin B (1986). A review of the role of sympathetic innervation of the ciliary muscle in ocular accommodation. *Ophthalmic Physiol Opt* 6(1):23–37.

Gilmartin B, Bullimore MA (1987). Sustained near-vision augments inhibitory sympathetic innervation of the ciliary muscle. *Clin Vis Sci* 1(3):197–208.

Gilmartin B, Hogan RE (1985). The role of the sympathetic nervous system in ocular accommodation and ametropia. *Ophthalmic Physiol Opt* 5:91–93.

Goss DA (1991). Clinical accommodation and heterophoria findings preceding juvenile onset of myopia. *Optom Vis Sci* 68(2):110–116.

Grunberg NE (1986). Stress and Vision. Oral presentation, College of Optometrists in Vision Development, Annual Meeting, San Diego, CA. Sound recording, Insta-Tape, Monrovia, CA, 1987.

Haines HF (1941). Normal values of visual functions and their application in case analysis. The analysis of findings and determination of normals, Part IV. *Am J Optom* 18(2):58–73.

Hendrickson H (1969). The vision development process. In: Wold RM (ed), *Visual and Perceptual Aspects for the Achieving and Underachieving Child*. Seattle: Special Child Publ, pp. 45–57.

Hess EH, Polt JM (1964). Pupil size in relation to mental activity during simple problem-solving. *Science* 143(3611):1190–1192.

Howell ER (1990). Differential diagnosis of accommodation/convergence disorders. Oral presentation, 1st International Congress of Behavioral Optometry, Monte Carlo, Nov. 5.

Judge SJ, Miles FA (1981). Gain changes in accommodative vergence induced by alteration of the effective interocular separation. In: Fuchs AF, Becker W (eds), *Progress in Oculomotor Research*. New York: Elsevier, pp. 587–594.

Kahneman D (1973). *Attention and Effort*. Englewood Cliffs, NJ: Prentice-Hall, pp. 1–49.

Kruger PB (1975). Luminance changes of the fundus reflex. *Am J Optom* 52(12):847–861.

Kruger PB (1977a). Changes in fundus reflex luminance with increased cognitive processing. *Am J Optom* 54(7):445–451.

Kruger PB (1977b). The role of accommodation in increasing the luminance of the fundus reflex during cognitive processing. *J Am Optom Assoc* 48(12):1493–1496.

Kruger PB (1980). The effect of cognitive demand on accommodation. *Am J Optom Physiol Opt* 57(7):440–445.

Lazarus RC (1969). *Patterns of Adjustment and Human Effectiveness.* New York: McGraw-Hill, pp. 161–208.

Libby WL, Lacey BC, Lacey JI (1973). Pupillary and cardiac activity during visual attention. *Psychophysiology* 10(3):270–294.

Malmo RB, Shagass C, Davis H (1950). Symptoms specificity and bodily reactions during psychiatric interview. *Psychosom Med* 12(6):362–376.

Malstrom FW, Randle RJ, Bendix JS, et al. (1980). The visual accommodation response during concurrent mental activity. *Percept Psychophysiol* 28(5):440–448.

Manas L (1958). The effect of visual training upon the ACA ratio. *Am J Optom Arch Am Acad Optom* 35(8):428–437.

Manas L (1965). *Visual Analysis.* 3rd ed. Chicago: Professional Press, pp. 32–38.

McCormack GL (1985). Vergence adaptation maintains heterophoria in normal binocular vision. *Am J Optom Physiol Opt* 62(8):555–561.

Miller RJ, LeBeau RC (1982). Induced stress, situationally specific trait anxiety, and dark focus. *Psychophysiology* 19:260–265.

Miller RJ, Takahama M (1987). Effects of relaxation and aversive visual stimulation on dark focus accommodation. *Ophthalmic Physiol Opt* 7:219–224.

Morgan MW (1948). Analysis of clinical data. *Optom Weekly* 39(34):1811–1818; 39(35):1843–1847.

Mountcastle VB (1974). *Medical Physiology.* Vol. 1, 13th ed. St. Louis: Mosby, pp. 788–792.

Nell V (1988). The psychology of reading for pleasure: Needs and gratifications. *Reading Res Qual* 23(1):6–48.

North R, Henson DB (1985). Adaptation to lens-induced heterophorias. *Am J Optom Physiol Opt* 62(11):774–780.

Nunnally JC, Knott PD, Duchnowski A, et al. (1967). Pupillary response as a general measure of activation. *Percept Psychophysiol* 2(4):149–155.

Ogle KN, Martens TG, Dyer JA (1967). *Oculomotor Imbalance in Binocular Vision and Fixation Disparity.* Philadelphia: Lea & Febiger, pp. 108–113, 175–184, 195–230.

Pelletier KR (1977). *Mind as Healer, Mind as Slayer: A Holistic Approach to Preventing Stress Disorder.* New York: Delacort.

Pribram K, McGuinness D (1975). Arousal, activation and effort in the control of attention. *Psychol Rev* 82(2):116–149.

Randle R, Roscoe SN, Petitt JC (1980). Effects of magnification and visual accommodation on aim-point estimation in simulated landings with real and virtual image displays. Moffett Field, CA: National Aeronautics and Space Administration, Ames Research Center, NASA Tech Paper 1635.

Schor CM (1979). The relationship between fusional vergence eye movements and fixation disparity. *Vision Res* 19:1359–1367.

Schor CM (1983a). Fixation disparity and vergence adaptation. In: Schor CM, Ciuffreda KJ (eds), *Vergence Eye Movements: Basic and Clinical Aspects.* Boston: Butterworth–Heinemann, pp. 465–516.

Schor CM (1983b). Analysis of tonic and accommodative vergence disorders of binocular vision. *Am J Optom Physiol Opt* 60(1):1–14.

Schor CM (1983c). Colorado Behavioral Vision Seminar. Estes Park, CO, September.

Schor CM (1986). The Glenn A. Fry Award Lecture: Adaptive regulation of accommodative vergence and vergence accommodation. *Am J Optom Physiol Opt* 63:587–609.

Schor CM (1988). Imbalanced adaptation of accommodation and vergence produces opposite extremes of the AC/A and CA/C ratios. *Am J Optom Physiol Opt* 65(5):341–348.

Schor CM, Narayan V (1982). Graphical analysis of prism adaptation, convergence accommodation and accommodative convergence. *Am J Optom Physiol Opt* 59:774–784.

Schor CM, Tsuetaki T (1987). Fatigue of accommodation and vergence modifies their mutual interactions. *Invest Ophthalmol Vis Sci* 28:1250–1259.

Selye H (1956). *The Stress of Life*. New York: McGraw-Hill.

Shepard CF (1941). The most probable "expecteds." *Optom Weekly* 32(19):538–541.

Skeffington AM (1928–74). Optometric Extension Program Continuing Education Courses, Santa Ana, CA: Optometric Extension Program Foundation.

Skeffington AM (1947). *Near Point Optometry*. Optometric Extension Program Continuing Education Courses, Santa Ana, CA: Optometric Extension Program Foundation, vol. 2, no. 4–12, Jan–Sept.

Skeffington AM (1950). *Near Point Optometry*. Optometric Extension Program Continuing Education Courses, Santa Ana, CA: Optometric Extension Program Foundation, 6(1):1–5, Oct.

Skeffington AM (1953). *A Modern Concept of Vision*. In: *Practical Applied Optometry*. Optometric Extension Program Continuing Education Courses, Santa Ana, CA: Optometric Extension Program Foundation, vol. 25, No. 9. Sept., pp. 85–96.

Skeffington AM (1964). *Introduction to Clinical Optometry*. Optometric Extension Program Continuing Education Courses, Santa Ana, CA: Optometric Extension Program Foundation, vol. 37, series 1, no. 2, Nov.

Stenhouse-Stewart DD (1945). Some observations on a tendency to near-point esophoria, and possible contributory factors. *Brit J Ophthalmol* 29: 37–42.

Toates FM (1972). Accommodation function of the human eye. *Physiol Rev* 52(4):828–863.

Vaegan JL (1979). Convergence and divergence show large and sustained improvement after short isometric exercise. *Am J Optom Physiol Opt* 56:23–33.

Wilson RM (1981). *Diagnostic and Remedial Reading for Classroom and Clinic*. 4th ed. Columbus, OH: Charles E. Merrill.

Yekta AA, Jenkins T, Pickwell D (1987). The clinical assessment of binocular vision before and after a working day. *Ophthalmic Physiol Opt* 7(4):349–352.

4

The Skeffington Model: Adaptations to Nearpoint Stress

In contrast to traditional models that attribute refractive, accommodative, and binocular disorders to genetic influence and random biologic variation, Skeffington (1928–74) held that these disorders commonly occur as end-products of environmental interaction, resulting either from interference with development or from nearpoint visual stress.

According to Skeffington, the characteristic visual stress response is a drive for convergence to localize closer than accommodation. This drive interferes with visual efficiency and must be resolved if near work is to be sustained comfortably. Unless this effector system mismatch is relieved, the individual is faced with a dilemma. If the subject accommodates for the plane of regard, convergence will localize nearer, resulting in double vision. If the subject converges for the plane of regard, accommodation will localize beyond this plane and vision will be blurred. The individual will see clearly, or singly, but not both. In the presence of such conflict, many individuals experience discomfort, visual inefficiency, and reduced comprehension. Many seek to avoid near work, and many initiate adaptive changes within the visual system (Skeffington 1964–65).

To localize accommodation and convergence in the same plane, the individual may initiate a variety of changes in the pattern of relationship between vergence and accommodation. These changes may ultimately become embedded as anomalies of refractive status and binocular function. Skeffington (1928–74) views conditions such as adventitious myopia, adverse high hyperopia, divergent squint, and various skews in binocular and accommodative function as adaptations by which the individual seeks to relieve the drive for convergence to localize closer than accommodation. These disorders are viewed not as primary conditions, but as end-products of adaptation to nearpoint stress–induced effector system mismatch. Ocular defects are held to occur when nearpoint stress is sustained and prolonged; they are unlikely to result from brief periods of transient visual stress with which the visual system is better able to cope (Flax 1985).

Properly prescribed low-plus nearpoint lenses relieve the drive for convergence to localize closer than accommodation. Such lenses allow the effector system mismatch to take place, yet bring focus to the same plane as alignment, thereby eliminating the source of difficulty and the need to adapt. Unless appropriate nearpoint lenses are provided or effective adaptation takes place, impaired visual achievement, avoidance, or discomfort results from the failure to adequately integrate convergence and accommodation (Skeffington 1964–65).

In the Skeffington model, vision is closely associated with information-processing and intellectual achievement. Although vision involves resolution, accommodation, and convergence, the process is broader than these mechanisms and involves perception, information-processing, and the integration of input from all senses with past experience and memory (Hendrickson 1969, 1976). Skeffington (1964–65) indicates that the nearpoint stress–induced mismatch between vergence and accommodation not only causes asthenopia, but that the effort to function in the presence of such a mismatch impairs high-level cognitive processing and reading comprehension. In making ocular adaptations such as myopia, the individual sacrifices lower-order visual abilities in the effort to restore visual efficiency and preserve higher-order information-processing ability.

Individuals may develop a variety of adaptations to resolve the effector system mismatch and reduce overconvergence. Myopia, development of a high exophoric buffer, and inhibition of accommodation are among the most common. Myopia serves to reduce accommodative demand and associated overconvergence, thus permitting focus and alignment to each localize at the plane of regard. Myopia is a highly effective adaptation, facilitating comfortable, efficient nearpoint function at the expense of distance acuity. Development of high exophoria and inhibition of accommodation are less effective; they serve to avoid overconvergence, but result in impairment of binocular function, intermittent suppression, visual inefficiency, and discomfort.

The path of adaptation taken by a particular individual depends on the significance to that individual of the functional limitations imposed by each adaptation, on environmental and genetic factors, and on the degree of plasticity in the visual system. The greater an individual's drive for achievement, the greater the likelihood of a myopic adaptation. In practice, many individuals demonstrate a combination of vision disorders (for example, myopia, high exophoria, accommodative insufficiency), suggesting that a variety of adaptive paths have been explored.

ASTHENOPIA, AVOIDANCE, AND ADAPTATION

The relation between vision disorders and asthenopia is complex. Many patients with functional vision problems experience significant discomfort; others do not. To understand this disparity requires consideration of the adaptive path that the individual has taken, as well as the various psychological factors involved.

Some individuals maintain adequate flexibility between vergence and accommodation, and are able to sustain near work comfortably and efficiently without symptoms. Such individuals demonstrate refractive and phorometric findings that approach expected levels, with maintenance of hyperopic and exophoric buffers.

Others, whose flexibility between accommodation and convergence is inadequate, whose exposure to near work is extensive, or whose intensity and concentration are very great, have difficulty with near work. They commonly demonstrate signs of overconvergence. Phorometric findings are typically constricted, since the mismatch between vergence and accommodation interferes with efficient binocular function. Such individuals frequently report symptoms associated with close work, including nearpoint blur, diplopia, headache, eyestrain, general tiredness, loss of place, inability to read for prolonged periods, impaired comprehension, print running together, blurred distance vision after near work, and difficulty focusing.

When close work causes discomfort and frustration, many individuals avoid near work as much as possible. They present with constricted prism vergence and accommodative findings, yet report no asthenopia, primarily because they avoid reading. When asked, they commonly report that they read little and do not like to read. They generally experience asthenopia when prolonged near work is unavoidable.

Such individual's lives frequently are shaped by their visual problems. Lack of interest in reading influences school achievement, career selection, and interest in higher education. Vision problems that cause disinterest in school may even predispose toward juvenile delinquency and criminality. A high incidence of vision disorders among juvenile delinquents has been reported (Dzik 1966; Dowis 1977; Kaseno 1982; Snow 1983).

Frequently, vision problems are not treated because patients are asymptomatic. It is important to recognize that uncorrected vision disorder may seriously limit achievement. The absence of asthenopia does not negate the presence of vision problems, since patients who avoid reading generally do not report symptoms. Treatment should be considered, even in the absence of asthenopia, when functional vision disorders exist that interfere with nearpoint efficiency or lead to avoidance of reading.

Although subjects who avoid reading as a consequence of functional vision disorder are frequently underachievers, such is not always the case. Some individuals who demonstrate patterns of avoidance are bright enough to achieve at adequate levels even though they limit reading to minimal levels. Such individuals often develop myopia or experience asthenopia when they reach a level of academic or vocational demand at which avoidance is impossible, as may occur when a child progresses in school; reaches high school, college, or graduate school; or works as an accountant, attorney, secretary, or computer operator.

A myopic adaptation usually permits efficient nearpoint function without asthenopia. Thus, the relationship between nearpoint stress and asthenopia is complex. Individuals may be asymptomatic because they have adequate binocular function, because they avoid reading, or because they develop myopia. The absence of asthenopia does not necessarily mean that visual function is adequate.

In this author's experience, patients who present with impaired accommodative and binocular findings, but without asthenopia, are generally asymptomatic either because they have developed myopia or because they avoid reading. When asthenopia is absent, many practitioners assume that existing visual problems are insignificant and do not require treatment. Recognition that patients with functional vision disorder may be asymptomatic because they avoid or adapt leads the clinician to consider treatment in such cases, to eliminate the need for continued avoidance or further development of adaptive vision disorder.

ADAPTIVE PATTERNS IN ACCOMMODATION AND CONVERGENCE

Skeffington (1964–65) indicates that in response to a drive for convergence to localize closer than accommodation, individuals may alter the innervational pattern to accommodation and/or convergence to avoid blur and diplopia. Depending on the specific adaptive pattern, the various phorometric findings become high or low in a variety of syndromes known as *case types*. The skewed phorometric findings are viewed, in the Skeffington model, not as the primary functional vision problem, but rather as products of adaptation to nearpoint stress.

These skews in accommodative and vergence findings do not achieve an optimum performance, or even a good performance as compared with the individual's potential. The changes in pattern reflect the best equilibrium that the individual can achieve. The only way in which optimal equilibrium can be restored is through the application of convex lenses, which allow identification to localize away and remove the need for distorted behavior (Skeffington 1950–51).

B1 and B2 Cases

Skeffington (1947, 1950–51) categorized the various patterns of skewed phorometric findings into syndromes. These syndromes, referred to as the B1, B2, and C case types, reflect differing patterns of response to the nearpoint stress–induced drive for convergence to localize closer than accommodation.

In prism vergence measures, the blur findings indicate the flexibility to shift vergence closer to or farther from the plane of regard without inducing an associated change in accommodation. In the presence of a drive for convergence to localize closer than accommodation, the base-out blur at near will be high and the base-in blur low. As base-out prism is added, the prism first serves to restore the equilibrium between vergence and accommodation; additional base-out prism then measures the degree to which vergence can shift closer before inducing a change in accommodation. The base-in blur at near will be low, since a portion of the available freedom to localize convergence beyond accommodation is used to overcome the tendency for convergence to localize closer (Skeffington 1947).

According to Skeffington, the characteristic response to the drive for convergence to localize closer than accommodation is an attempt to prevent diplopia by blocking or inhibiting the drive to converge nearer. When prism base-out is added beyond the blur point in the nearpoint base-out prism vergence test, the base-out break finding, and subsequently the base-out fusional recovery, are reduced as a result of this habitual, conditioned inhibition of convergence. This pattern of inhibiting convergence does not influence the prism base-in break and recovery findings, which remain high.

Thus, the usual response to nearpoint stress is typified by a characteristic pattern of nearpoint vergence findings: the base-out blur is high, but the base-out break and recovery are low; the base-in blur is low, but the base-in break and recovery are high. This syndrome is referred to as the *B1 case* (Skeffington 1947, 1950–51).

Skeffington indicates that not all individuals respond with this typical pattern. Some demonstrate the reversed pattern in which the base-in break and recovery at near (#17B, see Chapter 8) are low in relation to the base-out break and recovery (#16B). This pattern is referred to as the *B2 case*. The B2 pattern is viewed as a distortion of the B1 that results when the intensified impact of nearpoint visual activity drives the base-in break and recovery findings lower than the base-out.

Flax (1984) and Woolf (1963–64) suggest that the B1 and B2 case types result from different adaptive strategies used to maintain consistency between centering and identification despite the drive to center closer. They propose that the B1 pattern results when the individual attempts to restore centering to the plane of identification, while the B2 occurs when the individual attempts to bring the plane of identification closer to the plane of centering.

Flax (1984) relates the B1 and B2 patterns to dominance of the ambient and focal visual systems, respectively. For the B1 individual, he suggests, accurate localization is more important than discrimination. The B2 individual, in contrast, emphasizes identification and is more concerned with "what" than with "where."

Another response to the nearpoint stress–induced effector system disequilibrium, according to Skeffington, is the pattern of the C case type. In this case type, viewed by Skeffington as a noncharacteristic response that is probably biochemically based, the base-out breaks at distance and near are both low. The base-in break and recovery at distance, usually low in the B case type, remain unimpaired in the C type. According to Skeffington, the B case is the end result of a visceral dominance, and the C case is the end result when the individual's response occurs primarily in the skeletal system (Skeffington 1950–51).

ACCOMMODATION INSUFFICIENCY AND CONVERGENCE INSUFFICIENCY

Birnbaum (1985a) suggests that the conditions traditionally labeled *accommodative insufficiency* and *convergence insufficiency* constitute varieties of adaptation to nearpoint stress. Accommodative insufficiency, characterized by low PRA and/or low amplitude of accommodation, is traditionally viewed as a weakness of accommodation, or failure to develop adequate accommodative ability (Daum 1983). Convergence insufficiency, characterized by high exophoria at near, low positive fusional convergence, and receded convergence nearpoint, is traditionally attributed to weakness of convergence, or failure to develop adequate convergence skill (Cooper and Duckman 1978; Daum 1984). In contrast with these traditional explanations, Birnbaum claims that accommodative insufficiency and convergence insufficiency constitute adaptive patterns in which accommodation and convergence, respectively, are inhibited to reduce overconvergence during nearpoint visual activity.

Accommodative Insufficiency

Accommodative insufficiency has been attributed to ocular or systemic disease, lack of oxygen, toxemia, trauma, fatigue, excessive near work, and emotional factors (Hofstetter 1942). In the vast majority of cases, no pathology is present, and accommodative disorder is assumed to be functional in nature. The high incidence of functional accommodative disorder is often explained on the basis that the accommodative system has not evolved sufficiently to meet the extensive nearpoint demands imposed by society.

In contrast to traditional models that view accommodative insufficiency as a weakness of accommodation or a failure to develop adequate accommodative ability, Birnbaum (1985a) suggests that accommodative insufficiency occurs as a purposive inhibition of accommodative function, creating a lag of accommodation beyond the plane of regard to reduce associated overconvergence. Accommodative insufficiency is viewed as a product of nearpoint stress, not as the cause of the difficulty.

The subject who inhibits accommodation will respond poorly to phorometric probes which require localization of accommodation closer than convergence; thus, the PRA finding will be low. When inhibition is sufficiently conditioned, response to minus lenses is poor even monocularly, and monocular amplitude is reduced. Consistent with the concept that deficient accommodation results from near work, Yeow and Taylor (1991) report that accommodative amplitude declines more rapidly in video display users than in non-video display users.

Low monocular amplitude is quickly reversed with monocular accommodative rock training. This rapid improvement is consistent with the notion that low monocular amplitude reflects inhibition of previously developed function; if accommodation were organically weak or had failed to develop normally, such rapid improvement would not be expected. Indeed, in those few cases in which monocular amplitude does not normalize rapidly, neurological or psychogenic factors should be suspected (Birnbaum 1985a). The low PRA measure is slower to normalize, since it requires reversal of the basic nearpoint stress pattern of convergence localizing closer than accommodation (Birnbaum 1985a).

Convergence Insufficiency

Convergence insufficiency, like accommodative insufficiency, has been attributed to a broad variety of systemic and ocular causes. The systemic conditions include trauma, toxemia, endocrine disorder, vascular disease, encephalitis, drug intoxication, malnutrition, debility, hepatitis, mononucleosis, sinusitis, dental infection, anemia, anoxia, and heavy tobacco use. Several authors have attributed the disorder to psychogenic factors. Convergence insufficiency has also been attributed to a variety of ocular functions, including wide interpupillary distance, poorly developed accommodation, presbyopia, low AC/A ratio, poor sensory fusion ability, suppression, and mechanical factors related to the extraocular muscles (Cooper and Duckman 1978).

Although convergence insufficiency, like accommodative insufficiency, has been attributed to a myriad of etiologic factors, in the vast majority of cases there is no apparent organic cause. Most cases of convergence insufficiency are therefore considered to be functional in origin.

Skeffington (1947, 1950–51) held that the typical response to nearpoint stress—induced overconvergence is to build a higher exophoric buffer and to inhibit fusional convergence. Inhibition of fusional convergence gives rise to the B1 case type in which the base-out break and recovery measures at near are low. Birnbaum (1985a) points out the similarity of Skeffington's B1 case type to the condition traditionally labeled "convergence insufficiency," characterized by high exophoria and low positive relative convergence (PRC). Birnbaum suggests that most convergence insufficiency cases result not from a weakness of convergence or a failure to develop adequate convergence ability, but rather occur as the individual builds an exophoric buffer and inhibits fusional convergence in response to the nearpoint stress—induced drive for convergence to localize closer. Low PRC and convergence near point (CNP) findings result from reduced response to convergence stimulation as inhibition becomes conditioned.

In the context of the Skeffington model, Birnbaum (1985a) proposes that impaired convergence findings occur as the result of an adaptive process, rather than as a primary disorder. This is in contrast with traditional graphical analysis, in which the near phoria is considered a demand on fusional convergence and the base-out prism vergence measure is compared with nearpoint exophoria to determine the adequacy of fusional reserve. In the Skeffington model, this reserve-demand comparison does not exist; high exophoria and low base-out prism vergence measures are each viewed as the result of adaptive processes to reduce overconvergence.

Although exophoria may develop adaptively to buffer overconvergence, it is usually an inefficient adaptation. High exophores commonly demonstrate asthenopia or patterns of avoidance. In some cases, high exophoria may itself become a source of difficulty, interfering with binocular function and causing asthenopic symptoms (Forrest 1960a).

Clinical Observations

Several clinical observations suggest a tendency toward overconvergence in patients with convergence insufficiency, and are thus consistent with the notion that the convergence insufficiency pattern arises as an adaptive response to nearpoint stress (Birnbaum 1985a). Patients with exphoria under dissociated conditions often demonstrate eso-fixation disparity and an eso-associated phoria, suggesting a tendency toward overconvergence under fused conditions (Ogle et al. 1967).

Exophores frequently show an esophoric shift following brief periods of reading (Forrest 1960b, 1988), while performing cheiroscopic tracings and Van Orden Star patterns (Birnbaum 1985a), and during a series of repeated near-phoria measures (Birnbaum 1985b; Christenson et al. 1990). Such findings suggest the presence of an esophoric tendency during binocular visual tasks that require sustained attention, even though exophoria is measured under routine dissociated conditions (Birnbaum 1985a).

The PRA is commonly low in patients with convergence insufficiency. Since this test measures the ability to shift accommodation closer than convergence, a high finding would be expected in patients with true convergence weakness. That the PRA is commonly low is consistent with the idea that convergence insufficiency arises as an adaptive response to overconvergence. In the presence of an underlying tendency for convergence to localize closer than accommodation, it is more difficult to shift accommodation closer and the PRA tends to be low.

Signs of overconvergence are frequently observed during the treatment of patients with convergence insufficiency. During vision training, patients frequently show esophoria and eso-fixation disparity (Vaegan 1979; Schor 1983); esophoric posture on the Keystone Visual Skills test and cheiroscopic tracing; and constricted base-in prism vergence measures. The traditional explanation is that these findings result from overcompensation. However, it should be noted that esophores never "overcompensate" by showing underconvergence. An alternative explanation suggests that the esophoria demonstrated under binocular, fused conditions constitutes the underlying primary problem, and that constricted convergence measures are a product of inhibition to reduce overconvergence; during vision training, the inhibition of convergence rapidly diminishes and the basic tendency toward overconvergence becomes manifest. At this stage, nearpoint plus lens application is often indicated by the phorometric findings.

As with accommodative findings, convergence frequently improves so rapidly during treatment that the clinician may wonder why the patient did not learn these skills as a result of repeated exposure to near work. The convergence nearpoint and PRC findings often improve within a few treatment sessions (Cooper and Duckman 1978; Vaegan 1979; Daum 1984), more rapidly than would be expected if convergence insufficiency were the result of true convergence weakness. This is consistent with the notion that most cases of convergence insufficiency arise from functional inhibition, rather than from true weakness of convergence.

Organic Convergence Weakness

Occasional cases demonstrate true convergence weakness. Improvement is more difficult to achieve; gains are more limited and poorly retained. Such cases constitute perhaps 5% of the cases of convergence insufficiency, and are probably organic in origin. They may correspond to the C case type described by Skeffington (1950–51).

Cases of organic convergence weakness can usually be easily differentiated from the more common functional adaptive variety. An esophoric shift following tasks that require sustained concentration (for example, cheiroscopic tracing, reading for a brief period, repetitive near-phoria measures) is frequently found in functional cases of convergence insufficiency, but is never found in organic convergence weakness.

In cases of true convergence weakness, accommodative findings are generally normal. Functional convergence insufficiency cases frequently exhibit low accommodative measures, as inhibition of accommodation and inhibition of convergence occur simultaneously to reduce overconvergence.

In true convergence weakness, plus lenses always cause an increase in exophoria. In nearpoint stress–induced cases, exophoria may increase through the use of plus lenses, but often remains unchanged, suggesting that adaptation occurs to maintain a purposive exophoria. Many functional cases with high exophoria and receded CNP show immediate improvement in both measures when retested with low-plus lenses. In such cases, it appears that plus lens application permits better integration of accommodation and convergence, with an immediate decrease in exophoria and improved CNP.

RELATION BETWEEN ACCOMMODATIVE AND CONVERGENCE INSUFFICIENCY

In traditional models, convergence insufficiency and accommodative insufficiency are viewed as distinct, unrelated conditions. However, in practice, clinical differentiation between these disorders is often difficult or impossible, since many patients show impairment of both accommodative and convergence function (Cooper and Duckman 1978; Daum 1983, 1984).

Birnbaum (1985a) suggests that most cases of accommodative insufficiency and convergence insufficiency result from functional inhibition to reduce nearpoint stress–induced overconvergence. They arise from a common cause and frequently occur together, and thus do not represent truly different disorders. As a consequence, Birnbaum proposes *accommodation-convergence dysfunction* as a more appropriate term for this condition, which is among the most common adaptations to nearpoint stress.

HYPEROPIA

The distribution of the curve of refraction shows a marked peak not at emmetropia, but rather in low hyperopia. Hyperopia of 0.50 to 0.75 D is the most frequently occurring refractive state in humans (Borish, 1970). According to Skeffington to (1947, 1950–51, 1952a), this low hyperopia is desirable, since it provides a buffer, or operational latitude, in the presence of exogenous and endogenous factors that influence the accommodative system.

Skeffington views low hyperopia as an advantageous but expendable asset, which may be lost as a consequence of continued near work. Emmetropia, according to Skeffington (1952b), signals the loss of this operational freedom, or buffer. Emmetropia is not an ideal state, but is in and of itself evidence of the existence of a visual problem. When this process is continued, myopia develops. However, the survival value of distance visual acuity prevents its final surrender for many individuals; they stop at the brink and remain emmetropic, rather than continuing on to myopia.

Critics of the Skeffington model frequently raise the question, if low hyperopia is indeed optimal, why not prescribe low-minus lenses for emmetropes and overcorrect myopes, to artificially create low hyperopia? Such an approach is inappropriate, however, in this author's view, because even though excess minus lenses simulate hyperopia in their optical effect on accommodative demand, they do not provide the flexibility between effector systems that permits the retention of natural low hyperopia. Indeed, application of minus lenses to the individual with inadequate freedom between effector systems creates additional stress.

Skeffington views high hyperopia, greater than the normative 0.50 to 0.75 D, as an adverse adaptive response. He suggests that high hyperopia occurs as an extension of the survival range of identification in those cases in which autonomic activation to prepare for action persists to the extent that it becomes a detriment rather than a benefit (Skeffington 1952a, 1961).

Birnbaum (1985a) suggests that individuals who habitually inhibit accommodation to reduce overconvergence may embed this pattern and manifest high hyperopia. High hyperopia usually develops in infancy and early childhood, the period of life when the accommodation-convergence relationship is being formed. When there is a failure to develop adequate flexibility between these effector systems, adverse high hyperopia may occur adaptively, via conditioned inhibition of accommodation, to reduce overconvergence.

MYOPIA

In contrast to theories that view myopia as a product of random biologic variation, heredity, or excessive accommodation during near work, the Skeffington model sees myopia as an adaptation to nearpoint stress. Myopia resolves the drive for convergence to localize closer than accommodation by changing the inner optics of the eye so as to shift the range of identification inward, eliminate the effector system mismatch, and permit efficient near work (Skeffington 1950–51, 1952c). Birnbaum (1985a) suggests that myopia reduces the accommodation required to maintain clarity at near, and hence reduces associated overconvergence.

Consistent with the Skeffington model, clinical signs of overconvergence have been reported in early and progressive myopia. Goss (1991) presents data which indicate that prior to the onset of myopia, children who become myopic demonstrate a more esophoric or less exophoric near phoria and lower PRA than children who remain emmetropic. Birnbaum (1979, 1985a) similarly reports the clinical impression that incipient and progressing myopes typically demonstrate esophoria on the near-phoria test and a low PRA finding. The lower PRA indicates lack of ability to shift accommodation closer than convergence, and is commonly found in individuals with a tendency for convergence to localize closer (Birnbaum 1985a).

Myopia is viewed as the most effective adaptation to nearpoint stress, serving in most cases to obtain comfortable, efficient nearpoint function. Beginning myopes frequently report nearpoint asthenopic symptoms before the onset of myopia. These symptoms often disappear once myopia develops.

The path of adaptation selected by a particular individual reflects that individual's priorities. When it is most important to maintain achievement and binocular function, myopia is the adaptation of choice. Because myopia impairs distance visual acuity, other adaptive paths are often taken. These are less effective at near point, but preserve distance acuity. If these adaptations prove unsatisfactory, or become so as nearpoint demands increase, myopia may ultimately follow. Myopia frequently occurs when college or vocational requirements present demands for near work beyond that previously encountered.

Developmental and Acquired Myopia

Skeffington (1952c) does not believe that nearpoint stress is the sole cause of myopia. Rather, he hypothesizes three possible etiologies: congenital, developmental, and acquired.

Developmental myopia, according to Skeffington, occurs early in life, if cultural restraints interfere with the developmental process, during the stage reported by Getman and Bullis (1950–51) in which the child routinely tends to bring objects of interest inward for inspection, and demonstrates "against" motion with the retinoscope.

Myopia which is acquired during or following the school years, in contrast, is viewed by Skeffington as an adaptive outcome of nearpoint stress in which a functional problem becomes structural. Such myopes typically demonstrate the B1 or B2 pattern of vergence findings characteristic of response to nearpoint stress–induced overconvergence. Skeffington (1952c) indicates that acquired myopia can therefore be differentiated from congenital and developmental myopia in that, in acquired myopia, the vergence pattern will be that of the B case type.

Myopic Anisometropia and Astigmatism

Although myopia is usually similar in magnitude in both eyes, *myopic anisometropia* may develop when the maintenance of distance visual acuity is more important to the individual than retention of binocular function. In myopic anisometropia, the emmetropic or slightly myopic eye is used for distance vision. The more myopic eye is used for near point, reducing accommodative demand and associated overconvergence (Birnbaum 1985a).

The onset of myopia is frequently preceded by the development of low *against-the-rule astigmatism* (Hirsch 1964). Birnbaum (1978) hypothesizes that this astigmia may serve as an early adaptation. In the presence of a lag of accommodation during near work, accommodation is localized beyond the plane of regard. Against-the-rule astigmatism therefore produces vertically oriented blur circles, which permit resolution of the vertically oriented characters of our language with reduced accommodation, and hence with reduced overconvergence. Birnbaum suggests that against-the-rule astigmatism permits one to accommodate less while maintaining adequate resolution at nearpoint, with minimum loss of distance acuity. However, when nearpoint stress persists or visual efficiency is unsatisfactory, it is followed by myopia. Several cases have been reported in which low against-the-rule astigmatism reduced or disappeared following nearpoint plus lens prescription or vision therapy to treat accommodative dysfunction (Weisz 1978; Garzia and Nicholson 1988).

Apell and Streff (1962) view astigmatism not as a pre-myopic adaptation, but rather as one that serves to integrate more of the visual field. In contrast with the myope who emphasizes near space, and the hyperope who emphasizes far, the astigmat attempts to integrate near and far space simultaneously through change in the optics of the eye. The astigmat pays a price for this adaptation in terms of decreased resolution and skew in localization.

Divergent Squint

During sustained visual concentration at near, the visceral system becomes dominant, creating an inward shift of accommodation and an associated increase in convergence (Skeffington 1950–51). In time, the impairment in visual performance at near spreads to far, where the individual can maintain the pattern of greater innervation to accommodation in one of two ways: the subject may maintain convergence for far while allowing accommodation to move nearer, creating myopia; or, he or she may accommodate for distance and maintain the innervational pattern for reducing innervation for convergence, creating divergent squint. Myopia and divergent squint are viewed as alternative adaptations: the myope sacrifices visual acuity to preserve efficient nearpoint function and normal binocular vision; the divergent squinter ablates binocularity to preserve distance acuity.

In conflict with this view of divergent strabismus as an adaptation to nearpoint stress, Costenbader (1950) indicates that most cases of divergence excess have onset before the age of 1 year, and that only 5% of cases occur after age 5. In contrast, Jampolsky (1964) reports that exodeviation usually begins as an exophoria that deteriorates into intermittent and then constant exotropia, first at distance and later at near. His observation is more consistent with Skeffington's. However, this author has rarely observed such progression from convergence insufficiency to divergent squint.

Although the origin and course of divergent squint are thus uncertain, it is clinically observed that intermittent exotropes frequently demonstrate esophoria or less than the expected exophoria at near; esophoric shift on cheiroscopic tracing or on repeated near-phoria measures; eso-fixation disparity; and low PRA. These various indications of overconvergence, viewed in traditional models as paradoxical or as a result of overcompensation (Schor 1983), are consistent with the Skeffington model in which divergent squint is viewed as one potential adaptive outcome of a nearpoint stress—induced drive for convergence to localize closer than accommodation. Laboratory findings (Cooper et al. 1982) that divergence excess patients show abnormally high stimulus AC/A and moderately high response AC/A are consistent with these clinical observations of overconvergence tendency.

Flax (1968) notes that although it is difficult to reconcile a nearpoint stress etiology with a divergence excess of early onset, the analytical measurements of intermittent exotropes frequently parallel those of the B case type. At some point, initially or during the course of vision training, intermittent exotropes frequently demonstrate nearpoint esophoria, low base-in prism vergence measures, and indications of prescribable plus lens power at near point. Flat indicates that failure to prescribe appropriate near point plus lenses frequently leads to regression, with reversion to divergence excess after treatment is completed because the underlying nearpoint stress has not been resolved.

Thus, although the etiology of divergent squint is uncertain, and indeed cases may arise from various causes, in many cases clinical observations are consistent with a nearpoint stress model. One possible means to reconcile observations of overconvergence in divergence excess with data indicating early onset is to hypothesize that, in some cases, divergence excess may arise from nearpoint stress during early infancy, when the child is involved primarily with near space and the accommodation-convergence relationship is developing and fragile.

DETERMINANTS OF ADAPTIVE PATH

The path of adaptation taken by a particular individual, according to Skeffington (1950–51), is a product of individual need and of the relative value to the individual of the various aspects of visual function. None of the adaptive paths are optimal; each involves some sacrifice in visual function, compromising distance visual acuity, binocular vision, nearpoint efficiency, or information-processing capacity.

When the drive for achievement is great, Skeffington suggests a myopic adaptation is likely in which distance visual acuity is sacrificed to achieve maximum nearpoint efficiency. The individual who is unwilling to sacrifice distance acuity may compromise binocular function by developing divergent squint, anisometropia, or various skews in vergence and accommodative function. Many individuals explore a variety of adaptive paths and demonstrate multiple functional vision disorders. Other individuals, unwilling to tolerate impairment of either distance acuity or binocular function, either persevere with inefficient function, discomfort, and reduced information-processing ability, or avoid near work as much as possible.

Psychologic Factors

Although Forrest (1988) views near work as a trigger mechanism for myopia and other adaptive disorders, he believes that psychologic factors related to attitude, intensity, and central-peripheral visual information-processing preferences are the primary determinants of the path of adaptation taken by a particular individual. Forrest views myopia as a perceptual and psychologic barrier created to protect oneself from the world. He suggests that people who see themselves as victims and react with feelings of inadequacy are more prone to myopia, while those who react to feeling vulnerable by challenging and attacking the world are more likely to project attitudes outward and develop hyperopia.

Forrest (1988) cites central-peripheral organization as a key factor in the development of high phorias. He indicates that esophores and exophores each have difficulty simultaneously integrating information from center and periphery, but react in different ways. Exo-processors alternate attention between center and periphery according to the demands of the particular situation. However, they prefer a global perspective, and may develop a high exophoria or intermittent exotropia to facilitate global awareness. The eso-processor, in contrast, is highly central, preferring the greater depth and richness derived from a more restricted intake. Esophoric posture, in this view, facilitates peripheral detuning so that one can emphasize attention to detail.

Forrest (1988) suggests that those who are more rigid in their approach to the task are less able to maintain flexible visual operation and more likely to develop refractive deviations and visual/spatial skews. Excessive tension or rigidity during visual tasks generates lowered peripheral awareness and restricted, less flexible vergence and accommodative ranges, often with high AC/A and CA/C ratios. Thus, the analytical findings reflect both *psychologic* and *accommodation-convergence* factors.

Consistent with Forrest's (1988) notion that psychologic factors are important elements in nearpoint stress, numerous reports link vision disorders such as myopia, strabismus, and convergence insufficiency with personality and emotional status (Nawlatzki and Avrouskine 1957; Young 1967; Beckwitt 1971; Lanyon and Giddings 1974; Groffman 1978). Relationships between autonomic balance and personality have also been suggested, and measures of physiologic function have shown that myopes tend to exhibit sympathetic dominance (Gawron 1981, 1983). Birnbaum (1984) claims that autonomic reactivity, influenced by stress, intensity, emotional status, and personality, may be the physiologic mechanism by which these behavioral factors influence the development of vision disorders.

NEARPOINT STRESS AND STRESS-INDUCED ILLNESS

Noting models that suggest that systemic disease may arise from neuroendocrine changes associated with sustained stress, Birnbaum (1984) points out parallels between the concepts of nearpoint stress–induced vision disorder and stress-induced disease.

In response to stress, the body generates a pattern of widespread neuroendocrine changes. This pattern, characterized by activation of the sympathetic nervous system, evolved biologically to facilitate action in response to stressor agents such as enemies and predators. Fighting or fleeing from such biologic stressors generally serves to resolve the stress, at which time sympathetic activation subsides and the parasympathetic system acts to restore homeostasis (Cannon 1929).

In our society, however, emotional stress is pervasive and widespread. Psychologic stress generates the same pattern of sympathetic activation and altered neuroendocrine function as does biologic stress. However, in response to emotional stress there is usually no physical fight or flight. Most people maintain an enforced outward calm, stress persists, and the body's physiologic stress response continues unabated. Indeed, the hypothalamic centers receive the message that the body's response has been inadequate to relieve the stress, and the physiological stress response intensifies.

When emotional stress is prolonged or intense, repeated excitation creates a conditioned high level of stress activation that leads to altered physiology and ultimately to disease. Stress-induced illness, in this model, is held to occur as the end result of alteration in the innervational pattern to the various organs of the body, the specific illness depending on the pattern of neuroendocrine response characteristic of a given individual. Cardiovascular, endocrine, and gastrointestinal disease, cancer, rheumatoid arthritis, migraine, and respiratory disease have been linked to stress, emotional state, and personality (Malmo et al. 1950; Henry and Stephens 1977; Pelletier 1977; Everly and Rosenfeld 1981).

Skeffington's model of nearpoint stress has much in common with this concept. The nearpoint stress model holds that a variety of vision disorders occur adaptively to reduce an effector system mismatch which, according to Birnbaum (1984), arises from the activation of autonomic reflexes that are linked biologically to physiological arousal, fight-or-flight response, and attentional mechanisms, but are inconsistent with efficient performance during the sustained nearpoint task demands imposed by modern society. Birnbaum (1984) suggests that stress-induced illness and nearpoint stress–induced vision disorders are thus linked; each results from the activation of neuroendocrine reflexes that are biologically appropriate, but which are incompatible with conditions encountered in our society, pervasive psychological stress in the one case and extensive demands for sustained concentration at near in the other. In this context, adaptive vision disorders such as myopia and disorders of vergence and accommodation may be considered not only as nearpoint stress—induced vision disorders, but as varieties of stress-induced illness.

SUMMARY

During near work, vision will be blurred or double in the individual who is unable to resolve the drive for convergence to localize closer than accommodation. Properly prescribed low-plus nearpoint lenses restore equilibrium between vergence and accommodation. When such lenses are not prescribed, the individual may persevere with asthenopia and diminished information-processing ability, avoid near work, or adapt within the visual system to restore equilibrium as well as possible. In the attempt to adapt to nearpoint stress—induced overconvergence, individuals may develop myopia, adverse high hyperopia, exophoria, divergent squint, anisometropia, against-the-rule astigmatism, and various disorders of vergence and accommodation. Myopia is usually the most effective adaptation to restore nearpoint visual efficiency and relieve asthenopia. When an individual shows constricted vergence and accommodative findings but reports no asthenopic symptoms, it is likely that the patient has either developed a myopic adaptation or tends to avoid near work. The path of adaptation taken by a particular individual will vary with individual needs and may be influenced by psychologic factors. Birnbaum relates adaptive vision disorders to stress physiology and suggests that they be viewed as varieties of stress-induced illness.

SUGGESTED READING

Birnbaum MH (1985). Nearpoint visual stress: Clinical implications. *J Am Optom Assoc* 56(6): 480–490.
Skeffington AM (1928–74). Optometric Extension Program Continuing Education Courses. Santa Ana, CA: Optometric Extension Program Foundation.

REFERENCES

Apell RJ, Streff JW (1962). Compensatory lenses and the astigmatic patient. In: *Optometric Care and Guidance*. Optometric Extension Program Continuing Education Courses, Santa Ana, CA: Optometric Extension Program Foundation, April, pp. 39–46.
Beckwitt ML (1971). Stress and strabismus. *Ann Psychiatry* 9(1):11–29.
Birnbaum MW (1978). Functional relationship between myopia, accommodative stress, and against-the-rule astigmia: A hypothesis. *J Am Optom Assoc* 49(8):911–914.
Birnbaum MW (1979). Management of the low myopia pediatric patient. *J Am Optom Assoc* 50:1281–1289.

Birnbaum MH (1984). Nearpoint visual stress: A physiological model. *J Am Optom Assoc* 55(11):825–835.

Birnbaum MH (1985a). Nearpoint visual stress: Clinical implications. *J Am Optom Assoc* 56(6):480–490.

Birnbaum MH (1985b). An esophoric shift associated with sustained fixation. *Am J Optom Physiol Opt* 62(11):732–735.

Borish IM (1970). *Clinical Refraction.* 3rd ed. Chicago: Professional Press.

Cannon WB (1929). *Bodily Changes in Pain, Hunger, Fear and Rage: An Account of Recent Researches into the Function of Emotional Excitement.* New York: Appleton.

Christenson GN, Korth C, Marcolivio M (1990). An investigation of the "esophoric shift" and its relationship to parameters of the fixation disparity curve. *J Behav Optom* 1(7):179–182.

Cooper J, Ciuffreda K, Kruger PB (1982). Stimulus and response AC/A ratios in intermittent exotropia of the divergence-excess type. *Br J Ophthalmol* 66:398–404.

Cooper J, Duckman R (1978). Convergence insufficiency: Incidence, diagnosis and treatment. *J Am Optom Assoc* 49(6):673–680.

Costenbader FD (1950). The physiology and management of divergent strabismus. In: Allen JH (ed), *Strabismic Ophthalmic Symposium I.* St. Louis: Mosby, pp. 349–366.

Daum KM (1983). Accommodative insufficiency. *Am J Optom Physiol Opt* 60(5):352–359.

Daum KM (1984). Convergence insufficiency. *Am J Optom Physiol Opt* 61(1):16–22.

Dowis RT (1977). The effect of a visual training program on juvenile delinquency. *J Am Optom Assoc* 48(9):1173–1176.

Dzik D (1966). Vision and the juvenile delinquent. *J Am Optom Assoc* 37(5):461–468.

Everly GS, Rosenfeld R (1981). *The Nature and Treatment of the Stress Response: A Practical Guide for Clinicians.* New York: Plenum.

Flax N (1968). Oral presentation. San Jose Visual Training Conference, Aug. 24–25, Morro Bay, CA, transcript by Caryl Croisant.

Flax N (1984). A current look at the OEP B1 and B2 case typings. *J Optom Vis Dev* 15(1):10–21.

Flax N (1985). Functional case analysis: An interpretation of the Skeffington model. *Am J Optom Physiol Opt* 62(6):365–368.

Forrest EB (1960a). A modern philosophy of vision. III. The motor components of the visual process. *Optom Weekly* 51:17–20.

Forrest EB (1960b). A modern philosophy of vision. IV. The story of stress. *Optom Weekly* 51:332–334; 635–636.

Forrest EB (1988). *Stress and Vision.* Santa Ana, CA: Optometric Extension Program Foundation.

Garzia RP, Nicholson SB (1988). Clinical aspects of accommodative influences on astigmatism. *J Am Optom Assoc* 59(12):942–945.

Gawron VJ (1981). Differences among myopes, emmetropes and hyperopes. *Am J Optom Physiol Opt* 58(9):753–760.

Gawron VJ (1983). Ocular accommodation, personality and autonomic balance. *Am J Optom Physiol Opt* 60(7):630–639.

Getman GN, Bullis G (1950–51). *Developmental Vision.* Optometric Extension Program Continuing Education Courses, Santa Ana, CA: Optometric Extension Program Foundation, vol. 24.

Goss DA (1991). Clinical accommodation and heterophoria findings preceding juvenile onset of myopia. *Optom Vis Sci* 68(2): 110–116.

Groffman S (1978). Psychological aspects of strabismus and amblyopia—A review of the literature. *J Am Optom Assoc* 49(9):995–999.

Hendrickson H (1969). The vision development process. In : Wold RM (ed), *Visual and Perceptual Aspects for the Achieving and Underachieving Child*. Seattle: Special Child Publ.

Hendrickson H (1976). Vision development in man: A review. In: Greenstein TN (ed), *Vision and Learning Disability*. St Louis: American Optometric Association, pp. 21–47.

Henry JP, Stephens PM (1977). *Stress, Health and the Social Environment: A Sociobiologic Approach to Medicine*. New York: Springer-Verlag.

Hirsch MJ (1964). Predictability of refraction at age 14 on the basis of testing at age 6—Interim report from the Ojai longitudinal study of refraction. *Am J Optom Arch Am Acad Optom* 41(10):567–573.

Hofstetter HW (1942). Factors involved in low amplitude cases. *Am J Optom Arch Am Acad Optom* 19(7):279–289.

Jampolsky A (1964). Ocular deviations. *Int Ophthalmol Clin* 4:598.

Kaseno S (1982). *A Vision Therapy Project with Juvenile Delinquents*. Presented at Southern California Vision Forum. Sound recording, Santa Ana, CA: Optometric Extension Program Foundation.

Lanyon RI, Giddings JW (1974). Psychological approaches to myopia: A review. *Am J Optom Physiol Opt* 51(4):271–281.

Malmo RB, Shagass, Davis H (1950). Symptom specificity and bodily reactions during psychiatric interview. *Psychosom Med* 12(6):362–376.

Nawlatzki I, Avrouskine M (1957). Psychogenic factors in disturbances of ocular muscle balance: Exophoria with convergence insufficiency. *Acta Med Orient* 16(3):94–96.

Ogle KN, Martins TG, Dyer JA (1967). *Oculomotor Imbalance in Binocular Vision and Fixation Disparity*. Philadelphia: Lea & Febiger, pp. 108–113, 175–184, 195–230.

Pelletier KR (1977). *Mind as Healer, Mind as Slayer: A Holistic Approach to Preventing Stress Disorders*. New York: Delacorte.

Schor CM (1983). Fixation disparity and vergence adaptation. In: Schor CM, Cuiffreda KJ (eds), *Vergence Eye Movements: Basic and Clinical Aspects*. Boston: Butterworth–Heinemann, pp. 465–516.

Skeffington AM (1928–74). Optometric Extension Program Continuing Education Courses, Santa Ana, CA: Optometric Extension Program Foundation.

Skeffington AM (1947). *Near Point Optometry*. Optometric Extension Program Continuing Education Courses, Santa Ana, CA: Optometric Extension Program Foundation, vol. 2, no. 4–12, Jan–Sept.

Skeffington AM (1950-51). *Near Point Optometry*. Optometric Extension Program Continuing Education Courses, Santa Ana, CA: Optometric Extension Program Foundation, Oct. 1950–Sept. 1951.

Skeffington AM (1952a). Hyperopia. In: *Practical Applied Optometry*. Optometric Extension Program Continuing Education Courses, Santa Ana, CA: Optometric Extension Program Foundation, vol. 24, no. 11, Nov., pp. 97–108.

Skeffington AM (1952b). Emmetropia. In: *Practical Applied Optometry*. Optometric Extension Program Continuing Education Courses, Santa Ana, CA: Optometric Extension Program Foundation, vol. 24, no. 10, Oct., pp 87–96.

Skeffington AM (1952c). Myopia. In: *Practical Applied Optometry*. Optometric Extension Program Continuing Education Courses, Santa Ana, CA: Optometric Extension Program Foundation, vol. 24, no. 12, Dec., pp. 109–120.

Skeffington AM (1961). The case of the high hyperope who wanted to go higher— and did not. In: *Functional Optometry in Theory and Practice*. Optometric Extension Program Continuing Education Courses, Santa Ana, CA: Optometric Extension Program Foundation, vol. 33 no. 7, April, pp. 51–58.

Skeffington AM (1964–65). *Introduction to Clinical Optometry.* Optometric Extension Program Postgraduate Courses, Santa Ana, CA: Optometric Extension Program Foundation, vol. 37, Oct. 1964–Sept. 1965.

Snow R (1983). The relationship between vision and juvenile delinquency. *J Am Optom Assoc.* 54(6):509–511.

Vaegan (1979). Convergence and divergence show large and sustained improvement after short isometric exercise. Am *J Optom Physiol Opt* 56:23–33.

Weisz CL (1978). Induced against-the-rule astigmatism in accommodative disorders. *J Am Optom Assoc* 49:335–336.

Woolf D (1963–64). *Visual Function in Theory and Practice.* Optometric Extension Program Continuing Education Courses, Santa Ana, CA: Optometric Extension Program Foundation, series 1, no. 9, June 1964.

Yeow PT, Taylor SP (1991). Effects of long-term visual display terminal usage on visual functions. *Optom Vis Sci* 68(12):930–941.

Young FA (1967). Myopia and personality. *Am J Optom Physiol Opt* 44(3):192–201.

5

Vision, Posture, and Spatial Relations

Darrell Boyd Harmon, Ph.D. (1942), an educator and kinesiologist, found an increase in prevalence of visual problems with age among elementary school children, from 20% among those entering school to 80% after 5 years of elementary school. He found no such increase in children of migratory workers, who spent little time in school. Harmon therefore began to investigate factors in the school environment that cause vision disorder, and developed a model that emphasized relationships between vision, posture, and spatial relations (Harmon 1958). He postulated that a variety of refractive and oculomotor disorders develop to preserve efficient function and accurate spatial localization when individuals repeatedly sustain near work in adverse postures.

VISION AS A SPATIAL ANALYZER

Harmon (1958) views the retina as a quadrant system for spatial analysis. The fovea serves as a central reference point that divides the retina into temporal and nasal halves. The horizontal raphé divides the retina into superior and inferior halves. The resulting quadrant system, organized around the fovea as a central invariant, permits spatial projection and accurate localization of objects in space.

However, since the eyes move with respect to the head, the head moves with respect to the body, and the body moves with respect to objects in space, an object in space cannot be accurately localized based solely on retinal input. Accurate spatial localization requires knowledge of eye, head, and body position, as well as retinal information. Eye position information is derived from monitoring the efferent signals to the extraocular muscles and from proprioceptive input from these muscles (Steinbach 1986; Campos et al. 1988; Petito et al. 1988; Skavenski 1990; Nommay et al. 1991).

Accurate spatial localization requires that kinesthetic input from body, head, and neck be correlated with retinal input and with information as to eye position so that the location of an object perceived through the visual sense matches its actual location as verified by movement and touch. Duke-Elder (1942) notes a close correlation between the extraocular muscles, the labyrinths which record movements of head in space, and the muscles of the neck, which register movements of the head in relation to the trunk. Some 20% of the retinal fibers run to the superior colliculus rather than to the lateral geniculate body, and are associated with primitive photostatic reflexes related to posture and orientation in space (Duke-Elder 1942).

VISION AND POSTURE

According to Harmon (1958), posture relates not only to spatial judgements, but also to efficiency in performing a visual task. To perform any task, an individual must first come to balance with gravity, and then with the particular task at hand. This must be accomplished with minimal effort, or else it creates "noise on the line," which interferes with task performance and efficiency. Performing a task in a posture that is not optimally balanced requires an expenditure of energy that detracts from the ability to perform the task easily and efficiently.

Optimal Near-Work Posture

The optimal posture for near work, according to Harmon (1951, 1958), is one that minimizes tension and permits effective spatial localization. In this optimal posture, the lines connecting the midpoint between the two eyes, the midpoint between the points of the two elbows, and the midpoint between the second knuckles of the middle fingers of the two hands, form roughly an equilateral triangle, with its base inclined approximately 20 degrees from the horizontal (Figure 5.1). The trunk and head lean forward, the upper arms hang downward freely from the shoulders, the forearms move upward, and the hands move inward. These movements bring the forearms and the plane of regard into a plane parallel with that of the face, perpendicular to the line of sight (Figure 5.2). Consequently, the visual and gravitational space worlds match as nearly as possible, so that spatial distortion is minimal.

To maintain this optimal posture when reading, reading material must be inclined at approximately 20 degrees from the horizontal. For writing and drawing, a tilt-top desk or a desk accessory that provides a 20-degree incline must be used (Figure 5.3). In this optimal near-work posture, the distance from the eye to the task is equal to the distance from the point of the elbow (olecranon) to the second knuckle of the middle finger (Figures 5.1, 5.2, and 5.3). This distance, from olecranon to second knuckle, is referred to as the *Harmon distance*, and is held to constitute the physiologically optimal near working distance for a particular individual.

In this optimal near-work posture, the head and trunk are supported with minimal activity of the supporting muscles of the body, so that tension is mini-

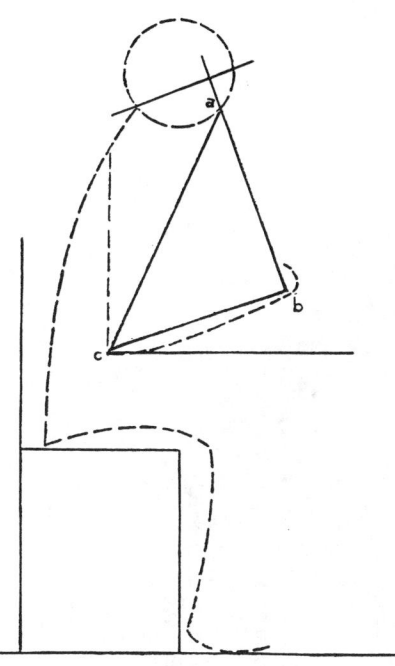

Figure 5.1 The posture physiologically optimal for near work is one in which the lines connecting the midpoint between the two eyes (a), the midpoint between the second knuckles of the middle fingers of the two hands (b), and the midpoint between the points of the two elbows (c), form roughly an equilateral triangle with its base inclined approximately 20 degrees from the horizontal. (From D.B. Harmon, *Notes on a Dynamic Theory of Vision,* 1958.)

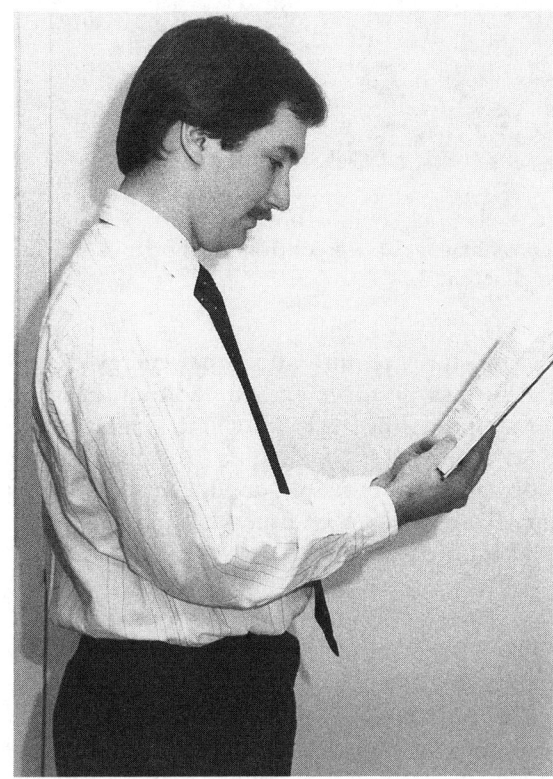

Figure 5.2 In the optimal near-work posture, the forearms and the plane of regard are brought into a plane parallel with that of the face, perpendicular to the line of sight.

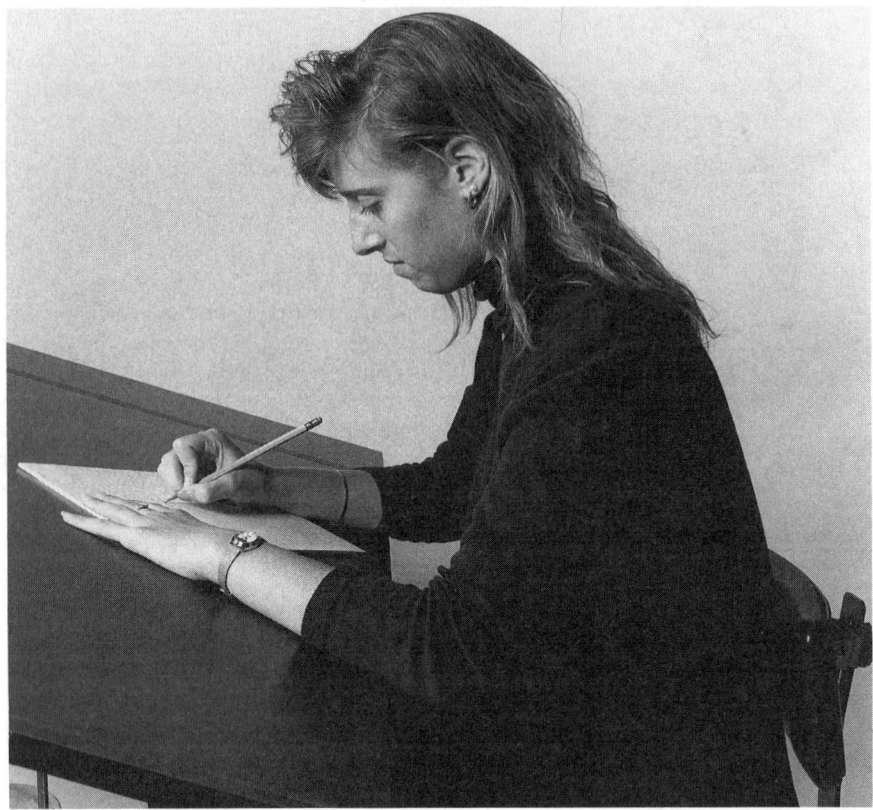

Figure 5.3 To achieve the posture physiologically optimal for near work, reading and writing material should be inclined approximately 20 degrees from the horizontal. A tilt-top desk can be used to achieve this inclination.

mized (Harmon 1951, 1958). Other postures require additional energy expenditure and hence detract from efficient task performance. In addition, Harmon (1951, 1958) indicates this posture is optimal because it facilitates manual manipulation; it maintains the two eyes as nearly as possible at the same distance from the task so as to facilitate binocular visual function; and it orients the body so that visual and postural coordinates approach each other as closely as possible, thus permitting a normal spatial frame of reference.

Physiologic Effects

Evidence has shown that the optimal near-work posture described by Harmon does indeed minimize tension and physiologic activation during near work. Harmon (1960) reported that subjects reading with proper nearpoint lenses showed reduced physiological activity of the body as compared with subjects reading with nonoptimal lenses. Differences in lens power as little as 0.12 D were sufficient to induce changes in electrocardiogram monitors, galvanic skin response, skin temperature, respiration, and body posture. Harmon claims that the proper nearpoint lens helps to promote optimal near-work posture, and that proper posture in turn influences physiological activity.

Pierce (1966–68, 1970) found that emmetropic college students reading with +0.50-D lenses showed reduced heart rate, electromyographic amplitude, and respiration rate, with improved reading rate on the task, as compared with a control group who read with plano lenses. Pierce suggests that these effects result from changes in posture and working distance induced by the lenses.

Greenspan (1970) also found changes in near-work posture and working distance with nearpoint plus lenses. Nearpoint working distance increased with plus lenses up to the power of the dynamic retinoscopy finding. Further, performance on a nearpoint task was optimal with lenses of this critical power, and decreased with higher- or lower-power lenses.

Effects of Adverse Posture

Children spend most of their time in school involved in reading, writing, and other near-vision tasks. Improperly designed furniture, inadequate lighting, glare, improper task placement, and intense application may lead to suboptimal near-work postures.

Children who are forced out of balance in their reflex efforts to adjust to poorly designed desks and seats, to exclude glare from their eyes, and to adjust to uneven patterns of brightness in the field of vision, tend to tilt and rotate their heads and bodies, placing the neck and back under stress. These stresses are intensified when the center of action in performing the task is very close. Conflicting activities are set up within the child that disturb visual perceptions related to the task, create adverse body stresses, and require excessive expenditure of energy, which in turn reduces efficiency in performing the task (Harmon 1951, 1958).

When the task is frequently repeated so that postural distortion becomes habitual, growth patterns are altered so as to relieve postural stress. The organism *grows along the lines of stress to reduce stress*: changes in tonicity are followed by structural warping, which serves to bring the individual into the compensatory posture, with reduced energy required to adjust to the task. As the child continues to function in adverse surroundings, the result is some combination of structural warping and diminished performance (Harmon 1951, 1958).

Spatial localization may also be adversely affected. Environmental factors such as glare, excess tension, and inappropriate desk size may cause a child to work with extreme body slant or head turn. Such postures create a mismatch between the spatial information derived from the visual and gravitational systems, thus interfering with spatial localization (Harmon 1951, 1958).

In the presence of such posture, a large compensatory version movement is required to achieve ocular alignment with the task. It is generally agreed that approximately 15 degrees is the maximum version movement that can be sustained for efficient, prolonged function. Tension and discomfort result from performing tasks in postures that require prolonged larger version movements (Harmon 1951, 1958).

In the optimal near-work posture described by Harmon (1951, 1958), the near-work material is inclined approximately 20 degrees from the horizontal. An optimal balance cannot be obtained when near work is performed on a flat surface. Under such conditions, visual and spatial coordinates do not match, tension and physiological activation are increased, and efficiency in task performance decreases.

When an inclined surface is not used, the child may maintain erect posture with the Y-axis of the body in a vertical position. In maintaining this posture, the cervical spine is rigidly erect and tension in the muscles of the neck is at a maximum. Further, gaze is depressed beyond that required for performance at a tilt-top desk. In this position of extreme gaze depression, lateral eye movements in the lower portion of the working field require the action of other extraocular muscles in addition to the horizontal recti. These angular stresses are incorrectly referred to the body frame of reference, falsifying spatial perception and increasing postural stress (Harmon 1951, 1958).

To reduce this demand for extreme gaze depression, the individual who is required to perform near work on a horizontal surface may lean forward excessively to establish a parallel relationship between the facial and work planes (Figure 5.4). This posture is deleterious in that it generates extreme tension in the upper back and neck, and promotes an excessively close working distance (Harmon 1951).

COMPUTERS AND ADVERSE POSTURE

Video display terminals frequently impose conditions that cause postural distortion. Adverse postures may be induced by improper task placement, inadequate viewing distances and angles, improper height and location of the display screen and keyboard, a need to view documents placed flat on the desk, poorly designed chairs, poor lighting, glare, inadequate contrast, and lenses that are poorly designed with regard to power and placement of the bifocal addition. Awkward posture leads to operator discomfort and inefficiency. Operators of video display terminals frequently complain of eyestrain, headache, and muscle pain in the neck, back, and shoulders (Miller 1984).

Grant (1987) indicates that convergence is easier during depressed gaze. The computer screen requires near vision and convergence in a situation in which gaze depression is considerably less than that required for other nearpoint tasks. Computer users may elevate the chin to achieve gaze depression, resulting in head, neck, and shoulder discomfort, or may focus on the target with the head in the primary position and gaze minimally depressed, in which case convergence is more difficult.

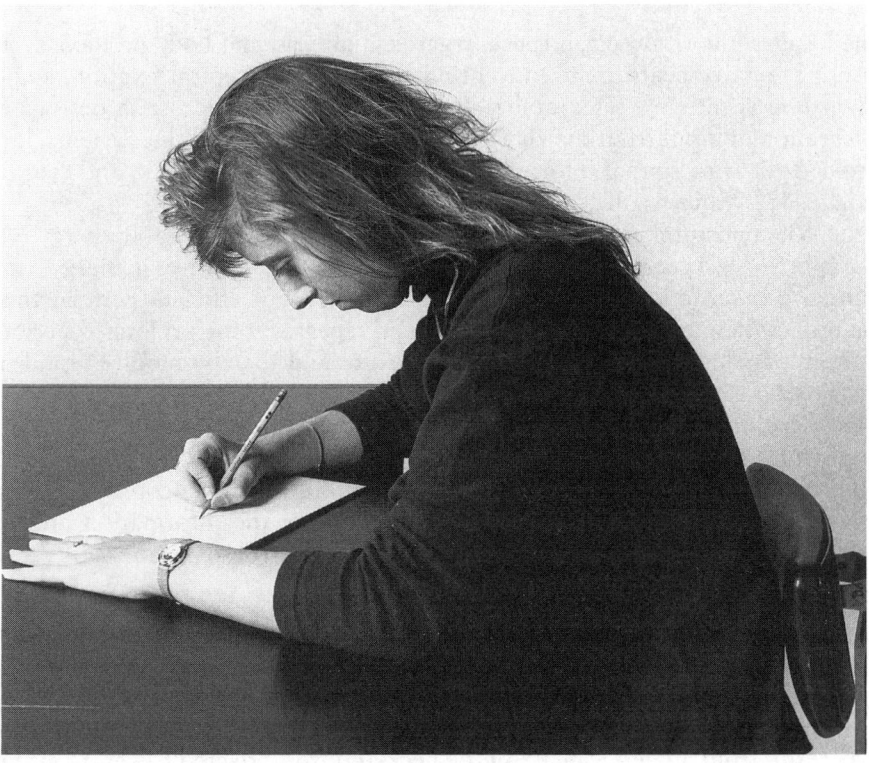

Figure 5.4 An alternative posture when a tilt-top desk is not used is to lean forward excessively to bring the face parallel to the work plane.

DEVELOPMENT OF OCULAR SKEWS

Working in an unbalanced posture requires excess energy and interferes with spatial localization and efficient task performance. According to Harmon (1958), the primary biologic function of vision lies in its spatial functions, rather than in optical or image clarity function. In our literate society, major consideration is generally given to factors of acuity and resolution. However, when postural distortion induced by adverse nearpoint working conditions interferes with the ability to match spatial inputs from the retinal and body bilateral systems, optical function and resolution, which are secondary in terms of biologic survival, may be sacrificed to preserve spatial localization. Myopia, hyperopia, astigmatism, anisometropia, and hyperphoria may develop to preserve spatial relationships in the presence of long-standing chronic postural distortion.

Accurate spatial localization is obtained by matching spatial information derived from the retinal projection system with that derived from the motor systems. When body skews are transient, perceptual compensation allows accurate localization of objects in space, regardless of head and body position, whether or not eye movements are used to bring an object into central fixation, and even when one is moving. This ability to perceptually compensate is derived from integration of input from the visual, kinesthetic, and labyrinthine systems, linking and coordinating spatial information from the head, neck, trunk, and eyes (Harmon 1958; Wallach 1985).

When postural distortion is habitual or chronic, considerable energy is used in ongoing perceptual compensation (Harmon 1958). The use of energy for perceptual compensation detracts from that available for efficient performance on the task. When adverse posture is sustained repeatedly for prolonged periods, it is more parsimonious to alter ocular structure and thereby modify visual input so as to match kinesthetic input directly, without need for intervening perceptual compensation.

Conditions such as myopia, hyperopia, astigmatism, hyperphoria, and anisometropia may develop, according to Harmon, as an outcome of persistent postural skews. These adaptations serve to reduce the information-processing necessary to match input from the visual and postural systems and thus facilitate efficient task performance.

MYOPIA, HYPEROPIA, ESOPHORIA, AND EXOPHORIA

Harmon (1958) suggests that myopia, hyperopia, esophoria, and exophoria may result from altered tonicity in the neck and trunk related to nearpoint working conditions. Since the neck serves as a transducer for feedback between eyes and trunk, the tonic state of the trunk and neck is reflected in the tonic status of the motor mechanisms of accommodation and convergence. Hypertonic, tense, statically held trunks or necks result in excessive feedback or gain to ocular mechanisms, transposing space toward the individual. When an individual works so intensely that body tension is increased, and when near work is performed repeatedly for sustained periods, myopia may develop in order that the input from the visual system match the kinesthetic input that space is transposed closer. In Harmon's terms, the organism grows along the line of stress to reduce stress. Myopia facilitates visual efficiency at near by permitting the individual to achieve a unified spatial percept with minimum need for perceptual compensation. Hypotonic functioning of neck or trunk with reduced feedback or gain at the eyes moves space away from the individual and leads to hyperopia (Harmon 1958). Esophoria and exophoria may similarly occur (Harmon 1958) as a result of increased or decreased tonicity in the neck and trunk, with consequent transposition of space toward or away from the individual.

ANISOMETROPIA

Functional asymmetries of the neck and trunk in which bilateral body or neck tonus is unequal cause rotation of the plane of regard in space and may lead to differences in functioning between the eyes (Harmon 1958). Suppression, anisometropia, astigmatism, cyclophoria, and hyperphoria may occur as a result. According to Harmon, body mechanics are a factor in approximately 70% of cases of hyperphoria, astigmatism, and anisometropia.

When a task is placed off-center, or when structural or functional posture skews are induced by a flat work surface, glare, or improper lighting, the face will no longer be parallel with the plane of the task. One eye will be closer to the task than the other, and the intensity of illumination between the eyes will differ. When the difference in illumination between the eyes exceeds 12%, suppression of vision in one eye will occur. If the postural skew is such that the deviation from parallelism is greater than 20 degrees, this 12% tolerance will be exceeded, leading to suspension of vision in the eye that receives lower illumination (Harmon 1958).

Intermittent suppression uses energy that would otherwise be available for information-processing, and interferes with efficient task performance. Consequently, when a task that induces postural asymmetry is frequently repeated and sustained, and when the demand for achievement is high, anisometropia may occur as a means of obtaining a match between visual and kinesthetic inputs, while maintaining efficient binocular performance without need for suppression. Anisometropia permits a high level of visual efficiency on the task at hand, even though it may interfere with binocular function and performance on tasks performed in other postures.

The organism, according to Harmon (1958), grows along the line of stress to reduce the stress. Adaptation will occur to relieve stress induced by adverse posture and to maximize efficient visual function in those tasks that impose greatest demand and that have greatest import to the individual.

Postural asymmetry is frequently induced by excess tension when writing. The intense child tends to grip the pencil tightly at the point, and then must tilt the head and move close to the page to see the pencil point (Figure 5.5). At working distances as close as 4 to 6 inches, a substantial difference in accommodative demand for the two eyes is generated. The development of anisometropia, with the closer eye becoming more myopic, eliminates the need for suppression due to unequal accommodative demand.

ASTIGMATISM

Astigmatism may also result from postural skews imposed by improper near working conditions. Head tilt and face rotation commonly occur when the individual is out of alignment with the task, serving to permit lateral eye movement along a line of print. Such head tilts cause rotation of the Y-axis of the optical system and induce cyclotorsion. If chronically repeated over long periods, cyclotorsion can result in cyclophoria and astigmatism. Astigmatism is viewed by Harmon as a means of optically changing the distribution of light on the retina to match visual with gravitational input with minimum need for perceptual compensation. Harmon (1958) notes that astigmats characteristically dem-

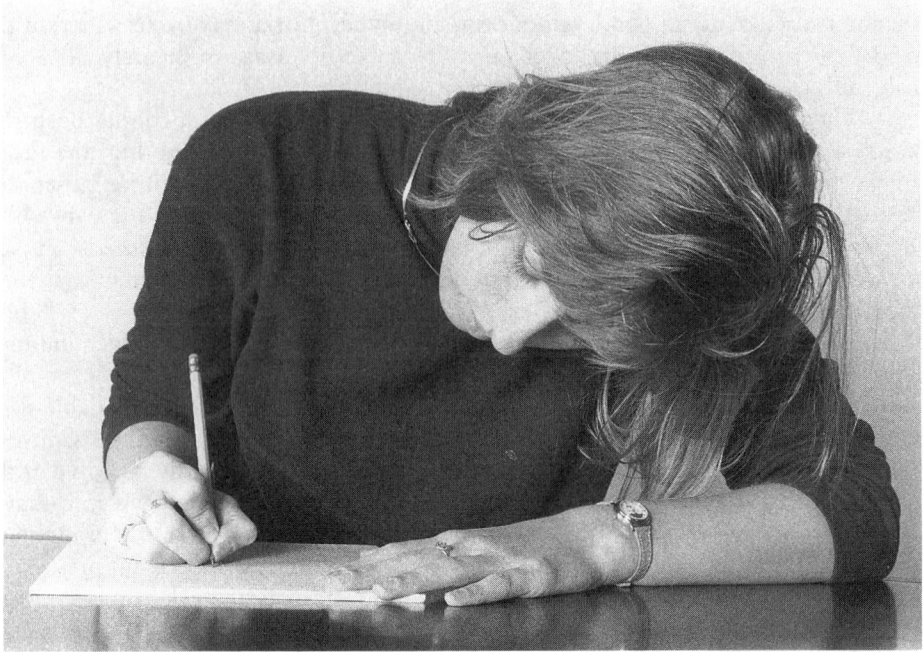

Figure 5.5 The intense individual who grips the pencil tightly near the point must tilt the head and move close to the page to see the point as she writes. This posture creates a difference in accommodative demand for the two eyes.

onstrate head tilts, and that in most cases the head tilt is functionally related to the off-center and rotated placement of near tasks and to the axis of astigmatism.

Head tilts are also seen with hyperphorias (Harmon 1958). Many functional hyperphorias are related to postural distortions accompanied by pelvic or shoulder tilts. Harmon indicates that small pelvic tilts arising from spinal curvature or trunk torsion which shorten a leg by as little as 1/8 inch, may induce significant hyperphoria.

Consistent with Harmon's (1958) notion that refractive disorders such as astigmatism and anisometropia can result from sustained ocular use in adverse posture, relationships between refractive status and posture during ocular use have been reported by Childress et al. (1970), Forrest (1980, 1981), and Harris (1988). Childress et al. (1970) report that individuals who center near work on their midline and position themselves directly in front of the television set show little astigmatism or anisometropia. Anisometropic individuals are generally those whose work involves greater visual demand on the side of the more myopic eye. Draftsmen, for example, do much of their work to the right of midline, and often show greater myopia in the right eye. Astigmatism that is unequal in magnitude in the two eyes is usually associated with asymmetric work posture in which the eye with the greater cylinder is farther away from the common near fixation point (Childress et al. 1970).

The axis of astigmatism tends to correlate with the direction of the visual demand. Secretaries whose work is spread across a desk and requires extensive horizontal scanning demonstrate a high incidence of with-the-rule astigmatism, while telephone operators, whose switchboards are located in a vertical plane requiring up-and-down scanning, tend to exhibit against-the-rule astigmatism. Childen who watch television for prolonged periods while lying in a prone position, looking toward the television, often show astigmatism at axes 75 degrees in the right eye and 105 degrees in the left; those who consistently watch television from one side are likely to show more myopia in the eye closer to the set and more astigmia in the eye farther away (Childress et al. 1970).

Forrest (1980, 1981) relates astigmatism to the patterns of eye scan, head scan, and head posture in habitual use during predominant visual tasks. He found that differential use of eye and head movement in different meridians is a key element in the development of astigmatism.

Little or no astigmatism occurs when eye and head movement preferences are similar in all meridians. However, when an individual regularly moves the eyes rather than the head while scanning in one meridian, and moves the head more than the eyes when scanning the meridian 90 degrees away, astigmatism develops with the minus cylinder axis in the meridian of greatest eye scan. The meridian in which eye scan is minimum is likely to be the most myopic. *With-the-rule astigmatism* relates to preference for eye scanning in the horizontal meridian, and *against-the-rule astigmatism* to a preference for eye scanning in the vertical. The magnitude of astigmatism is greatest when the difference between eye movement and head movement patterns in the different meridians is more substantial (Forrest 1980, 1981).

Oblique astigmatism and anisometropic astigmatism also correlate with posture and scan patterns (Forrest 1980, 1981). Forrest reports that parallel oblique astigmatism (for example, axis 75 degrees in each eye) is caused by persistent obliquity in visual scan pattern. Such obliquity may be associated with a persistent head tilt, or with task demands that are consistently obliquely oriented. Symmetrical oblique astigmatism (for example, axis 75 degrees in one eye, 105 degrees in the other) occurs when an individual persistently scans above or below the primary plane (for example, lying prone on the floor and looking up to watch television tends to produce intorted axes of astigmatism). When anisometropic astigmatism is found, the eye with greater astigmatism is usually the one that is positioned farther from habitual tasks, peering across the midline to view the task. According to Forrest (1980, 1981), these effects of head posture and oblique scan patterns are superimposed on those that result from the differential use of head and eye movement patterns in different meridians.

Forrest (1980) reports that the clinician can frequently predict an individual's characteristic pattern of head posture, eye scan, and head scan from knowledge of the individual's astigmatism. Further, changes in astigmatism in a given individual can usually be related to work changes that lead to altered patterns of eye movement, head movement, and head posture.

When an individual moves the eyes more than the head in one meridian, but emphasizes head scan in the meridian 90 degrees away, the pull of the extraocular muscles on the globe will differ in the various meridia. Similarly, oblique eye scan patterns generate forces on the eyeball that differ from those induced when eye movements are primarily horizontal or vertical. Forrest (1981) suggests that the differential pull of the extraocular muscles on the globe in the various meridia is the mechanism by which astigmatism results from these eye movement patterns. However, he notes that keratometer measures do not show the same consistency with patterns of ocular use as do measures of total ocular astigmatism (Forrest 1984).

Forrest (1984) reports that treatment regimens that alter patterns of head scan, eye scan, and head posture can effectively reduce astigmatism, regardless of the age of the patient. Such treatment regimens incorporate changes in working posture, task placement, and head and eye movement practices, as well as the use of exercises that emphasize eye movements in the direction in which the patient habitually tends to minimize visual scan.

Harris (1988) reports that symphony musicians, who work in asymmetric postures for long periods of time and whose scan patterns are dictated by their position in the orchestra and by the constraints imposed by their particular instruments, show patterns of astigmatism and anisometropia consistent with those predicted by the models of Harmon and Forrest.

These reports of Childress et al. (1979), Forrest (1980, 1981, 1984), and Harris (1988) support Harmon's (1958) thesis that ocular disabilities can result from postural skews. Harmon holds that the ability to adapt, to change as a product of use, is a fundamental property of organic matter. Harmon's model is based on the premise, attributed by Harmon (1958) to the biologist Julian Huxley, that the structure of a biologic system can be altered throughout life, within genetic limits, as a result of the manner in which the system is put to use.

The organism grows along the line of stress to reduce stress. Structure is altered to preserve function and achieve economy of effort. Altered structure, in turn, further influences function. A structural change that serves adaptively to facilitate function in the presence of a particular persistent stress may interfere with function in other situations for which the adaptive structural change is counterproductive.

Ocular anomalies such as hyperphoria, astigmatism, and anisometropia, which serve to facilitate information-processing in the presence of task-induced postural distortion, may nevertheless impair acuity or binocular function and constitute a handicap in the performance of tasks at other distances with different postural demands.

The notion that environmental interaction plays a major role in the development of both ocular structure and visual function is a fundamental tenet of functional and behavioral optometry. This premise underlies the work of Getman (1950–51; 1957–58), who emphasized the importance of adequate experience in visual development, and of Skeffington (1928–74) and Harmon (1958), who respectively emphasized the significance of culturally imposed near work and the role of ocular use in adverse postures as factors which generate stress on the visual system, interfere with visual efficiency, and lead to adaptive changes in both visual function and ocular structure.

SUMMARY

Harmon postulates that for any particular task, there is an optimal posture that minimizes bodily tension and facilitates efficient performance. When an individual is required to perform a task under adverse working conditions, postural distortions are induced that increase the energy required to maintain balance and detract from that available for task performance. In addition, perceptual compensation is required to match visual and gravitationally derived spatial coordinates. Under such conditions, visual efficiency and information-processing ability are affected adversely. Individuals who work in adverse postures for sustained periods may develop ocular skews such as myopia, hyperopia, anisometropia, astigmatism, and hyperphoria to preserve spatial relationships and compensate for induced bodily skews, in effect sacrificing lower level optical function to minimize interference with higher level cognitive functions. Studies are reviewed that link astigmatism and anisometropia to patterns of ocular use.

SUGGESTED READING

Harmon DB (1958). *Notes on a Dynamic Theory of Vision.* 3rd rev. ed. Austin, TX: author.

REFERENCES

Campos EC, Chiesi C, Maccaferri M (1988). Possible role of ocular proprioception in space perception: Analysis of the effect of surgery on strabismic patients. In: Jovicevic B (ed), *Pediatric Ophthalmology and Strabismus.* Belgrade, Yugoslavia: Jugoslovenska Revija, pp. 93–101.

Childress ME, Childress CW, Conklin RM (1970). Possible effects of visual demand on refractive error. *J Am Optom Assoc* 41(4):348–353.

Duke-Elder WS (1942). *Textbook of Ophthalmology.* Vol 1. *The Development, Form, and Function of the Visual Apparatus.* St. Louis: Mosby.

Forrest EB (1980). Astigmatism as a function of visual scan, head scan and head posture. *Am J Optom Physiol Opt* 57(11):844–860.

Forrest EB (1981). A new model of functional astigmatism. *J Am Optom Assoc* 52(11):889–897.

Forrest EB (1984). Eye scan therapy for astigmatism. *J Am Optom Assoc* 55(12):894–901.

Getman GN, Bullis G (1950–51). *Developmental Vision.* Optometric Extension Program Continuing Education Courses, Santa Ana, CA: Optometric Extension Program Foundation, vol. 24.

Getman GN, Kephart NC (1957–58). *Developmental Vision.* Optometric Extension Program Continuing Education Courses, Santa Ana, CA: Optometric Extension Program Foundation, vol. 30.

Grant AH (1987). The computer user syndrome. *J Am Optom Assoc* 58(11):892–901.

Greenspan SB (1970). Effects of children's nearpoint lenses upon body posture and performance. *Am J Optom Arch Am Acad Optom* 47(12):982–990.

Harmon DB (1942). Some preliminary observations on the developmental problems of 160,000 elementary school children. *Med Woman's J* 49(3):75–82.

Harmon DB (1951). *The Coordinated Classroom*. Grand Rapids, MI: American Seating Co.

Harmon DB (1958). *Notes on a Dynamic Theory of Vision*. 3rd rev. ed. Austin, TX: author.

Harmon DB (1960). *Nearpoint Lenses and Physiological Activity: A Movie*. Produced by the author, Austin, TX.

Harris P (1988). Visual conditions of symphony musicians. *J Am Optom Assoc* 59(12):952–959.

Miller SC (1984). Meeting the eye care needs of video display terminal operators. *J Am Optom Assoc* 55(8):611–618.

Nommay D, Vercher J, Gauther GM (1991). Localization of targets in humans: The role of ocular muscle proprioception. In: Schmid R, Zambarbieri D (eds), *Oculomotor Control and Cognitive Processes*. Amsterdam: Elsevier, pp. 21–28.

Petito GT, Greenwald I, Fox CR, et al. (1988). A model of spatial localization and its application to strabismus. *Am J Optom Physiol Opt* 65(2):108–117.

Pierce JR (1966–68). Research on the relationship between nearpoint lenses, human performance and physiological activity of the body. In: *Research Reports and Special Articles Pertaining to Vision and Its Care*. Optometric Extension Program Continuing Education Courses. Series 1, no. 1–12, Oct. 1966–Sept. 1967; series 2, no. 1–5, Oct. 1967–Feb. 1968, Santa Ana, CA: Optometric Extension Program Foundation.

Pierce JR (1970). A study of the relation between performance and physiological activity as a function of nearpoint working distance and posture. PhD dissertation, University of Portland, OR.

Skavenski AA (1990). Eye movement and visual localization of objects in space. In: Kowler E (ed), *Eye Movements and Their Role in Visual and Cognitive Processes*. Amsterdam: Elsevier, pp. 263–287.

Skeffington AM (1928–74). Optometric Extension Program Continuing Education Courses, Santa Ana, CA: Optometric Extension Program Foundation.

Steinbach MJ (1986). Muscles as sense organs. *Arch Ophthalmol* 104:1148–1149.

Wallach H (1985). Perceiving a stable environment. *Scientific Am* 252:118–123.

PART II

Case Analysis and Functional Lens Prescription

The basic concepts that underlie the Skeffington and Harmon models differ significantly from those underlying graphical analysis and traditional reserve-demand systems of case analysis. Harmon and Skeffington view nearpoint visual stress and resultant vision disorders as products of interaction with the environment. According to Skeffington, reading and related nearpoint tasks present demands that are incompatible with our biologic heritage. Harmon emphasizes the impact of improper posture and adverse working conditions. Therapeutic intervention based on these concepts emphasizes nearpoint lens application, guidance, and environmental manipulation. The goals include prevention of vision disorders and remediation of existing dysfunction.

Graphical analysis and reserve-demand case analysis systems, in contrast, consider accommodation-convergence disorders to be the result of hereditary influences, random biologic variation, and a variety of systemic factors that influence innervation to the oculomotor system. Little credence is given to the role of the environment and near work as causative factors. In contrast to approaches based on the concepts of Skeffington and Harmon, the potential for prevention is rarely considered.

Approaches to case analysis and management vary with these differing conceptual frameworks. Graphical analysis, Sheard's criterion, and Percival's criterion are based on the phoria and prism vergence measures, which are held to reflect fusional demand and compensatory fusional reserve. Adherents of these systems are likely to prescribe lenses or prisms to reduce fusional demand in asthenopic patients, and to initiate vision therapy in those cases in which lens and prism application appears unlikely to be effective. Newer systems emphasize the importance of evaluating binocular function under fused (rather than dissociated) conditions, and therefore assess the adequacy of vergence function through analysis of forced vergence fixation disparity curves. OEP analysis, derived from Skeffington's nearpoint stress model, is based on the notion that many functional vision disorders arise as adaptations to a hypothesized drive for convergence to localize closer than accommodation, and emphasizes the use of low-plus lenses for near work to relieve the effector system mismatch.

In each of these approaches, systems for case analysis are designed to identify those patients needing care, to determine the optimal lens prescription, and to assess the need for vision therapy. Dynamic retinoscopy procedures and supplementary performance tasks yield additional information regarding optimal lens prescription and need for vision therapy. The case history is fundamental to all systems for case analysis, providing information regarding the patient's symptoms and performance, which the practitioner can in turn relate to the examination findings to determine the need for care.

The case history is discussed in Chapter 6. Graphical and fixation disparity approaches to case analysis are described in Chapter 7. The 21-point OEP analytical routine and OEP case analysis are presented in Chapter 8. Various other case analysis approaches, methods for nearpoint retinoscopy, and other tests for determination of the optimal nearpoint lens prescription are discussed in Chapter 9. Reports of the efficacy of low-plus lenses for nearpoint use are summarized in Chapter 10.

6

Case History

Regardless of the method of case analysis adopted by a particular clinician, the case history is a key element in the evaluation procedure. Through the case history, the practitioner determines the patient's symptoms and complaints, degree of interest and involvement in near-vision tasks, academic achievement, and special interests and needs. The reported symptoms and performance deficits are then related to the examination findings. Inability to relate the examination findings to symptoms and real-life performance deficits, and to predict accurately the benefits of therapy and the adverse effects of neglecting treatment, leaves the patient with little reason to undergo care.

TAKING THE CASE HISTORY

The examiner should generally begin the case history by asking whether the patient is experiencing any visual difficulty. After eliciting the chief complaint and any secondary symptoms the examiner should explore specific areas related to nearpoint visual function, including clarity and comfort during near-vision tasks, school achievement, interest in reading, and occupational and avocational visual demands.

Patients should be asked about clarity and comfort during both distance and near-vision tasks. Can the patient read comfortably? Is the print clear? Does it stay clear during prolonged nearpoint application? How long can the patient actually read or study before the eyes feel tired or strained, or before headache occurs? Although many patients report that they experience asthenopia only after prolonged reading, further questioning sometimes reveals that they read very little, and consider 10 minutes of reading to be a long time. Clarity and comfort should also be evaluated for distance vision tasks such as watching television and movies, driving, and viewing chalkboard material.

Because many individuals with functional vision disorders dislike and avoid reading, patients should be questioned regarding their interest in reading, whether they like to read, and how much they actually read. Patients with functional vision disorder who report no asthenopia but read very little should not be considered asymptomatic, since their lack of interest in reading may well result from their vision disorder.

The practitioner must not simply elicit the chief complaint, but should investigate the full gamut of symptoms commonly associated with functional vision disorder. When symptoms are reported, the examiner should evaluate the nature, severity, frequency, duration, and precipitating circumstances of each symptom. The examiner must consider the relative likelihood of various possible causes for these symptoms, and formulate tentative hypotheses to be confirmed or rejected as the examination proceeds.

The case history does not end with the initial questions, but continues throughout and following the examination to assess the manner in which the problems detected affect the patient. It frequently happens that the doctor finds a visual problem even though no symptoms have been reported in the initial case history. In such cases, the examiner should consider what symptoms or performance deficits (including avoidance) might be expected to accompany the visual problem, and specifically ask the patient about such symptoms; the patient will frequently recognize symptoms that he or she had not thought to mention initially.

Patients may neglect to mention significant symptoms unless the clinician makes specific inquiry. Symptoms may go unreported because they are overshadowed in the patient's mind by the chief complaint. The patient may simply overlook other symptoms when the case history is taken. Even symptoms as obvious and severe as diplopia may be unreported if they are so long-standing that the patient accepts their presence as natural. Poor reading achievement, avoidance, and disinterest in reading may go unreported if the patient does not perceive them as visually related.

The practitioner should therefore inquire about a broad range of potential visually related symptoms, in addition to those volunteered by the patient. Common symptoms of functional vision disorders include blurred vision at distance or near; print blurs after reading a short time; distance vision blur after reading; difficulty shifting focus from near to far; squinting; eyes turn or cross; double vision; headaches; eyestrain; eyes tire or hurt; general or ocular fatigue; inability to read for a long time; eyes red, irritated, tearing; rubs eyes or blinks frequently; strains, frowns, grimaces, or shows other signs of tension while reading; closes or covers one eye; reads or writes with head close to page; tilts head when reads or writes; poor posture when reads or writes; moves head while reading; poor school achievement; not working to potential; poor reading ability; poor word recognition; reads word-by-word; confuses similar letters or words; reverses letters or words; skips, rereads, or omits words; reads or works slowly; uses finger or marker to keep place while reading; loses place frequently when reading or copying from chalkboard; makes errors in copying from chalkboard to desk; poor reading comprehension; avoids near tasks; dislikes reading; and short attention span.

SOURCES OF ASTHENOPIA

Visual discomfort or asthenopia is a subjective experience that arises from both psychologic and physiologic factors, and hence does not always correlate closely with oculomotor findings. Symptoms of visual fatigue are usually localized in the eyes or head, but may be much more diffuse on occasion (Bartley 1942).

Nearpoint asthenopic symptoms are traditionally attributed to the effort required to overcome vision disorders such as accommodative or convergence insufficiency. However, it is well established that the sensory processes and motor functions that subserve vision have high thresholds for physiological impairment (Bartley and Chute 1947; Pigion and Miller 1985). It is therefore likely that asthenopic symptoms arise not primarily from demands on accommodation and convergence per se, but rather from the conflict and frustration that result from visual inefficiency. Bartley (1942) and Bartley and Chute (1947) suggest that asthenopic symptoms commonly arise not from fatigue of the ocular structures, but rather as a function of the organism as a whole, becoming localized in the eyes when visual function is inadequate so that performance on visual tasks drops below a level satisfactory to the individual.

Forrest (1988) emphasizes that a diligent, intense, focal approach to near work exacerbates the visual stress response. In this author's experience, individuals who are high-driving, intense, and focal are more likely to experience asthenopia, both because of the heightened visual stress response and because the resulting visual inefficiency is particularly frustrating to those who are highly achievement-oriented. Even in the absence of overt visual problems, asthenopia may ensue when goals for achievement are so high as to be unobtainable, when nonvisual factors limit achievement, or when an individual is so intense in near-work application as to generate tension and fatigue.

LEARNING-RELATED PROBLEMS

Optometrists frequently see children whose chief complaint is learning or reading difficulty. Vergence, accommodative, and ocular motility disorders commonly interfere with reading efficiency, comfort, and comprehension. Visual-perceptual disorders are more likely to interfere with acquisition of word recognition skills (Flax 1970). In evaluating a child with reading or learning difficulty, the optometrist must obtain information regarding the specifics of the academic problems, to determine whether learning difficulty may be related to the child's visual status. It is frequently advisable that the optometrist obtain this information from the classroom teacher, reading or resource room teacher, or school psychologist.

School achievement should be probed whenever evaluating a child. Is the child doing well in school? Does she like to read? Is she a good reader? If not, what specific reading difficulties does she have? Is phonetic decoding ability adequate? Does the child confuse similar looking words, forget familiar words, or make numerous small word errors? Is reading comprehension adequate? Do comprehension and efficiency break down with time? In what grade did reading difficulty begin? Does she get special help in reading? Does she do well in other subjects? Spelling? Math? Handwriting? Is there difficulty copying from the chalkboard, or frequent loss of place or skipping words or lines when reading?

Birth and developmental history should also be explored when examining a child with learning difficulty. Visual-perceptual disorders and deficient visual information-processing abilities are frequently accompanied by lags in motor or speech development that may be functional or organic in origin. A report of premature birth, complications during pregnancy or delivery, or illness or abnormality during early childhood may signal an organic basis.

USE OF CHECKLISTS

Checklists of symptoms relevant to children's vision disorders are incorporated in "A Teacher's Guide to Vision Problems," published by the American Optometric Association, and in "Does Your Child Have a Learning-Related Vision Problem?" and "Educator's Guide to Classroom Vision Problems," pamphlets produced by the Optometric Extension Program Foundation. These checklists, designed to assist parents and teachers in detecting vision disorders, are also suitable for use by the optometrist, providing a comprehensive list of potential visual signs and symptoms related to classroom performance. Reviewing such a list with the patient helps to ensure that problems are not overlooked.

These checklists, and more extensive questionnaires developed by individual optometrists, are frequently used as preexamination case history forms. Such forms, to be completed by the parent and/or teacher, are mailed when the appointment is made and returned either prior to or on the date of the examination. Such forms allow the practitioner to review the information before beginning the examination, permitting faster, more comprehensive case history-taking and facilitating the identification of areas to be probed in depth. A very thorough case history checklist, developed by Daniel Woolf, O.D., and Joseph A. Viviano, O.D., is illustrated in Table 6.1.

Following the examination, a telephone call to the teacher or other educator working with the child, followed by a written report, is effective in communicating optometric findings and recommendations. The thoughtful doctor will make recommendations, when indicated, for special seating, use of large-print materials, frequent rest periods during near work, use of finger or marker to keep place, and specific teaching methodologies, based on the individual child's visual status. Such communication is helpful for the child and is an effective practice development technique, since it conveys the doctor's interest and concern to educators.

Table 6.1 Case history checklist designed by Drs. Daniel Woolf and Joseph A. Viviano, Summitt, NJ. (Reprinted with permission.)

OPTOMETRIST'S CHECKLIST FOR EDUCATORS AND PARENTS
Designed and tested by Drs. Daniel Woolf and Joseph A. Viviano

Name _____

This checklist of symptoms of visual problems observed at school and at home will help us understand how the child performs visually in his daily activities. Please mark symptoms which occur frequently with <u>two</u> checks, those which occur occasionally with <u>one</u> check. Please use first open column.

	Date			

Reading
Fatigue with reading or comprehension drops with time ..				
Confusion of similar words or letters				
Omits words				
Short attention span while reading				
Difficulty keeping place while reading				
Holds head too close to book				
Slow reading or word-by-word reading				
Skips or rereads lines				
Uses finger or marker as a pointer				
Avoids reading				
Says the words aloud or lip reads				
Reverses words or letters				
Difficulty remembering what has been read				
Difficulty remembering newly learned words				
Poor sitting posture and position while reading				
Excessive head turning while reading				
Frowning, excessive blinking, scowling, squinting, or other facial distortions while reading				
Rubs eyes during or after reading				
Tilts head to one side				
Turns head so as to use one eye only				
Closes or covers one eye				

Writing and Other Desk Tasks
Holds head too close to desk when writing				
Gross postural defects while seated at desk				
Restlessness while working at desk				
Difficulty copying from chalkboard or book				
Squints or blinks looking up at chalkboard				
Tilts head to one side				
Turns head so as to use one eye only				
Omits or repeats letters, words, or phrases				
Poor eye-hand coordination, including poor writing				
Writes neatly but too slowly				
Reversals persisting in grade 2 or beyond				
Weight on the writing arm				
Does not use other hand to hold paper				

Table 6.1 *Continued*

	(1)	(2)	(3)
Immature pencil grip	___	___	___
Poor finger movement in writing	___	___	___
Draws with short sketchy lines	___	___	___
Turns paper to draw lines in different directions	___	___	___
Body Posture and Space Awareness			
Unusual awkwardness	___	___	___
Frequent tripping or stumbling	___	___	___
Body rigidity while looking at distant objects	___	___	___
Thrusts head forward or backward while looking at distant objects	___	___	___
Confuses right and left directions	___	___	___
Appearance of Eyes			
Crossed eyes—turning in or out	___	___	___
Watering or bloodshot eyes	___	___	___
Red-rimmed, crusted, or swollen lids	___	___	___
Frequent styes	___	___	___
General Behavior			
Short attention span	___	___	___
Dislike for tasks requiring sustained visual concentration	___	___	___
Nervousness, irritability, or restlessness after maintaining visual concentration	___	___	___
Inattentiveness, daydreaming	___	___	___
Unusual fatigue after completing a vision task	___	___	___
Frequent signs of frustration	___	___	___
Tension during close work	___	___	___
Avoids close work	___	___	___
Questions for Children			
Does your vision get blurry at any time?	___	___	___
Can you make it clear?	___	___	___
Do you ever see objects double?	___	___	___
Do you have headaches, dizziness, or feel sick to your stomach when you use your eyes, or do you get carsick?	___	___	___
Do letters and lines "run together" or words "jump"?	___	___	___
Do your eyes ever feel hot or itch?	___	___	___
Does light bother your eyes?	___	___	___
Do you know where to catch a pop-up fly ball, how far to throw a ball, where the ball is going to be?	___	___	___
	(1)	(2)	(3)

Reported by:

Column (1) _____ Position _____
Column (2) _____ Position _____
Column (3) _____ Position _____

VIDEO DISPLAY TERMINAL CASE HISTORY

Asthenopic complaints are frequently associated with use of video display terminals (VDTs). The case history, therefore, should routinely include questions regarding use of video displays:

- Does the patient use a computer or video display? How frequently, and for how long?
- Does the patient experience eyestrain, visual fatigue, general tiredness, headache, neckache, or backache while working at the VDT?
- Are lighting, contrast, glare control, seating, and positioning of the unit adequate and comfortable?
- Where is the VDT positioned with respect to the patient? What is the working distance? Height? Lateral placement?
- What other visual demands are placed on the patient while working on the VDT? Where is the material to be copied? Are there other office machines that must be viewed to input data? Where are they located? Are there distance vision demands? Each of the visual demands at the work station must be analyzed with regard to the working distance, height and lateral placement.

Margach (1982) provides an extensive case history form to assist in gathering information regarding visual complaints, visual demands, and design of the VDT work station. Such data permit the optometrist to prescribe lenses suitable for the specific needs of the VDT operator, and to guide the patient regarding control of ergonomic factors that effect visual efficiency.

SUMMARY

The case history provides information as to the patient's symptoms and complaints, academic achievement, ability to perform efficiently in relation to real-world visual demands, and degree of interest and involvement in near work. Case history is generally taken at the beginning and amplified throughout the evaluation, and may involve the use of checklists and interviews with teachers and other professionals in addition to questions directed toward the patient and parents.

SUGGESTED READING

Borish IM (1970). *Clinical Refraction*. 3rd ed. Chicago: Professional Press.
Manas L (1965). *Visual Analysis*. Chicago: Professional Press.

REFERENCES

Bartley SH (1942). A factor in visual fatigue. *Psychosom Med* 4:369–375.
Bartley SH, Chute E (1947). *Fatigue and Impairment in Man*. New York: McGraw-Hill.

Flax N (1970). Problems in relating visual function to reading disorder. *Am J Optom* 47:366–372.

Forrest EB (1988). *Stress and Vision*. Santa Ana, CA: Optometric Extension Program Foundation.

Margach CB (1982). Video display terminals. In: *Literature and Research Review*. Optometric Extension Program Continuing Education Courses, Santa Ana, CA: Optometric Extension Program Foundation, vol. 54, series 7, no. 7, April; vol. 55, series 8, no. 1–3, Oct.–Dec.

Pigion RG, Miller RJ (1985). Fatigue of accommodation: Changes in accommodation after near work. *Am J Optom Physiol Opt* 62(12):853–863.

7

Graphical and Fixation Disparity Analysis

Graphical analysis is a method of plotting clinical measures of vergence and accommodation to determine the range of stimuli through which an individual is able to maintain clear, single binocular vision. Graphical analysis does not mandate the use of any particular system for interpretation of the findings; rather, graphical display enhances the visibility of the relationship between the various findings, permitting the utilization of various systems and rules for analysis (Hofstetter 1983; Goss 1986).

The relationship between the phorometric findings is portrayed in the form of a parallelogram (Figure 7.1). Convergence findings are plotted on the abscissa (x-axis) and accommodative findings on the ordinate (y-axis). The findings typically plotted are the dissociated phorias at distance and near; the base-in and base-out prism vergence blur, break, and recovery measures at distance and near; the plus and minus lens to blur findings; the amplitude of accommodation; and the convergence near point.

The demand line is an oblique line across the graph connecting the points that represent, for each distance in space, the stimulus to accommodation and stimulus to convergence. This line was described by Donders (1864) in the earliest graphical representation, and is frequently referred to as *Donders' line.*

To construct the graph, the phoria measures at distance and near are plotted, and connected by a line called the *phoria line.* The distance phoria positions the graph on the convergence scale (abscissa), and the AC/A ratio specifies its slope.

The base-in and base-out to blur, break, and recovery are similarly plotted, as are the plus and minus to blur findings. One line is drawn connecting the base-out to blur values at distance and near, and another connecting the base-in to blur values. These lines represent the right- and left-hand limits of the zone of clear, single binocular vision. The parallelogram is completed on the bottom by the baseline of the graph and at the top by a horizontal line drawn across the graph at the level equal to the amplitude of accommodation (Borish 1970; Goss 1986).

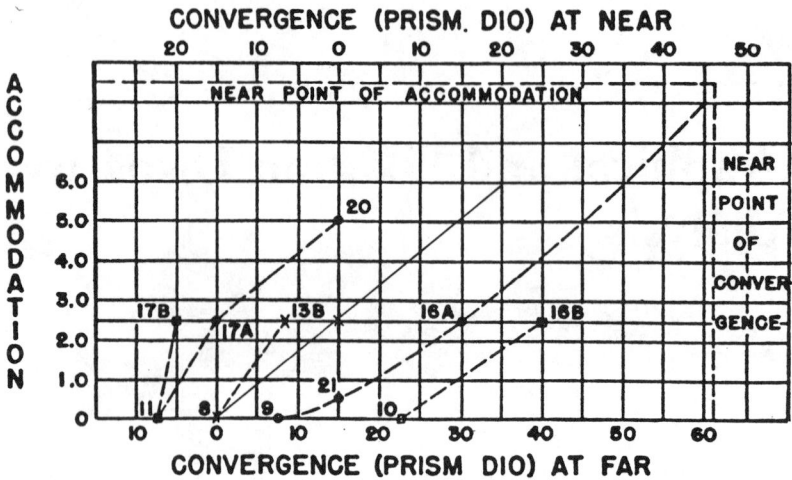

Figure 7.1 A typical graph for display of phorometric findings, derived from the work of Glenn Fry, O.D., Ph.D. Convergence findings are plotted on the x-axis and accommodative findings on the y-axis. (Modified from Borish, IM, *Clinical Refraction*, Chicago: Professional Press, 1970, Fig XXI-5, p. 883. Reprinted with permission of Butterworth–Heinemann, Boston.)

Various criteria may be used to analyze the findings. In addition to its clinical utility in determining the need for prism, lens, and orthoptic application, graphical display of the phorometric findings makes it easier to identify potentially spurious findings. Graphical analysis has also been used as a tool to research the relationship between accommodation and convergence (Hofstetter 1983).

CRITERIA FOR COMFORT

Donders (1864) was the first to use a graphical form to portray the relationship between accommodation and convergence. He graphed the limits of accommodation that could be elicited at given levels of convergence, and postulated that accommodation could be comfortably sustained at a given fixation distance only if PRA was greater than negative relative accommodation (NRA). Landolt (1886) added the ranges of relative convergence to the graph, and proposed that not more than one third of the absolute range of convergence could be maintained without asthenopia.

Percival's Criterion

Percival (1928) postulated that the middle third of the zone of clear, single binocular vision is an area or zone of comfort. For an individual to be comfortable at a given fixation distance, Donder's demand line, the line that connects points of equal demand for accommodation and convergence (for example, 3 diopters of accommodation and 3-m angles of convergence), should fall within this zone, that is, within the middle third of the range of relative convergence. If it does not, prism, lens power change, or vision training is indicated.

To determine whether Percival's criterion has been met, the base-in and base-out blur limits are added to determine the total width of the zone of clear, single binocular vision, and this width is divided by 3 to determine the width of the zone of comfort. If either the base-in or base-out blur is less than the width of the comfort zone, Percival's criterion has not been met. Prism prescription, with the base toward the higher limit, may be used to move the demand line within the middle third (Goss 1986).

Thus, for example, given a base-out blur of 12^Δ and a base-in blur of 3^Δ, the total width of the zone of clear, single binocular vision would be $12 + 3 = 15^\Delta$, and the zone of comfort would be $15 \div 3 = 5^\Delta$. Since the base-in blur is smaller than the width of the comfort zone, prism base-out is indicated to move the demand line within the middle third. A 2^Δ base-out prism would satisfy Percival's criterion, since through the prism the base-out blur would become 10^Δ and the base-in blur 5^Δ; the width of the comfort zone would remain $15 \div 3 = 5^\Delta$, but the base-in blur would now barely fall within this zone (Figure 7.2).

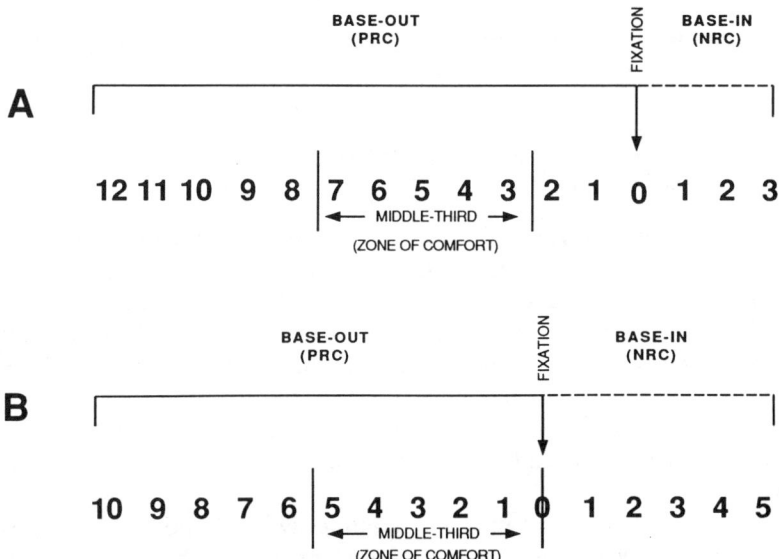

Figure 7.2 (A) Given a base-out blur of 12^Δ and a base-in blur of 3^Δ, the point of fixation falls outside the zone of comfort and Percival's criterion is not satisfied. (B) Through a 2^Δ base-out prism, the base-out finding will decrease 2^Δ and the base-in finding will increase 2^Δ, shifting the fixation point barely within the zone of comfort and thereby satisfying Percival's criterion. (Modified from I.M. Borish, *Clinical Refraction*, 3rd ed. Chicago: Professional Press, 1970, p. 877. Reprinted with permission of Butterworth–Heinemann, Boston.)

Sheard's Criterion

Sheard (1928, 1930) added the phoria line to the graph, suggesting that it, rather than Donder's demand line, represents the real demand or starting point for fusional vergence. He postulated that to maintain comfort, the fusional reserve (compensating vergence) should be at least twice as great as the fusion demand (phoria). The base-out prism blur should be at least twice the exophoria; when esophoria exists, the base-in prism blur should be at least twice the esophoria. When discomfort exists, the failure to meet these criteria indicates the need for prism application, modification of lens prescription, or orthoptics (Borish 1970; Grisham 1983; Goss 1986).

Sheard's criterion may be expressed as a formula for prism prescription for patients with discomfort presumed to be caused by heterophoria:

$$\text{Sheard prism} = \frac{2(\text{phoria}) - \text{compensating vergence blur}}{3}.$$

Thus, for a patient who showed 8^Δ exophoria at near with a base-out to blur at near of 10^Δ, the Sheard prism would be:

$$\frac{2(8) - 10}{3} = 2^\Delta \text{ base-in.}$$

If the patient were symptomatic, a 2^Δ base-in prism would be indicated as the minimum necessary to satisfy Sheard's criterion (Grisham 1983).

Clinical Use and Validity of Sheard's and Percival's Criteria

Sheard's and Percival's criteria have been used for many decades as "rules of thumb" to guide in the prescription of lenses and prisms, and the training of symptomatic patients. These criteria were derived clinically and empirically. Hofstetter (1971) traces the Sheard criterion to "a moment of scientific wistfulness" when "Sheard used the analogy of 'money in the bank' to describe why the binocular fusional reserve ought to be about double the fusional demand to assure the patient of comfort." He then traces the elevation of this notion to "a guideline," "a rule of thumb," "a criterion," "Sheard's criterion," and finally, "Sheard's law."

Thus, while Sheard's criterion is commonly used and has a long tradition, it is important to recognize that it is a concept, rather than a well-documented fact. In recent years, studies have been undertaken to assess the validity of Sheard's and Percival's criteria, to determine whether they in fact predict asthenopia, and to determine the effectiveness of prism prescriptions derived from them.

Arner et al. (1956) found no significant correlation between asthenopia and either Sheard's or Percival's criteria. In contrast, Sheedy and Saladin (1977, 1978) found that Sheard's criterion serves as an effective predictor of asthenopic symptoms among exophores, and that Percival's criterion correlates better with the presence or absence of asthenopic symptoms among esophores.

There is little evidence that Sheard's and Percival's criteria for prescribing prism have clinical validity. Worrell et al. (1971) studied the effectiveness of prisms prescribed on the basis of Sheard's criterion. They found that prism corrections were subjectively preferred over glasses without prism for esophoria at distance, but not esophoria at near or exophoria at distance. For those with exophoria at near, prism glasses were preferred over non-prism glasses by presbyopes, but not prepresbyopes. Prism prescriptions for exophores were less effective than convergence training. Dalziel (1981) reported that, in patients with convergence insufficiency, vision training that improved base-out prism vergence to a level which satisfied Sheard's criterion was effective in relieving asthenopia.

Goss (1986) suggests that, to satisfy Sheard's and Percival's criteria in cases of convergence insufficiency, vision training to increase base-out fusion reserve is the method of choice. Base-in prism prescription for near is an alternative. Minus lens power is generally not added, since the AC/A is low. In contrast, in convergence excess, the AC/A is high and a bifocal addition is effective in reducing the esophoria and thereby satisfying the criteria.

In contrast with the relatively low prism prescriptions usually indicated by Sheard's and Percival's criteria, Lie and Opheim (1985, 1990) and Hasse (1980) recommend full prism correction in cases of heterophoria with asthenopic symptoms, with an increase in prism if the deviation increases. They view prism-induced increases in heterophoria not as adaptive, but rather as a result of underlying latent heterophoria. They report that asthenopic symptoms are resolved and long-term stability achieved (following stepwise successive recorrection when necessary) in most patients. However, in some cases where heterophoria is converted to heterotropia, surgery is required.

Clinicians are typically wary of prescribing prism, since some patients adapt to recreate the original heterophoria (McCormack 1985), others obtain no relief from symptoms, and still others experience disturbing spatial distortion. Functionally oriented practitioners generally prefer vision therapy as a treatment option, believing it better to remediate visual dysfunction with training than to simply relieve fusional demand with prism, especially since many patients with high heterophoria show both accommodative and vergence disorders. Vision therapy generally offers greater potential to improve visual efficiency.

Morgan's Syndrome Analysis

Morgan (1944a) developed a system of analysis based on the pattern of relationships among the various phorometric measures. He organized the findings into two groups. Group A includes the amplitude of accommodation, PRA, exophoria at near, and base-in vergences at distance and near. In general, these measures reflect the ability to stimulate accommodation and the flexibility to shift accommodation nearer than vergence. Group B findings include the base-out blur and break at near; dynamic retinoscopy; fused cross-cylinder; and the NRA. These tests probe the tendency for accommodation to lag behind vergence, and the ability to shift convergence nearer than accommodation.

In general, the tests within each group tend to vary together, running high or low as a group, although within each group the correlation is not perfect, so that not all tests covary in the expected manner. In cases of accommodative disorder, the group A tests tend to be low and the group B tests high. In cases of convergence insufficiency, the tests in group A tend to be high, and those in group B tend to be low.

Morgan (1944a) suggests that accommodative disorders and convergence disorders each be further subdivided into three divisions depending on whether the AC/A is low, normal, or high. Treatment options in these cases include lens power change, prism prescription, and vision training. The AC/A ratio helps to determine which method is applied, since it predicts the effect that indicated plus or minus lenses will have on the findings. When the AC/A is low, according to Morgan, maximum plus is usually accepted at near. However, when the gradient is high, the maximum plus will tend to interfere in the accommodation/convergence relationship to a greater degree and may not be acceptable.

Grisham (1983) identifies vergence dysfunction by comparing prism vergence, heterophoria, and accommodative measures with clinical standards based on Morgan's (1944a) data for the general population (Table 7.1). When any of the measures fall outside of the low tail of the first standard deviation for the

Table 7.1 Morgan's norms for phoria, prism vergence, and relative accommodation findings

	Mean	*SD*
Distance phoria	1 exophoria	±2ᐃ
Base-out blur	9ᐃ	±4ᐃ
Base-out break	19ᐃ	±8ᐃ
Base-out recovery	10ᐃ	±4ᐃ
Base-in break	7ᐃ	±3ᐃ
Base-in recovery	4ᐃ	±2ᐃ
Near phoria	3 exophoria	±5ᐃ
Monocular cross-cylinder	+1.00 D	±0.50 D
Binocular fused cross-cylinder	+0.50 D	±0.50 D
Base-out blur	17ᐃ	±5ᐃ
Base-out break	21ᐃ	±6ᐃ
Base-out recovery	11ᐃ	±7ᐃ
Base-in blur	13ᐃ	±4ᐃ
Base-in break	21ᐃ	±4ᐃ
Base-in recovery	13ᐃ	±5ᐃ
PRA	−2.37 D	±1.12 D
NRA	+2.00 D	±0.50 D

(Modified from M.W. Morgan, Jr., Analysis of Clinical Data, *Am J Optom Arch Am Acad Optom*, 21(12): 477–491, © The Am Acad of Optom, 1944.)

general population, binocular dysfunction is suspected. Treatment (lenses, prisms, and/or vision therapy) is indicated if the identified deficiency represents a practical problem for the patient. Grisham identifies three general categories of vergence dysfunction: (1) deficient horizontal fusional vergences in the absence of significant heterophoria; (2) high heterophorias with normal fusional vergence abilities; and (3) high heterophorias with abnormal prism vergence responses.

Duane-White Syndromes

The Duane-White categorization of vergence anomalies is widely used (Duane 1897; White 1941; Tait 1951; Borish 1970). The system classifies anomalies of convergence and divergence as convergence insufficiency, convergence excess, divergence insufficiency, and divergence excess (see Chapter 1). In practice, the differentiation between these syndromes is not always clear.

The Duane-White syndromes are derived from the concept of a phoria as a latent strabismus, and tend to be associated with traditional notions of etiology, assuming that binocular vision disorders result from abnormal innervation to the extraocular muscles caused by genetic or random biologic influences, rather than from environmental interaction. Nevertheless, regardless of the model adopted by a particular practitioner, the system is extremely useful to quickly describe the clinical picture for a given patient.

FIXATION DISPARITY

In recent years, interest has increased in the use of fixation disparity in the analysis of binocular vision disorders. Proponents favor the use of fixation disparity because, in contrast with phoria/vergence analysis, it permits the evaluation of the oculomotor system under binocular fused conditions.

Fixation disparity is a very small misalignment of the two eyes, usually measuring less than 10 minutes of arc, which is present during binocular fusion. Sensory fusion occurs because the deviation is so small that the disparate images of the fixation point fall within Panum's area.

Although there is general agreement that fixation disparity arises from stress on the vergence system, the exact nature and role of fixation disparity are uncertain. Mallett (1964) and Ogle et al. (1967) view fixation disparity as a vergence lag arising from failure to fully compensate for heterophoria. However, heterophoria and fixation disparity occur in opposite directions in approximately 25% of cases (Saladin and Sheedy 1978).

Schor (1980) holds that fixation disparity provides a stimulus to the fusional vergence system and serves to compensate for the decay of fast-fusional vergence innervation. When vergence adaptation is inadequate to relieve stress on the fusional vergence system, fixation disparity serves as a steady-state error to stimulate fast-fusional vergence (see Chapter 1). These explanations are not necessarily incompatible. Fixation disparity may, in a given patient, result from failure to fully compensate for heterophoria, from need for a steady-state stimulus for the fusional vergence system, or both (Dowley 1989).

Testing Fixation Disparity

Instruments used to assess fixation disparity generally present a binocularly fused target and a pair of polarized vernier lines, each of which is seen by one eye only. When these vernier lines are physically aligned, the patient with fixation disparity will perceive them as misaligned, the degree of misalignment indicating the magnitude of fixation disparity.

Instruments used to evaluate fixation disparity include the Disparometer (Sheedy 1980); the Wesson fixation disparity card (Wesson and Koenig 1983); the Mallett unit (Mallett 1964, 1966); the American Optical vectograph target (Grolman 1971); the Borish nearpoint chart (Borish 1978); and the Bernell nearpoint analysis slide no. 554A (Bernell Corp). The Disparometer and the Wesson card each permit the direct measurement of fixation disparity and can be used to assess changes in fixation disparity with prism- (and lens-) induced changes in vergence demand. The other instruments permit the detection of fixation disparity, but do not measure it directly; they measure the associated phoria by determining the amount of prism that must be added to achieve subjective alignment of the vernier lines and reduce fixation disparity to zero.

The Disparometer (Figure 7.3) consists of a rotatable disk that contains a series of vernier lines with varying degrees of misalignment. If the presence of

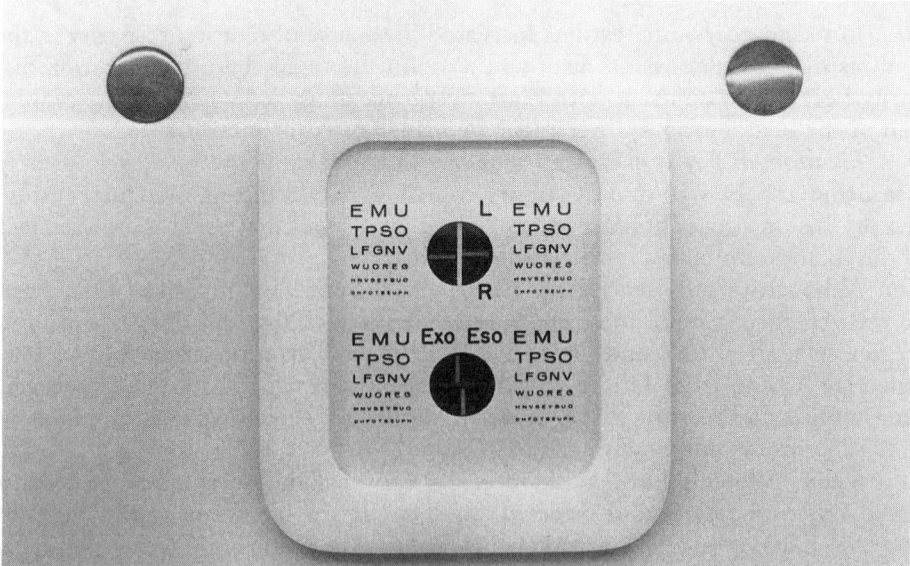

Figure 7.3 Front view of the disparometer. The upper target is used to measure vertical and the lower to measure lateral fixation disparity. (Photo courtesy of Dr. James Sheedy.)

fixation disparity is indicated by the subjective report of misalignment when the vernier lines are actually aligned, the disk is rotated to find the pair of lines that the patient perceives to be aligned. The physical separation of the lines designates the amount of fixation disparity, and is read directly from the instrument.

The Wesson fixation disparity card (Figure 7.4) presents a central fused square within which are located a black arrow, seen by one eye, and a series of colored lines, seen by the other. If the patient reports that the black arrow points to the red center line, there is no fixation disparity. In the presence of fixation disparity, the black arrow is displaced from the central red line; the degree of displacement is measured as the amount of fixation disparity present.

The Disparometer and the Wesson fixation disparity card can each be hand-held or attached to a phoropter nearpoint rod. Each instrument can be used to introduce varying degrees of prism and to measure the degree of fixation disparity for each prism power, and thus generate a forced vergence fixation disparity curve. Such curves provide useful information for the analysis of binocular vision; hence, these instruments are advantageous compared with those that only permit measurement of the associated phoria. Yaeger and Boltz (1986) describe

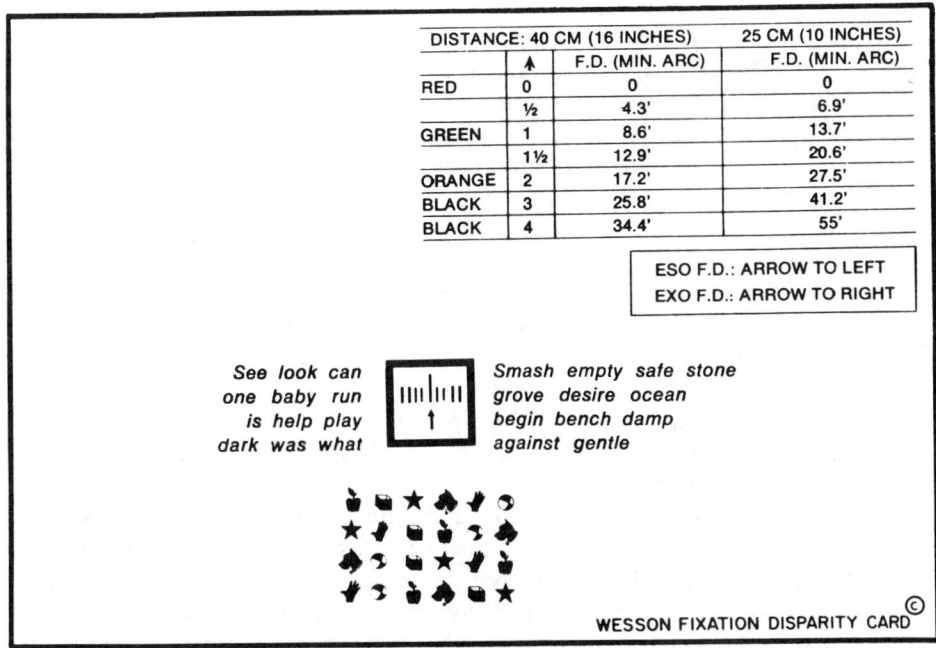

DISTANCE:	40 CM (16 INCHES)		25 CM (10 INCHES)
	↟	F.D. (MIN. ARC)	F.D. (MIN. ARC)
RED	0	0	0
	½	4.3'	6.9'
GREEN	1	8.6'	13.7'
	1½	12.9'	20.6'
ORANGE	2	17.2'	27.5'
BLACK	3	25.8'	41.2'
BLACK	4	34.4'	55'

ESO F.D.: ARROW TO LEFT
EXO F.D.: ARROW TO RIGHT

See look can one baby run is help play dark was what

Smash empty safe stone grove desire ocean begin bench damp against gentle

WESSON FIXATION DISPARITY CARD ©

Figure 7.4 The Wesson fixation disparity card. Within the central fused square, polarization is such that the arrow is seen with one eye and a series of colored lines by the other. The displacement of the black arrow from the long central red line indicates the magnitude of fixation disparity, determined from the table at the upper right. (Reprinted with permission of Dr. Michael Wesson.)

a computer program to measure fixation disparity and generate forced vergence fixation disparity curves.

Forced Vergence Fixation Disparity Curves

Forced vergence fixation disparity curves are generated by forcing vergence through the use of base-in and base-out prisms, and measuring the fixation disparity associated with each vergence demand level. As base-in prism is added, a demand is created for negative fusional vergence; alignment tends to lag slightly behind this demand, creating an eso-fixation disparity that increases as base-in prism demand is increased. Similarly, when base-out prism is added, fixation disparity tends to increase in the exo direction (Ogle et al. 1967; Sheedy 1980).

Graphical representation of these data provides useful information regarding binocular function (Figure 7.5). The vergence demand introduced by prism is indicated on the horizontal axis, base-in to the left and base-out to the right. Fixation disparity is plotted on the vertical axis, with esodisparity above and exodisparity below the horizontal.

There are four characteristics of a forced vergence fixation disparity curve (Sheedy 1980):

1. Fixation disparity

    The vertical or y-intercept of the curve is a measure of fixation disparity present without induced prism stress.
2. Associated phoria

    The horizontal axis intercept (x-intercept) is a measure of the associated phoria, the prism required to reduce fixation disparity to zero.
3. Curve type

    Fixation disparity curves are classified by shape into four characteristic types (Figure 7.6) (Ogle et al. 1967). The type I curve is a sigmoid curve with a near-vertical extension at each end, which indicates that fixation disparity increases rapidly as the limits of fusional vergence range are approached, and that this increase in fixation disparity is about equal for increases in base-in and base-out fusional vergence demand.

    The type I curve is the most common, occurring in approximately 60% of the population. It is most often associated with an asymptomatic patient and is considered the most "normal" curve, although the presence of a type I curve does not necessarily indicate that binocular function is adequate. The other curve types occur less frequently and are more often associated with asthenopia (Sheedy and Saladin 1978; Sheedy 1980).

    The type II curve, commonly associated with esophoria, is one in which adaptation to base-out prism is greater than that to base-in, so that fixation disparity increases to a much greater degree for base-in

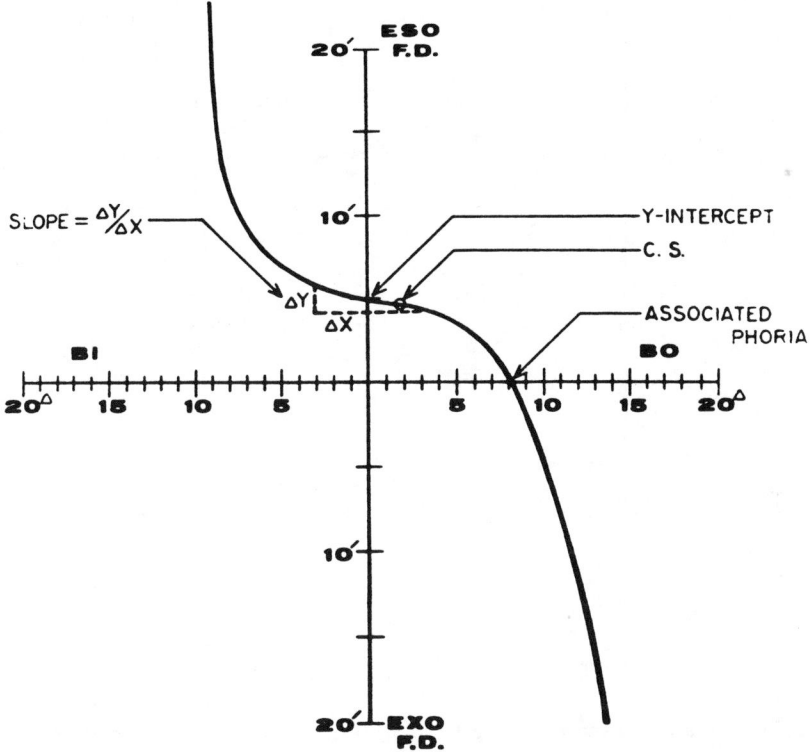

Figure 7.5 Forced vergence fixation disparity curve indicates the magnitude of fixation disparity induced by base-in and base-out vergence demand. The y-intercept of the curve indicates the magnitude of fixation disparity present in the absence of prism-induced vergence demand. The x-intercept indicates the associated phoria. The slope is commonly derived using a best-fit straight line in the range of 3△ base-in to 3△ base-out. The center of symmetry (C.S.) is the flattest portion of the central region of the curve. (From Goss, DA. *Ocular Accommodation, Convergence, and Fixation Disparity,* Fig. 13-4. New York: Professional Press, p. 132, 1986. Reprinted with permission of Butterworth–Heinemann, Boston.)

than for base-out fusional demand. The type II curve occurs in approximately 25% of the population.

The type III curve, commonly associated with exophoria, is one in which adaptation to base-in prism is greater than that to base-out. Consequently, fixation disparity increases to a much greater degree for base-out than for base-in fusion demand. The type III curve occurs in approximately 10% of the population.

The type IV curve is associated with abnormal binocular vision, and is found in 2% to 5% of the population. Type IV patients show very narrow fusional vergence ranges; near the limits of fusional ver-

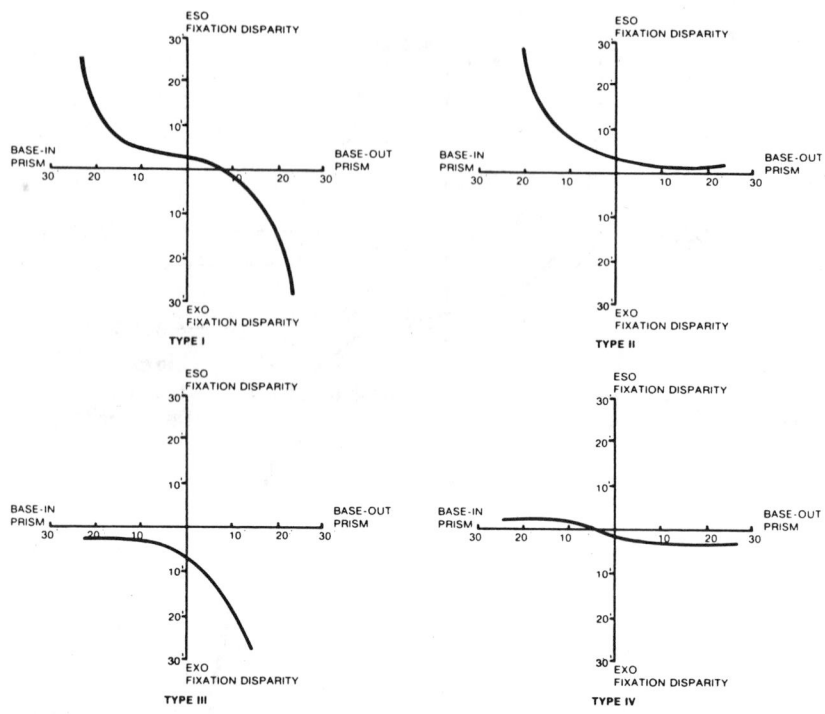

Figure 7.6 Fixation disparity curve types. (From J.E. Sheedy, Actual measurement of fixation disparity and its use in diagnosis and treatment, *J Am Optom Assoc* 51(12): 1079–1084, 1980. Reprinted with permission.)

gence, they do not show increased fixation disparity, but rather break into diplopia.

4. Slope of the curve

A reciprocal relationship exists between fixation disparity and vergence adaptation. When vergence adaptation is good, little fixation disparity is manifest. The presence of fixation disparity implies an inadequate adaptation mechanism.

This relationship is reflected in the slope of the fixation disparity curve. A flat slope indicates an ability to adapt to prism-induced stress without increasing fixation disparity, and thus indicates that vergence adaptation is adequate. A steep slope indicates that fixation disparity increases rapidly with prism-induced vergence, and suggests that prism adaptation is not operating effectively to reduce vergence stress. A slope of greater than 45 degrees is considered relatively steep; a slope less than 45 degrees is considered flat (Sheedy and Saladin 1977).

The slope of the fixation disparity curve varies in the different areas of the curve. "Slope" generally refers to the area of the curve that reflects habitual functioning: that is, the slope of the curve in the area where it intersects the y-axis, indicating zero-induced prism demand; or the area of the curve between the y-axis and x-axis intercepts (between zero-induced prism demand and the associated phoria). The slope may be derived using a best-fitting straight line through points in the range of fusional demand of approximately 3^Δ base-out to 3^Δ base-in (Saladin and Sheedy 1978; Sheedy and Saladin 1983; Goss 1986).

Clinical Utilization of Fixation Disparity Data

Fixation disparity data are fairly effective in discriminating symptomatic from asymptomatic individuals. Asthenopic symptoms are more frequent when the degree of fixation disparity is greater, when the shape of the curve is other than type I, and when the slope is steep (Arner et al. 1956; Sheedy and Saladin 1977, 1978). Duwaer (1983) reports that variability in instantaneous fixation disparity measures, reflecting instability of binocular alignment, correlates more closely with asthenopia than does slope of the fixation disparity curve or magnitude of fixation disparity.

Prism is often prescribed by determining the associated phoria, the prism required to reduce fixation disparity to zero. The associated phoria is graphically represented as the x-axis intercept of the fixation disparity curve, and constitutes the amount of fusional vergence that has not been replaced by prism adaptation (Ogle et al. 1967; Mallett, 1969, 1974; Schor 1983a).

Another method that has been advocated is to prescribe that prism which shifts the flattest area of the fixation disparity curve to the y-intercept. The patient habitually functions on the portion of the curve that intersects the y-axis; since the flattest area of the curve represents the range of vergence demand over which prism adaptation is most effective, it is desirable that this area of the curve intersect the y-axis. The central area of the flattest portion of the curve is known as the center of symmetry. When a steep portion of the fixation disparity curve intersects the y-axis, but the curve shows a flatter portion elsewhere, advocates of this method advise that enough prism be prescribed to shift the flat portion of the curve so that the center of symmetry intersects the y-axis (Sheedy 1980; Sheedy and Saladin 1983).

The fixation disparity curve usually flattens before the x-intercept. Less prism is generally required to shift the flat area to the y-intercept than to neutralize the associated phoria (Sheedy 1980). Therefore, prism prescriptions determined on this basis are usually smaller in degree. In addition, Sheedy indicates that prism prescriptions based on shifting the flat area of the curve are generally more successful.

When the fixation disparity curve has no flat portion, Sheedy and Saladin (1983) recommend the use of vision therapy to flatten the slope. Vergence training serves to increase the rate and amplitude of prism adaptation, and hence to flatten the slope of the fixation disparity curve. Sheedy and Saladin report that vergence training is effective in reducing the slope of type I and (with greater difficulty) type III fixation disparity curves, but that the slope of type II curves typically does not change. In type II curves, characteristic of esophores who demonstrate greater fixation disparity for divergence than for convergence demands, lenses and prisms are the treatment of choice. Plus lenses or bifocals are recommended when there is esophoric fixation disparity at near.

Accommodation/Convergence Interactions

During binocular fused viewing, mutual interactions between accommodative-convergence and convergence-accommodation act to increase the demand on fusional vergence and accommodation (see Chapter 1). As a result, these demands are greater under binocular conditions than would be predicted on the basis of the target distance and dissociated phoria (Schor and Narayan 1982; Schor 1983a, 1983b).

The values of the AC/A and CA/C ratios must be determined before the effect of these mutual interactions can be quantified and used in clinical case analysis. The gradient AC/A ratio is determined clinically by taking the near-phoria measure with and without a +1.00-diopter lens addition. The AC/A ratio, the change in convergence associated with 1 diopter of accommodation, is the difference between these two phoria measures (Morgan 1944b).

The CA/C ratio, the change in accommodation associated with a unit change in convergence, is clinically determined using either dynamic retinoscopy or binocular cross-cylinder methods to monitor accommodation as the stimulus to convergence is changed. Monocular estimate method (MEM) retinoscopy or the binocular fused cross-cylinder test is performed with and without 6^Δ base-in prism before the eyes. The change in accommodation obtained with 6^Δ base-in is the accommodation associated with a 1-m angle of convergence, assuming a 60-mm interpupillary distance and a 16-inch fixation distance, and hence indicates the CA/C (Schor and Narayan 1982).

A low spatial frequency difference of Gaussian (DOG) target does not stimulate significant reflex accommodation, and hence serves as a useful target in determining the CA/C ratio. The patient fixates the DOG target, a 1-m angle vergence change is induced with Risley prisms, and the change in accommodation is determined retinoscopically (Tsuetaki and Schor 1987).

Since the accommodation induced by a 1-m angle of convergence is usually small in degree, the accuracy of these methods may be increased by using 12^Δ base-in prism instead of 6^Δ assuming that 12^Δ base-in is within the patient's capacity to fuse. The change in accommodation that occurs with 12^Δ base-in represents the convergence-accommodation associated with 2-m angles of convergence, and is divided by 2 to give the CA/C ratio.

Once the AC/A and CA/C ratios have been determined, the mutual interactions between vergence and accommodation can be quantified. The following equations are used to compute the demands on fusional convergence and accommodation under binocular conditions (Schor and Narayan 1982):

$$\text{Cd (fusional convergence demand)} = \frac{\text{phoria at near}}{1 - (AC/A \times CA/C),}$$

$$\text{Ad (total accommodative demand)} = (Cd \times CA/C) + 2.50 \text{ D.}$$

For a patient who shows 6^Δ esophoria at near, an AC/A ratio of 4:1, and a CA/C ratio of 0.5/6:

$$Cd = \frac{6}{1 - (4 \times 0.5/6)} = 9^\Delta,$$

$$Ad = (9 \times 0.5/6) + 2.50 \text{ D} = 3.25 \text{ D.}$$

This patient will require 9^Δ of fusional divergence to compensate for the 6^Δ esophoria, and will require 3.25 D of accommodation, 0.75 D greater than the 2.5-D stimulus to accommodation.

These heightened demands are even greater when the AC/A is high. For example, given the same patient, but with an AC/A of 8:1:

$$Cd = \frac{6}{1 - (8 \times 0.5/6)} = 18^\Delta,$$

$$Ad = (18 \times 0.5/6) + 2.50 = 4.0 \text{ D.}$$

Even though the near phoria is 6^Δ esophoria, as a result of AC/CA interaction this patient with an 8:1 AC/A will require 18^Δ of fusional divergence and a total of 4.0 D of accommodation, 1.5 D greater than the accommodative stimulus.

The effect of these mutual interactions can also be determined graphically (Figures 7.7 and 7.8). The AC/A line is drawn through the near reference point, the intersect of the stimuli to accommodation and convergence. The CA/C line is drawn through the associated near phoria. The intersection of the AC/A and CA/C lines indicates the demand on fusional vergence and accommodation under binocular, fused conditions. The amount of fusional vergence required for binocular alignment is indicated by the horizontal vector of the distance from the intersection of the AC/A and CA/C lines to the associated near phoria. The additional accommodation required is indicated by the distance from the intersection of the AC/A and CA/C lines to the stimulus to accommodation line (Schor and Narayan 1982; Schor 1983a, 1983b).

The interactions between vergence and accommodation that increase demand under binocular, fused conditions may be neutralized with prisms or lenses. Either the prism power which corrects the associated near phoria, or the nearpoint lens addition which compensates the convergence accommodation error induced by fusional divergence to correct the associated near phoria, will serve to eliminate subsequent mutual interaction (Schor and Narayan 1982; Schor 1983a, 1983b).

In the examples given above, either a +0.50 add or a 6^Δ base-out prism correction would effectively eliminate AC/CA interactions. The lens and prism corrections required would be identical for the two patients, even though they

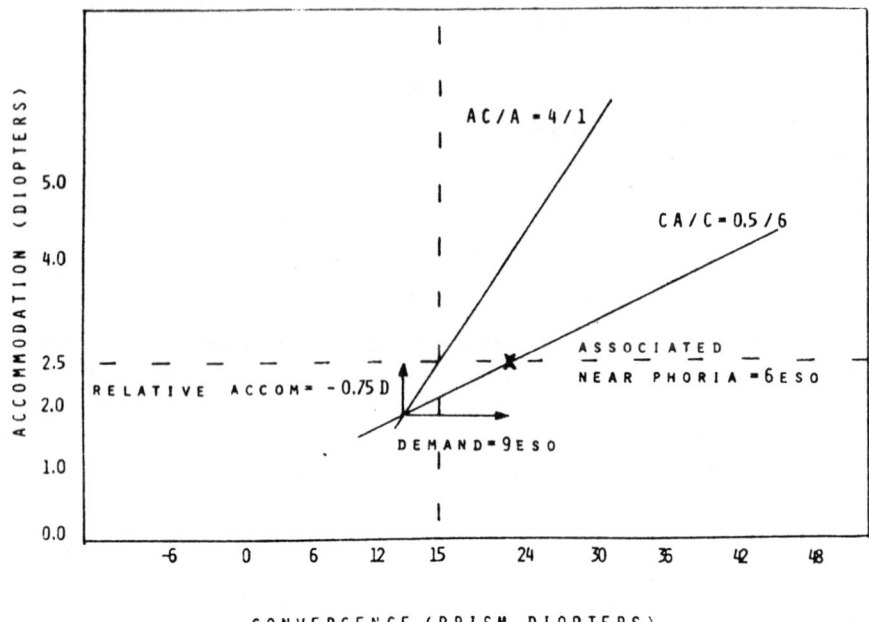

Figure 7.7 The CA/C line is drawn through the associated phoria (X). The AC/A line is drawn through the intercept of the two dotted lines indicating the stimuli to accommodation and convergence presented by a fixation target at 16 inches. For an individual with normal AC/A (4/1) and CA/C (0.5 D/6$^\Delta$) ratios, the intersection of the AC/A and CA/C lines indicates that 0.75 diopters of relative accommodation (in addition to the 2.5 diopters required for the 16-inch fixation distance) and 9$^\Delta$ of fusional divergence will be required to correct a phoria of 6$^\Delta$ associated esophoria. (From C.M. Schor, Analysis of tonic and accommodative vergence disorders of binocular vision, *Am J Optom Physiol Opt* 60(1):1–14, © The Am Acad of Optom 1983. Reprinted with permission.)

have markedly different AC/A ratios. For each patient, a 6$^\Delta$ base-out prism eliminates the need for fusional vergence to correct the associated phoria, and hence terminates the mutual interaction. Similarly, a +0.50-diopter nearpoint lens addition compensates the convergence accommodation error induced by the 6$^\Delta$ of fusional divergence required to correct the associated phoria, so that reflex accommodation is unnecessary and further mutual interaction is eliminated. Since the CA/C ratio is typically low, the power of the plus lens addition required to neutralize accommodation/convergence interaction is usually low, regardless of whether the AC/A ratio is high or low (Schor and Narayan 1982; Schor 1983a).

Proximal Vergence and Associated Measures

Wick (1985) reports that proximal vergence is an important part of the near-vergence response. Under binocular, fused conditions, proximal convergence is significantly greater than estimated on the basis of dissociated measures,

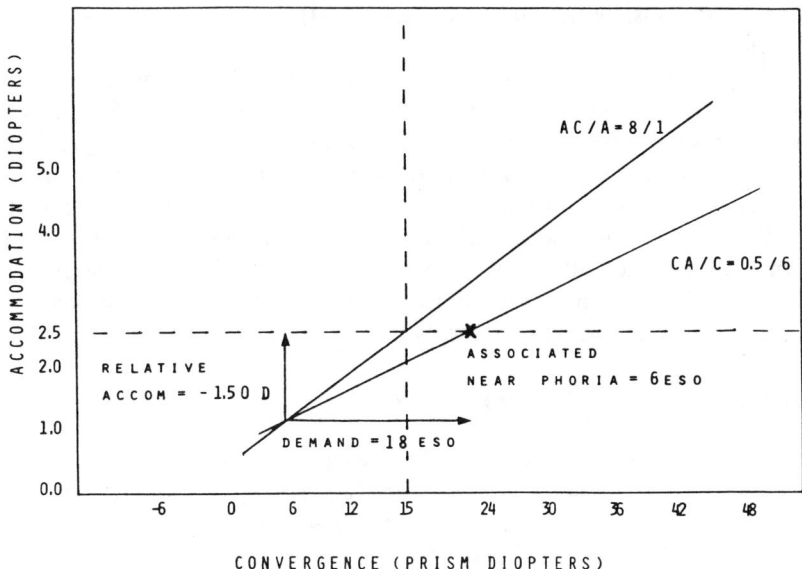

Figure 7.8 When the AC/A ratio is high, the demands on accommodation and convergence each become very large. In this figure, the associated phoria and CA/C values are the same as those depicted in Figure 7.7; the only change is that the AC/A is high (8/1). The intersection of the AC/A and CA/C lines indicates increased demand on both accommodation (1.5 D) and fusional divergence (18ᐃ) required to correct the 6ᐃ associated phoria when the AC/A is high. The demands on accommodation and convergence each increase as the AC/A increases and the slopes of the AC/A and CA/C become parallel. (From C.M. Schor, Analysis of tonic and accommodative vergence disorders of binocular vision, *Am J Optom Physiol Opt* 60(1):1–14, © The Am Acad of Optom 1983. Reprinted with permission.)

contributing much more to the total near-vergence response than does accommodative vergence.

Proximal vergence may be calculated from the following formula:

$$PV = (p.d. \times 2.5) - h + H,$$

where p.d. is the interpupillary distance, h is the near phoria through +2.5-diopter lenses, H is the distance phoria, and esophoria is minus and exophoria is plus. Dissociated proximal vergence is determined using dissociated phoria values in the calculation, and the associated proximal vergence is determined using associated phoria measures (Wick 1985).

The associated AC/A ratio is determined by graphically representing the changes in fixation disparity induced by various lens and prism powers, and then determining the prism and lens values that induce equal amounts of fixation disparity. This method is held to give the vergence change associated, under binocular conditions, with a unit of accommodation, and hence the associated AC/A (Ogle et al. 1967).

Wick and London (1987) urge that forced vergence fixation disparity curves, fixation disparity, associated phoria, fixation disparity–derived AC/A, proximal vergence, and CA/C responses be used in graphical analysis in preference to traditional dissociated measures, so that the graph portrays the relation between findings obtained under binocular conditions. A criterion for comfort analogous to Sheard's criterion, but based on fusional demand under binocular conditions as determined by calculations of accommodation/convergence interaction, was slightly more effective in differentiating symptomatic from asymptomatic patients than was the traditional Sheard's criterion (Daum et al. 1989).

PRESCRIBING VERTICAL PRISM

Traditionally, practitioners have been extremely cautious about prescribing vertical prism. Many clinicians have carefully prescribed prism only to have the patient experience discomfort and reject the new glasses. In other cases, patients not only accept the glasses, but actually "eat up" the prism, showing an increase in vertical phoria. Many clinicians, concerned that patients will reject prism glasses or increase their vertical phorias as a result of wearing them, prescribe vertical prism only when absolutely necessary to resolve diplopia or asthenopia.

In contrast with traditional models that attribute hyperphoria to innervational anomalies and to oculomotor paresis, Harmon (1958) suggests that hyperphoria may arise functionally when abnormal head posture is induced by adverse environmental conditions. Hyperphoria that arises to improve visual efficiency during sustained near-vision tasks performed in adverse posture may become habituated and create difficulty when the patient assumes other postures. Patients often compensate by developing small head tilts during everyday visual conditions.

Many patients with small vertical phorias compensate by adopting a slight head tilt. This compensatory head posture typically becomes habituated, so that the patient is not even aware of it. It is generally an effective adaptation, since such patients are typically asymptomatic and often demonstrate good binocular function.

Patients who compensate for small vertical phorias with a slight head tilt generally measure significantly less vertical when tested in free space than is found in the refractor. Behind the refractor, the head is straightened to align with the instrument and the full vertical phoria is measured. In free space, the patient assumes the compensatory head posture, and the vertical phoria measure is reduced, often to zero. Prism prescribed on the basis of the refractor measure is thus frequently greater than the vertical phoria that exists during habitual free space conditions. Such a prism prescription will typically induce symptoms where none existed before, and is frequently rejected.

Patients who are well compensated with slight head tilt are usually asymptomatic and seldom require vertical prism prescription. When vertical prism is indicated to relieve discomfort or diplopia, prescription should never be based solely on the refractor findings. To reduce the likelihood of rejection, the practitioner should first verify the existence and amount of vertical phoria in free space. Generally, the prism prescribed should not exceed that measured in free space.

The vertical phoria in free space can be determined with a trial frame using a Maddox rod with trial case prisms or prism bar; by performing an alternate cover test while using vertical prisms to create horizontal alignment of the images; or with a hand-held Maddox rod/Risley prism combination. The latter method is the least cumbersome.

Measures in free space should be obtained in straight-ahead gaze at far point and on downward gaze at near point, as well as in any other directions of gaze that are significant for the particular patient. In some cases, as a result of noncomitancy or prismatic effect of anisometropic spectacles, anisophoria may require differing vertical prism corrections in different fields of gaze.

Borish (1970) uses a subjective method to determine the acceptance of vertical prism. In the presence of vertical imbalance, binocular visual acuity may be slightly compromised as imperfect fusion causes a slight blur. Borish recommends that while binocularly viewing a row of letters of best visual acuity, the patient's reaction be obtained with the prism placed with its base in the correct orientation, as well as in other orientations. If the patient reports an improvement in acuity or a feeling of greater comfort only with the prism in the indicated direction, a placebo effect is ruled out and Borish considers that prism should be prescribed.

In contrast with patients who reject vertical prism, some patients with hyperphoria "eat up" vertical prism and demonstrate an increase in vertical phoria following use of vertical prism. It has been assumed in such cases that a latent hyperphoria exists, and that the brief suspension of fusion during the phoria test is not sufficient to reveal the true imbalance. Marlow (1932) and Roy (1956) advocate the use of prolonged occlusion to identify the full extent of the phoria.

Borish (1970) suggests that the full vertical phoria may not be manifest until several prism prescriptions have been worn over a period of years. The fact that vertical prism may have to be increased from one examination to another, he suggests, does not indicate an increase in the true deviation, but rather that the full extent of the deviation, previously concealed, is becoming manifest.

In contrast with this notion of a latent hyperphoria that becomes manifest when prism is prescribed, the increase in phoria that often follows prism application has more recently been attributed to prism adaptation. After prismatic neutralization of a vertical (or lateral) phoria, many patients adapt to restore the phoria (and fixation disparity) to the value that existed previously (Schubert 1943; Ogle and Prangen 1953; Carter 1965; Schor 1983a).

Carter (1965) indicates that in patients with normal binocular vision and adequate sensory fusion, prism adaptation is normal. Such patients are typically asymptomatic. Prism prescription should generally be avoided for hyperphores with good prism adaptation, since adaptation to restore the original vertical phoria is likely. Patients lacking adequate fusion are likely to demonstrate poor prism adaptation and to be asthenopic. Such patients are more likely to benefit from prism application, since they are unlikely to adapt to the prism.

The slope of the vertical fixation disparity curve provides an indication of the capacity for prism adaptation. Rutstein and Eskridge (1985) report that patients with reduced ability to adapt to vertical prism demonstrate steeper slopes of the vertical fixation disparity curve than do those with good adaptation. Such patients have greater difficulty compensating for vertical heterophoria and often experience visual discomfort. They are more likely to require vertical prism correction, and less likely to show increases in required prism due to adaptation.

That many individuals respond to prism by adapting to restore previously existing heterophoria (Ogle and Prangen 1953; Carter 1965) implies that such heterophoria has value to the individual, and is consistent with Harmon's notion of hyperphoria as a purposeful adaptation. If hyperphoria facilitates performance in the presence of head tilt or other postural distortion induced by adverse working conditions, it may be expected that if neutralizing prism is prescribed, patients with normal binocular vision and adequate prism adaptation will adapt to restore the original, purposive hyperphoria. Such patients are typically asymptomatic.

Thus, it is generally the asymptomatic hyperphore who either rejects or "eats up" vertical prism, since prism prescription interferes with the compensation or adaptation he has made. Rejection of vertical prism and prism-induced increase in vertical phoria can usually be avoided by prescribing vertical prism only when indicated to relieve diplopia or discomfort. Hyperphoria in symptomatic patients is less likely to be adaptive in origin, and prism prescription is likely to be well accepted.

Various methods are used to determine the amount of vertical prism to be prescribed. Giles (1960) advises prescribing two thirds of the measured phoria for distance and three quarters for near vision. Morgan (1960) and Posner (1951) suggest fully correcting the vertical deviation. Marlow (1932) and Roy (1956) not only fully correct the phoria, but use prolonged occlusion to elicit the full deviation.

Some practitioners feel that minor deviations can be ignored, while others believe that vertical imbalances as small as $\frac{1}{4}^\Delta$ are significant and should be compensated with vertical prism (Borish 1970). When the imbalance indicated by the phoria disagrees with that indicated by the vertical vergence measures, Borish (1970) advocates that the amount of prism prescribed should be that which equalizes the vertical vergences:

$$\frac{\text{(base-down to break)} - \text{(base-up to break)}}{2} = \text{correcting prism.}$$

Current authorities generally advise vertical prism prescription based on fixation disparity measures. The most common recommendation is to correct the associated phoria by prescribing that vertical prism which reduces vertical fixation disparity to zero (Grosvenor 1975; Sheedy 1979; Schor 1983a; Eskridge and Rutstein 1986; Goss 1986).

Rutstein and Eskridge (1983) describe vertical fixation disparity curves as straight lines, indicating a linear relationship between vertical vergence demand and vertical fixation disparity. Petito (1986) demonstrates that vertical fixation disparity curves may have a sigmoid shape with a flattened zone indicating a zone of prism adaptation; the sigmoid shape and flattened zone become evident only when very small prism increments (0.5^Δ) are used to generate the curves. Petito suggests that for patients with vertical imbalance who demonstrate sigmoid fixation disparity curves, the center of symmetry (center of the flattened zone of prism adaptation) may indicate a prism value more acceptable than that indicated by the associated phoria, if the two differ.

SUMMARY

Traditional methods of case analysis use various criteria to determine the need for prisms, added lens power, or vision therapy to relieve asthenopia induced by high heterophoria, inadequate fusional vergence reserves, and accommodative dysfunction. Graphical analysis is used to facilitate assessment. The current trend is to analyze binocular vision through the use of findings obtained under fused rather than dissociated conditions, including the assessment of forced vergence fixation disparity curves, vergence adaptation, and mutual interactions between vergence and accommodation during binocular viewing.

SUGGESTED READING

Borish IM (1970). *Clinical Refraction*. 3rd ed. Chicago: Professional Press.

Goss DA (1986). *Ocular Accommodation, Convergence and Fixation Disparity: A Manual of Clinical Analysis*. New York: Professional Press.

Schor CM, Ciuffreda KJ (eds) (1983). *Vergence Eye Movements: Basic and Clinical Aspects*. Boston: Butterworth–Heinemann.

REFERENCES

Arner RS, Berger SI, Braverman G, et al. (1956). The clinical significance of the effect of vergence on fixation disparity—A preliminary investigation. *Am J Optom* 33:399–409.

Borish IM (1970). *Clinical Refraction*. 3rd ed. Chicago: Professional Press.

Borish IM (1978). The Borish nearpoint chart. *J Am Optom Assoc* 49(1):41–44.

Carter DB (1965). Fixation disparity and heterophoria following prolonged wearing of prisms. *Am J Optom Arch Am Acad Optom* 42:141–152.

Dalziel CC (1981). Effect of vision training on patients who fail Sheard's criterion. *Am J Optom Physiol Opt* 58:21–23.

Daum KM, Rutstein RP, Houston G, et al. (1989). Evaluation of a new criterion of binocularity. *Optom Vis Sci* 66(4):218–228.

Donders FC (1864). *On the Anomalies of Accommodation and Refraction of the Eye*. Translation by W.D. Moore. London: New Sydenham Society.

Dowley D (1989). Fixation disparity. *Optom Vis Sci* 66(2):98–105.

Duane A (1897). *A New Classification of the Motor Abnormalities of the Eye Based upon Physiological Principles, Together with Their Symptoms, Diagnosis and Treatment*. New York: JH Vail.

Duwaer AL (1983). New measures of fixation disparity in the diagnosis of binocular oculomotor deficiencies. *Am J Optom Physiol Opt* 60(7):586–596.

Eskridge JB, Rutstein RP (1986). Clinical evaluation of vertical fixation disparity. Part IV. Slope and adaptation to vertical prism of vertical heterophoria patients. *Am J Optom Physiol Opt* 63(8):662–667.

Giles GH (1960). *The Principles and Practice of Refraction*. Philadelphia: Chilton.

Goss DA (1986). *Ocular Accommodation, Convergence and Fixation Disparity: A Manual of Clinical Analysis*. New York: Professional Press.

Grisham D (1983). Treatment of binocular dysfunctions. In: Schor CM, Ciuffreda KJ (eds), *Vergence Eye Movements: Basic and Clinical Aspects*. Boston: Butterworth–Heinemann, pp. 605–646.

Grolman B (1971). Binocular refraction-fixation disparity. *Optician* 162(4195):16–19.

Grosvenor T (1975). Clinical use of fixation disparity. *Optom Weekly* 66:1224–1228.

Haase HJ (1980). Binoculare korrektion. Die methodik und theorie von HJ Haase. Dusseldorf: Willy Schrinkel.

Harmon DB (1958). *Notes on a Dynamic Theory of Vision*. 3rd rev. ed. Austin, TX: Author.

Hofstetter HW (1971). Objects in optometric education. *J Am Optom Assoc* 42(6):544–549.

Hofstetter HW (1983). Graphical analysis. In: Schor CM, Ciuffreda KJ (eds), *Vergence Eye Movements: Basic and Clinical Aspects*. Boston: Butterworth–Heinemann, pp. 439–464.

Landolt E (1886). *The Refraction and Accommodation of the Eye and Their Anomalies*. Translation by Culver CM. Philadelphia: JB Lippincott (cited in Borish, 1970, p. 877.)

Lie I, Opheim A (1985). Long-term acceptance of prisms by heterophorics. *J Am Optom Assoc* 56:272–278.

Lie I, Opheim A (1990). Long-term stability of prism correction of heterophorics and heterotropics: A 5 year follow-up. *J Am Optom Assoc* 61(6):491–498.

Mallett RFJ (1964). The investigation of heterophoria at near and a new fixation disparity technique. *Optician* 148:547–551.

Mallett RFJ (1966). A fixation disparity test for distance use. *Optician* 152(3927):1–8.

Mallett RFJ (1969). Fixation disparity in clinical practice. *Aust J Optom* 52:97–109.

Mallett RFJ (1974). Fixation disparity — Its genesis in relation to asthenopia. *Ophthalmic Optician* 14:1159–1168.

Marlow FW (1932). The technique of the prolonged occlusion test. *Am J Ophthalmol* 32:320–323.

McCormack GL (1985). Vergence adaptation maintains heterophoria in normal binocular vision. *Am J Optom Physiol Opt* 62:555–561.

Morgan MW (1944a). Analysis of clinical data. *Am J Optom Arch Am Acad Optom* 21(12):477–491.

Morgan MW (1944b). The clinical aspects of accommodation and convergence. *Am J Optom Arch Am Acad Optom* 21(8):301–313.

Morgan MW (1960). Anomalies of the visual neuromuscular system of the aging patient and their correction. In: Hirsch MJ, Wick RE (eds), *Vision of the Aging Patient*. Philadelphia: Chilton, pp. 113–145.

Ogle KN, Martens TG, Dyer JA (1967). *Oculomotor Imbalance in Binocular Vision and Fixation Disparity*. Philadelphia: Lea & Febiger.

Ogle KN, Prangen A (1953). Observations of vertical divergences and hyperphorias. *Arch Ophthalmol* 49:313–334.

Percival AS (1928). *The Prescribing of Spectacles*. Bristol, England: Wright.

Petito GT (1986). Nonlinear forced vertical vergence fixation disparity curves and their clinical significance. *Am J Optom Physiol Opt* 63(11):908–914.

Posner A (1951). The prescribing of prisms for hyperphoria. *Am J Ophthalmol* 34(2):197–199.

Roy RR (1956). Headaches and binocular stress. *Optom Weekly* 47(41):1815–1818; 47(42):1871–1874.

Rutstein RP, Eskridge JB (1983). Clinical evaluation of vertical fixation disparity. Part I. *Am J Optom Physiol Opt* 60:688–693.

Rutstein RP, Eskridge JB (1985). Clinical evaluation of vertical fixation disparity. Part II. Adaptation to vertical prism. *Am J Optom Physiol Opt* 62:585–590.

Saladin JJ, Sheedy JE (1978). A population study of relationships between fixation disparity, heterophorias and vergences. *Am J Optom Physiol Opt* 55(11):744–750.

Schor CM (1980). Fixation disparity: A steady state error of disparity-induced vergence. *Am J Optom Physiol Opt* 57:618–631.

Schor CM (1983a). Fixation disparity and vergence adaptation. In: Schor CM, Ciuffreda KJ (eds), *Vergence Eye Movements: Basic and Clinical Aspects*. Boston: Butterworth–Heinemann, pp. 464–516.

Schor CM (1983b). Analysis of tonic and accommodative vergence disorders of binocular vision. *Am J Optom Physiol Opt* 60(1):1–14.

Schor CM, Narayan V (1982). Graphical analysis of prism adaptation, convergence accommodation and accommodative convergence. *Am J Optom Physiol Opt* 59:774–784.

Schubert G (1943). Grundlagen der beidaugigen motorishen koordinaation. *Pflugers Arch Ges Physiol* 247:279–291.

Sheard C (1928). Zones of ocular comfort. *Trans Am Acad Optom* 3:113–129.

Sheard C (1930). Zones of ocular comfort. *Am J Optom* 7(1):9–25.

Sheedy JE (1979). *Fixation Disparity Curves*. Columbus, OH: Vision Analysis.

Sheedy JE (1980). Actual measurement of fixation disparity and its use in diagnosis and treatment. *J Am Optom Assoc* 51(12):1079–1084.

Sheedy JE, Saladin JJ (1977). Phoria, vergence and fixation disparity in oculomotor problems. *Am J Optom Physiol Opt* 54(7):474–478.

Sheedy JE, Saladin JJ (1978). Association of symptoms with measures of oculomotor deficiencies. *Am J Optom Physiol Opt* 55(10):670–676.

Sheedy JE, Saladin JJ (1983). Validity of diagnostic criteria and case analysis in binocular vision disorders. In: Schor CM, Ciuffreda KJ (eds), *Vergence Eye Movements: Basic and Clinical Aspects*. Boston: Butterworth–Heinemann, pp. 517–540.

Tait EF (1951). Accommodative convergence. *Am J Ophthalmol* 34:1093–1107.

Tsuetaki TK, Schor CM (1987). Clinical method for measuring adaptation of tonic accommodation and vergence accommodation. *Amer J Optom Physiol Opt* 64(6):437–449.

Wesson MD, Koenig R (1983). A new clinical method for direct measurement of fixation disparity. *South J Optom* 1(10):48–52.

White JW (1941). The screen test and its modifications. *Am J Ophthalmol* 24:156–160.

Wick B (1985). Clinical factors in proximal vergence. *Am J Optom Physiol Opt* 62(1):1–18.

Wick B, London R (1987). Analysis of binocular visual function using tests made under binocular conditions. *Am J Optom Physiol Opt* 64(4):227–240.

Worrell BE, Hirsch MJ, Morgan MW (1971). An evaluation of prism prescribed by Sheard's criterion. *Am J Optom Arch Am Acad Optom* 48:373–376.

Yaeger MD, Boltz RL (1986). Computerized fixation disparity measurement. *Am J Optom Physiol Opt* 63(8):654–661.

8

Optometric Extension Program Analysis

OEP analysis is based on the Skeffington model of nearpoint stress (Skeffington 1928–74; Birnbaum 1985a). Phoria, vergence, accommodative, and refractive measures are viewed as adaptive end-products of a nearpoint stress–induced drive for convergence to localize closer than accommodation.

Phoria and fusional vergence measures are not viewed as fusional demands and reserves, and are not compared with one another. Rather, the patient's findings are compared with expected findings to determine whether they are high or low. High and low findings are grouped into patterns, or *case types*. Guidelines for therapeusis are based on the case type and the degree to which the pattern is ingrained, or embedded (Skeffington 1928–74; Manas 1965; Emery 1968–70; Lesser 1969; Hendrickson 1989).

The OEP system of case analysis differs significantly from other models in its assumptions regarding the etiology of vision disorders and the effect of time on their course and development; its interpretation of the significance of phoria and vergence measures; and its approach toward nearpoint lens application, vision training, management of asymptomatic patients, and prevention of vision disorders (Margach 1976). These differences are summarized as follows:

1. Etiology of vision disorders

   Traditional models generally attribute vision disorder to random biologic variation and genetic influence. The OEP model recognizes that genetic tendencies influence visual development, but considers environmental interaction as the major etiologic factor. Vision disorders are viewed as developmental or stress-induced (Kraskin 1968, 1981). Developmental vision disorders arise from interference with development and consequent failure to develop adequate visual abilities. Stress-induced vision disorders arise from breakdown of previously established skills due to stress on the visual system, especially that imposed by the near-work demands of our culture. The major role attributed to environmental influence leads

121

to therapeutic efforts to control these factors in order to prevent and remediate vision disorder.

2. Stability of phoria and prism vergence measures

In traditional graphical analysis, phoria and prism vergence measures are viewed as relatively static and stable. Variations are attributed to accommodative fluctuation and to response error (Hirsch and Bing 1948; Morgan 1955). OEP analysis views these findings dynamically. Changes in phoria and prism vergence measures are expected, and are held to result from nearpoint stress and subsequent adaptation (Birnbaum 1985a, 1985b).

3. Time factors in the development of vision disorders

The influence of time is not a consideration in traditional graphical systems. In contrast, the OEP model predicts ongoing change as a visual problem persists through time. Assessment of temporal factors and their implications for therapeusis is a key element of OEP analysis (Skeffington et al. 1945–51; Manas 1965).

Temporal factors considered in the OEP model include adaptation, deterioration, and embedding. Adaptive changes in refractive and phorometric findings occur in response to the nearpoint stress—induced drive for convergence to localize closer than accommodation. As adaptation proceeds through time, and the individual seeks to maintain equilibrium and function despite the effector system mismatch, the pattern of relationship among the various analytical findings changes in characteristic patterns referred to as *stages of deterioration*. *Embedding* occurs when stress is prolonged and the organism seeks to rebuild skills to a level that permits satisfactory function. The analytical findings rebound from the lower measures found immediately following the impact of nearpoint stress, but remain below expected levels. This process of reorganization thus permits continued function, although there is an increase in rigidity and loss of flexibility .

4. Significance of emmetropia and orthophoria

While traditional approaches view emmetropia and orthophoria as ideal, OEP theory holds that low degrees of hyperopia and exophoria are desirable and necessary to buffer accommodation and convergence against changes in innervation to the autonomic and central nervous systems, respectively. OEP analysis views emmetropia and orthophoria as signs of developing problems, rather than as optimal or perfect conditions.

5. Significance of low nearpoint phoria

In traditional graphical analysis, low heterophoria is generally ignored, since it does not impose significant fusional demand. In contrast, OEP analysis views nearpoint heterophoria less than the expected 6^Δ exophoria as a sign of nearpoint stress. Individuals with esophoria, orthophoria, or exophoria less than 6^Δ at near are assumed to lack an adequate exophoric buffer, and are considered likely to demonstrate overconvergence during intense, sustained nearpoint demands. Such individuals are thus held to be at greater risk for the development of nearpoint stress–induced vision disorders.

6. Relationship between phoria and prism vergence measures

Traditional graphical systems assess the relationship between fusional demand (phoria) and reserve (compensating prism vergence) to determine whether the fusional reserve is adequate to permit comfortable, single binocular vision. This reserve-demand concept does not exist in OEP analysis. A phoria is not compared with the "opposing" prism vergence. The near phoria is viewed as a product of nearpoint stress–induced overconvergence (which tends to produce esophoria at near) and subsequent adaptation to restore an exophoric buffer. Exophoria is seen not as a fusional demand, but as an adaptive response to buffer overconvergence.

OEP analysis does not regard prism vergence findings as measures of the ability to overcome a phoria, but as indicators of the quality of binocular vision. Nearpoint stress–induced effector system mismatch interferes with binocular efficiency, resulting in a reduction of prism vergence measures below the expected level.

Prism vergence measures have three components: blur, break, and recovery. *Blur* is a function of the flexibility between vergence and accommodation. Prism vergence tests create a progressive demand to shift ocular alignment closer or farther than the plane of accommodation. When little flexibility exists, the addition of even low prism causes a simultaneous accommodative shift with resultant blur. Low blur findings thus indicate an inadequate flexibility bond between accommodation and convergence.

Break is an indicator of the quality of binocular function, rather than of muscle strength, since extraocular muscle strength is far greater than the highest prism vergence measures. Break measures will be adequate or high when fusion ability is good. Low breaks occur when effector system mismatch interferes with efficient binocular function, with consequent impairment of ability to maintain fusion as demand is progressively increased during prism vergence tests.

Recovery is a more subtle indicator of the quality of binocular function. Fusional recovery requires a jump vergence movement to restore fusion, and hence demands a high level of binocular integration. Even mild interference with binocular function will produce a low recovery finding.

Reduced prism vergence findings are thus among the earliest signs of interference with binocular function. Constricted blur, break, or recovery findings indicate the presence of nearpoint stress–induced vision disorder.

7. Relationship between distance and nearpoint findings

Traditional graphical analysis regards distance phoria and prism vergence findings as measures of oculomotor balance at distance; findings taken at near are related to nearpoint visual function (Borish 1970). Criteria for comfort at distance and near are analyzed independently, and therapeutic measures are applied at the distance indicated. Thus, in some cases, the mandate of graphical analysis might be for prism application or lens modification for distance only.

In contrast, OEP analysis views vision disorders as beginning at near point and spreading to distance. Impaired distance findings are held to reflect a breakdown in binocular function as a result of nearpoint stress. Management is likely to involve vision training and nearpoint lens prescription, rather than prism application at distance (Skeffington 1945–51).

Birnbaum (1985a) suggests that near and distance phoria measures relate to the processes of stress activation and recovery from stress, respectively. Near phoria is viewed as a product of stress activation and adaptation in response to nearpoint stress. Distance vision involves recovery from stress. The distance phoria is held to reflect the habituated level of equilibrium that is reached following repeated cycles of stress exposure and recovery as the individual shifts fixation from near to distance in everyday life.

8. Behavioral influences on phoria and vergence measures

While traditional models view phoria and vergence findings strictly in terms of muscular imbalance and fusional reserve, theorists associated with OEP believe that behavioral factors related to spatial organization and cognitive-perceptual style play a role.

a. Effect of poor spatial judgement

Difficulty making spatial judgements is often reflected in inaccurate and unreliable responses to phoria, vergence, and cross-cylinder tests, and even to subjective refraction. Individuals who give poor responses on such tests often demonstrate difficulty in academic performance and in everyday tasks that require the ability to localize accurately in space.

b. Phorias and spatial localization

Skeffington (1953) and Getman (1970–71) relate phorias to spatial localization, suggesting that esophores tend to localize objects as closer and exophores as farther than their actual location. As a patient shifts fixation from far to near and back, according to Getman, inaccurate spatial localization manifests as undershooting and overshooting, which requires corrective adjustment to secure accurate fixation; these corrective adjustments correlate with the phoria measures at distance and near.

Phorias may reflect areas of spatial preference. Individuals more involved with and interested in near space may be more likely to exhibit esophoria, and those more interested in distance space are more likely to demonstrate exophoria. Skeffington (1972) believes that esophores and exophores differ in the way in which they organize space, esophores tending to relate specific areas in space to themselves, while exophores are more likely to relate specific areas in space to total space.

c. Phorias and cognitive-perceptual style

Several authors have proposed relationships between phoria direction and cognitive-perceptual style. Forrest (1976) suggests that esophoric and exophoric deviations result from an inability to integrate central and peripheral information. The high exophore copes by alternating attention between center and periphery according to the demands of the situation, preferring to derive as much information as possible from broad areas of space. The high exophore may even develop a tropia to facilitate peripheral information processing. The esophoric deviator, in contrast, is highly central. Deviating one eye inward serves to reduce the binocular field of vision, and hence aids in constricting peripheral awareness and emphasizing figure.

Birnbaum (1978a) relates phoria direction and visual information-processing style to cerebral hemispheric organization. He suggests that if, as hypothesized by Forrest (1976), esophores and esotropes tend to be highly central, attending primarily to detail and building a space world through sequential analysis, this may relate to a general overemphasis on left hemisphere function and analytical processing; similarly, if exodeviation relates to a more peripheral approach to visual-spatial processing, this may reflect the more diffuse, global, simultaneous style of the right hemisphere. In support of this notion, Birnbaum (1981) found that, among 7- to 10-year-old strabismic boys, esotropes perform better than exotropes on analytical tasks.

d. Behavioral aspects of fusional vergence measures

Vergence findings also may be viewed in relation to organismic behavior. The reach-grasp-release sequence involves processes basic to the acquisition of visual information. *Reach* involves selecting stimuli for attention; *grasp* involves sustained attention on the selected stimulus; and *release* involves the shift of attention to a newly selected stimulus (Getman and Kephart 1957).

Adequacy of reach, grasp, and release may be reflected in the prism vergence measures. Viewed in this context, the blur, break, and recovery findings are functions of the grasp, release, and reach processes, respectively. Fusional recovery thus reflects not only the quality of binocular function, but also the ability to visually select and seek new information (reach). The blur findings indicate the ability to sustain visual attention (grasp). The break findings reflect the ability to "let go" in order to move on to a new stimulus (release). Low break findings indicate a tendency to release too quickly; high breaks indicate a tendency to overhold (Smith 1973).

Vergence findings may also reflect the degree to which individuals are more global or more detail-oriented. Independent of actual differences in quality of binocular function, detail-oriented individuals may notice change sooner and hence report lower blurs and breaks than global individuals. A consistent absence of blur findings is characteristic of the global individual who fails to notice and discriminate fine differences. High blur and break findings do not always indicate excellent binocular function, but may also be present in the global individual who does not notice and attend to detail, or the very passive individual who is slow to respond.

9. Primacy of distance or nearpoint lens correction

In traditional graphical systems, the lens correction that neutralizes the refractive error is primary. Modification of this lens formula, or prescription of lenses specific for near use, is considered in pre-presbyopes only if ocular discomfort exists or is anticipated. In contrast, OEP analysis emphasizes determination and prescription of the optimal nearpoint lens correction, since functional vision disorders are thought to result from nearpoint stress.

10. Attitude toward nearpoint lens application and vision training

Although Sheard's criterion and graphical analysis systems provide guidelines for the application of lenses, prisms, and vision training to relieve discomfort, many traditional practitioners infrequently apply such guidelines. Traditional practitioners often ignore "minor" symptoms, attributing them to tension or to overwork. They infrequently prescribe low-plus nearpoint lenses, and tend to avoid prism prescriptions. Patients are typically referred for vision therapy only when symptoms are severe and referral cannot be avoided. Vision training is viewed as a last resort, to be advised only when all other means are exhausted.

In the OEP model, nearpoint lens prescription is viewed as desirable to reduce nearpoint stress—induced effector system mismatch. Case analysis is performed to determine whether such lenses will be accepted. When analytical findings indicate plus lens prescription, such lenses are advised even when symptoms are minimal or absent; the goal is to improve performance and to prevent vision disorder, as well as to relieve discomfort. Vision therapy is viewed not as a last resort, but as a commonly used treatment tool to improve visual function to a degree not possible with lenses alone.

When vision therapy is undertaken, treatment regimens designed by functional practitioners are likely to be broader in scope, more extensive, and lengthier than treatment programs prescribed by their traditional colleagues. Treatment programs based on graphical analysis are generally limited to vergence range extension to compensate high heterophoria, and are often home-based or limited to few office visits. Functional vision therapy regimens frequently encompass visual-perceptual-motor development and visual information-processing ability as well as remediation of deficient eye movement, accommodative, and binocular skills. Such treatment programs tend to be lengthier and to include both office-based and home therapy.

11. Use of prism correction

Graphical analysis, Percival's and Sheard's criteria, and analysis of fixation disparity data frequently give rise to recommendations for prism prescription. However, as a practical matter, even proponents of traditional systems often tend to avoid prism prescription, primarily out of concern that the patient will "soak up the prism" and demonstrate progressive increase in heterophoria. This can be avoided, according to Goss (1986), by having the patient read for a few minutes with the proposed prism correction. A significant change in phoria indicates the presence of prism adaptation and contraindicates prism prescription. Nevertheless, many practitioners, concerned about efficacy and stability, view prism prescription warily.

Prism prescription is never an outcome of OEP analysis, since prism is not among the therapeutic options. OEP practitioners generally avoid prism prescription not only from fear of prism adaptation, but also because high heterophoria is seen as a product of nearpoint stress, rather than as a primary problem. In this view, to prescribe prism is to treat the symptom, rather than the cause of the problem. Prism prescription does little to develop more adequate visual abilities. Most functional practitioners prefer vision therapy to prism prescription, since therapy offers greater potential to improve visual function.

12. Asymptomatic patients

In traditional graphical analysis, the presence of asthenopia, diplopia, or blur not corrected by refraction is a prime requisite for therapeutic intervention. Graphical analysis systems developed in relation to zones of comfort and relief from asthenopia. Case analysis is seldom applied, nor is treatment offered, unless ocular discomfort is present or expected.

The Skeffington model holds that nearpoint stress may lead to avoidance of close work. Patients who restrict near work may report little asthenopia, yet require treatment to eliminate vision disorders that interfere with near-work enjoyment and lead to avoidance.

Asthenopia is also frequently absent in patients who make a

myopic adaptation to nearpoint vision disorder. OEP practitioners are likely to initiate care in such cases, to relieve nearpoint stress and attempt to prevent further adaptation. The OEP model therefore dictates that the practitioner perform a complete visual analysis even in the absence of asthenopic symptoms, and consider treatment of existing vision disorder when indicated to eliminate potential causes of avoidance and to prevent the development of adaptive vision disorders.

13. Prevention

Traditional models attribute refractive and phorometric status primarily to genetic influence and to random biologic variation. Consequently, there is little basis for preventive care. Concepts of prevention are applied in relation to eye disease, but not with regard to vision care.

Optometrists schooled in the Skeffington model emphasize the influence of environmental factors, especially near work, in the development of vision disorders. Various skews in refractive, accommodative, and vergence findings are held to result from adaptation to nearpoint stress. OEP analysis is used to determine the appropriate regimen to provide optimal function at near and prevent further adaptation and deterioration.

THE OPTOMETRIC EXTENSION PROGRAM 21-POINT ANALYTICAL EXAMINATION

In OEP analysis, the basic diagnostic battery is a series of procedures that is commonly referred to as the *analytical examination, analytical refraction, analytical sequence, analytical routine,* or simply as the *analytical* or the *21-point examination.* Interpretation of the analytical findings allows the optometrist to determine the status of a visual problem; to determine whether lens application will be sufficient to restore adequate function, or whether optometric vision training is necessary; and to determine the appropriate lens prescription (Skeffington 1945–51; Manas 1965; Emery 1968–70; Lesser 1969; Hendrickson 1989).

The analytical sequence was introduced by Skeffington in the 1920s and expanded in the 1930s (Skeffington 1928, 1931, 1941–50). It is an organized, standardized method for gathering optometric data. The tests are performed in a specified sequence, and are commonly referred to by number rather than by name. The sequence of tests, the number by which each is known, and their expected values, are given in Table 8.1.

OEP analysis can be properly performed only if the tests have been administered in the standard sequence using standard OEP procedure. In OEP analysis, findings are compared with expecteds. Variations in procedure reduce the validity of this comparison and subsequent analysis. Communication with other prac-

Table 8.1 OEP test sequence and expected values

	Case Findings	Expecteds
#1	Ophthalmoscope	neg
#2	Ophthalmometer O.D., O.S.	
#3	Hab. phoria dist.	.50 exo
#13A	Hab. phoria near	6 exo
#4	Distance retinoscopy	
#5	Retinoscopy 20″	
#6	Retinoscopy 40″	
#7	Basic formula (subj.)	
#8	Induced phoria	.50 exo
#9	True adduction (first blur)	7 to 9
#10	Convergence	19/10 minimum
#11	Abduction	9/5 minimum
#12	Vertical phorias and ductions	Ortho & equal ductions
#13B	Induced phoria through #7	6 exo
#14A	Unfused cross cyl.	
#15A	Induced phoria	
#14B	Fused cross cyl.	
#15B	Induced phoria	
#16A	Base-out to blur-out	15
#16B	Pos. fus. res.	21/15 minimum
#17A	Base-in to blur-out	14
#17B	Neg. fus. res.	22/18 minimum
#18	Vertical phorias and ductions, near	Ortho & equal ductions
#19	Analytical amp. (accommodation)	5.00 minimum
#20	Minus to blur-out	−2.25 to −2.50
#21	Plus to blur-out	+1.75 to +2.00

Reprinted with permission from Lesser SK (1969). *Introduction to Modern Analytical Optometry*, rev. ed., first publ. 1935. Santa Ana, CA: Optometric Extension Program Foundation.

titioners requires a mutual understanding of the manner in which the tests were performed.

Since standard OEP procedure differs in some respects from refractive and phorometric techniques described by Borish (1970), Carlson et al. (1990), and others, the OEP methods are described here in detail. Illumination for distance tests is obtained with standard projectors. Nearpoint findings are taken at 16 inches, with the instrument set for the near pupillary distance, with adequate illumination, approximately 18 footcandles, except for the #14A, #15A, and #14B findings, which are taken with reduced illumination at approximately 2 footcandles. Phoria measures are taken from the base-in side by first turning in excess base-in prism. Tests are often referred to by number rather than by name. The standard sequence and procedure is as follows (Skeffington 1941–50; Manas 1965; Lesser 1969; Hendrickson 1989):

#1 Ophthalmoscopy

#2 Ophthalmometry

#3 Habitual lateral phoria at distance

    With the habitual distance prescription in place, the patient fixates a vertical line of 20/20 letters. A 6^Δ base-up prism is placed in front of the left eye. The measuring prisms are positioned before both eyes and turned to 12^Δ or 15^Δ base-in. Next, the prism is reduced, and the patient is asked to report when the images are aligned. If there is no convenient method for using measuring prisms binocularly, an alternate procedure is to place the vertical separating prism before the left eye and the measuring prism before the right.

#13A Habitual lateral phoria at near

    This finding is taken at 16 inches, with the patient's habitual nearpoint prescription in place, or plano if none has been worn. The procedure is the same as for the #3 finding. The fixation target is a vertical row of reduced 20/20 letters. The patient is instructed to keep the letters clear at all times.

#4 Distance retinoscopy, 6 m (20 feet)

    The patient fixates a large group of letters on the distance test chart. The examiner scopes at his customary working distance, usually 20 inches, attempting to align himself as nearly as possible with the visual axis.

    The examiner places enough plus lens power before the eye being scoped to create "against" motion in all meridians. With the other eye, which has no working lens placed before it, the patient observes the smallest identifiable letters. The examiner gradually reduces plus before the eye being tested until "neutral" is obtained in one meridian. Cylinder is introduced to neutralize "against" motion still observed in other meridians. The lens power in the instrument is reduced by +2.00 D sphere to compensate for the 20-inch working distance, and the procedure is repeated for the other eye.

It is standard practice to recheck the right eye finding after the left eye has been neutralized. If there is a significant difference, each eye is rechecked until the findings are stable.

#5 Retinoscopy at 20 inches (50 cm)

With the #4 distance retinoscopy finding still in the instrument, the patient fixates a group of small letters in close proximity to and in the plane of the retinoscope. The patient is asked to read the various letters to ensure fixation. The examiner, scoping on the midline of the patient at a 20-inch working distance, adds enough plus to the distance retinoscopy finding to create "against" motion in all meridians in both eyes, then gradually reduces plus until neutrality is reached. The total lens power in the instrument is then recorded as the #5 finding. No deduction is made.

#6 Retinoscopy at 40 inches (1 m)

The procedure is the same as that for the #5 finding, except that the examiner and fixation target are 40 inches from the patient. Begin with the #5 lens finding in place. This generally gives against motion at 1 m. Plus lens power is gradually reduced until neutrality is reached. The total lens power in the instrument is then recorded as the #6 finding. This finding is commonly omitted unless the patient is having difficulty at some intermediate distance, in which case the test is made at that distance, rather than at 1 m.

#7 Subjective (basic formula)

Any standard method is satisfactory, as long as it is completed binocularly, coming "out of the blur." The essential steps are

1. Determine the subjective cylinder finding for each eye by any satisfactory method and check it by another method.
2. Balance the two eyes for the target distance, with spheres, by any standard method.
3. Restore binocularity and increase plus binocularly until acuity is slightly less than 20/40.
4. Slowly reduce plus binocularly until the patient can just read a good 20/20, reading most or all of the 20/20 line and perhaps some of the easier 20/15 letters.

This finding is recorded as the #7 subjective measure. This maximum plus finding is *not* the lens that gives best acuity, and should not be thought of as the distance prescription. Rather, this maximum plus is viewed as the basic formula of the analytical routine, and it is through this maximum plus that subsequent tests in the routine are performed.

#7A Maximum plus to best distance visual acuity

The plus of the #7 is reduced binocularly to the maximum plus (or minimum minus) that gives best acuity. This finding is recorded, and is equivalent to the classical subjective finding.

#8 Induced lateral phoria at distance

The procedure is the same as that for the #3 habitual lateral phoria, except that this phoria is taken through the #7 finding.

#9 Base-out to first blur at distance

The patient views a vertical row of 20/20 letters on the distance chart. A +0.25 D sphere is added before both eyes, causing a slight blur. This is called to the patient's attention as an example "blur." The +0.25 D spheres are then removed. Base-out prism is slowly turned in equal amounts before the two eyes until the patient reports blur. The test is taken to the first recognizable blur, not to complete blur out. If no blur occurs, the finding is recorded as "x."

#10 Base-out to break and recovery at distance

After the first blur (#9) is obtained, the examiner continues to turn base-out prism before the two eyes. The patient is asked to report the moment the target doubles, clears, or moves to one side. (Clearing or moving of the target is interpreted as "suppression.") After the break point is determined, enough base-out prism is added to sustain diplopia and prevent fusion recovery. The base-out is slowly reduced until the images go back together; this is the recovery point. If base-in prism is required to obtain recovery, it is recorded as a negative value.

#11 Base-in to break and recovery at distance

This test is the same as #10, except that it is executed with base-in prism.

#12 Vertical phoria and ductions at distance

The vertical phoria may be determined using any standard technique. The vertical ductions are always taken after, never before, the farpoint lateral ductions.

#13B Lateral phoria at near through the #7 basic formula

This finding is taken in the same manner as the #13A, except that the #7 is in place.

#14A Unfused cross-cylinder

Using a finely ruled cross-line grid oriented at 90 and 180 degrees as a target, with reduced illumination, the examiner places enough vertical dissociating prism equally before both eyes, base-down before the right and base-up before the left, to cause the patient to see two completely separated targets.

The patient is asked if the vertical and horizontal lines in the upper target are equally clear and distinct. If they are not, the cylinder before the right eye is altered to equalize the lines, if possible. This is repeated for the lower target.

Cross-cylinders are placed before both eyes with the minus cylinder axes (red dots) vertical. Plus lens power is added binocularly until the vertical lines are blacker in both targets. The patient's attention is directed to the upper target, and the plus is reduced until the two sets of lines are equally black and clear. This is repeated for the lower target. The examiner then returns to the upper target and adjusts the lens power, if necessary; if alteration is needed, the examiner returns to the lower target and adjusts, if necessary. This procedure is continued until no further change is indicated. The maximum plus that yields equality of the lines is recorded. If the lines cannot be made equal, the minimum plus that leaves the vertical lines blacker is recorded. The #14A finding is recorded as the gross sphero-cylindrical lens combination in the instrument.

Cross-cylinder tests theoretically measure the accommodative posture which results when, due to the presence of the cross-cylinders, perfect focus cannot be obtained. The validity of the test for a particular patient can be assessed by repeating the test with the axes reversed. Reversal of the "blacker" response is expected. Failure to obtain reversal indicates that the patient is simply accommodating for one or the other set of lines, and establishes that the test is not valid.

#15A Lateral phoria through unfused cross-cylinder

With the #14A finding and the cross-cylinders in place, with reduced illumination, a lateral phoria measure is obtained using the cross-line grid as a target.

#14B Binocular fused cross-cylinder

With the #14A finding and cross-cylinders in place, the prisms are removed and the procedures of the #14A are repeated with the patient viewing a single, fused cross-line target. Typically, the vertical lines are blacker, since the test is begun through the #14A lens powers. Plus is reduced until the lines are equally black and distinct. If the patient reverses from vertical to horizontal, and thus has no "equality" lens, the most plus that makes the horizontal lines blacker is recorded as the #14B finding. The #14B finding is recorded as the "gross" sphero-cylindrical lens combination in place.

#15B Lateral phoria through fused cross-cylinder

The #15B phoria is taken with the #14B lenses in place, with the cross-cylinders removed and with standard nearpoint illumination, using a vertical row of 20/20 letters as a target.

Control Lens for Subsequent Findings

The phorometric findings will vary depending on whether they are taken through the #7, #7A, #14B, or some other lens formula. It is standard practice in the OEP analytical examination to use the #7 as the control lens through which to take the #8 through #14B findings. For emmetropes and nonpresbyopic hyperopes, the #7 is also used as the control for subsequent nearpoint findings. For myopes, nearpoint findings are taken through the lens correction habitually used for nearpoint; this is frequently either plano or less minus than the #7. For presbyopes, nearpoint findings are usually taken through the #14B net.

#16A Base-out to blur-out (positive relative convergence)

With a vertical line of 20/20 letters in place at 16 inches and rotary prism before each eye, prism base-out is binocularly added until the print is so blurred that the patient can longer read any of the letters. The total prism in place is the #16A finding. If no blur occurs, the finding is recorded as "x."

#16B Base-out to break and recovery (positive fusional reserve)

Continuing from the blur-out point, prism base-out is added binocularly until the patient reports that the target doubles, clears, or moves to one side. The base-out prism is then increased to prevent a spontaneous reversion to fusion. Prism base-out is binocularly reduced until the two targets become one. The break and recovery findings are recorded as the #16B.

#17A Base-in to blur-out (negative relative convergence)

This finding is taken in the same manner as the #16A finding, except that prism base-in is used.

#17B Base-in to break and recovery (negative fusional reserve)

This finding is taken as a continuation of the #17A, in the same manner as the #16B, except that base-in prism is used.

#18 Vertical phorias and ductions at near

These tests are performed in the same manner as the #12 finding, except at 16 inches, using a horizontal row of letters as the target.

#19 Analytical amplitude (accommodation)

A card with standard reading material, size 0.62m or J4, is placed at 13 inches. Plus spheres are binocularly reduced or minus spheres added to the control lens until there is a definite, sustained, noticeable blur. This is not a blur-out, which would prevent the patient from reading the type, but a blur of such degree as to make reading difficult.

The #19 finding is determined by adding 2.5 D (the accommodation assumed to be required for 13 inches, after allowing for lag of accommodation) to the minus lens power, over and above the #7, which the patient can clear before this first sustained blur.

#20 Minus to blur-out (positive relative accommodation)

The patient views 20/20 reduced Snellen test type at 16 inches, through the control lens. Plus is binocularly reduced or minus added until the patient is totally unable to read the print. The #20 finding is 0.25 D less than the minus lens power added to complete blur-out.

#21 Plus to blur-out (negative relative accommodation)

This finding is taken in exactly the same manner as the #20 finding, except that plus lens power is added to blur-out.

Procedural Differences

The standard procedure used to gather the data of the OEP 21-point analytical examination (Lesser 1969; Hendrickson 1989) differs in several important respects from the traditional methods described by Borish (1970), Carlson et al. (1990), and others. In performing distance retinoscopy, Borish (1970) recommends that both eyes be fogged. Carlson et al. (1990) describe a procedure using the streak retinoscope in which fogging lenses are not used. In the OEP analytical sequence, standard procedure is to fog only the eye that is being scoped.

In traditional methods, the subjective is performed to best acuity, and this finding is used as a tentative correction through which the phorometric findings are taken. In the OEP sequence, the subjective (#7) is recorded as the maximum plus that gives good 20/20 (rather than best visual acuity), and it is through this finding that the phorometric tests are performed. In OEP procedure, the plus of the #7 is reduced, if necessary, to give best acuity, and this finding is recorded separately as the #7A. As a result of these procedural differences, the distance retinoscopy finding obtained by traditional methods may differ from the OEP finding, and the OEP subjective #7 finding frequently differs from the traditional subjective to best acuity.

In traditional models, the retinoscopic finding is expected to match the subjective refraction. Differences are attributed to measurement error, response error, and optical factors. In OEP analysis, the #4 distance retinoscopy and the #7 subjective, obtained through procedures that differ from the traditional, are viewed as different measures, reflecting the conditions and demand levels under which they are taken. OEP analysis holds that differences between the #4 and #7 findings reflect differences in visual status, rather than artifacts of testing; consequently, these differences play a significant role in case analysis.

Similarly, traditional and OEP procedures for obtaining phorometric findings differ significantly. In traditional methods, the phoria is usually measured from both the base-in and base-out directions, and the findings averaged (Borish 1970; Carlson et al. 1990). In the OEP analytical routine, phoria findings are always taken from the base-in side. This serves to minimize esophoric measurement bias in a system in which great significance is attributed to the presence of esophoria.

Practitioners using traditional and OEP methodology may use differing criteria to take blur findings in the relative convergence and accommodation tests. Borish (1970) points out that the first blur is more valuable for analytical purposes (since it indicates the point at which one function cannot be further stimulated without activating the other), but that the first blur is more difficult to define than the blur-out. The choice as to which to use is left to the clinician, with the admonition only to be consistent. In OEP analysis, the base-out blur at distance (#9) is taken to the first recognizable blur; the blur findings at near (#16A, #17A, #20, #21) are all taken to blur-out.

The sequence of taking the tests may differ between OEP and traditional methods. In the OEP sequence, the base-out tests are taken before the base-in, and the minus to blur is taken before the plus to blur. Borish (1970), describing traditional methodology, follows the same sequence. In contrast, Eisenberg (1974) recommends a sequence followed by many traditional practitioners in which inhibitory findings (those taken through plus or through prism base-in) are taken before stimulatory findings (those taken through minus or prism base-out). Since the findings may be influenced by preceding tests (Borish 1970), differences in sequence may lead to differences in the findings.

Differences in phorometric findings induced by these procedural differences are compounded if the findings are taken through different lenses. Traditional methods generally use the subjective to best acuity as the base lens through which to obtain phorometric data in prepresbyopes. In the OEP analytical sequence, the #7 (maximum plus to first good 20/20) is used as the nearpoint control lens when examining prepresbyopic hyperopes and emmetropes; the habitual near-point lens is used for myopes.

The method for taking the amplitude of accommodation also differs between traditional and OEP routines. Traditional procedures usually use Donders' method: a fine target is moved toward the eye until it is blurred, and the distance from the target to the eye at that point is converted into diopters. The test is performed both monocularly and binocularly. In contrast with this push-up method, the OEP analytical amplitude (#19) is performed with minus lenses to the first sustained blur, and is taken only binocularly.

As a consequence of these procedural differences findings may vary among practitioners.

One advantage of the OEP procedure is the standardization it imposes with regard to technique. Illumination, target material, instructional set, sequence, and end point of each test are clearly specified, permitting replicability of findings and communication among practitioners.

Another significant difference between OEP and traditional methods of phorometric testing lies in the selection of tests to be performed. In traditional models, the distance vergence findings have little significance unless the patient has asthenopic symptoms associated with distance viewing. Consequently, these findings are frequently omitted. Similarly, the vergence in the same direction as the phoria (for example, base-in vergence in exophoria) has no role in traditional analysis and is often neglected. Indeed, if the patient is asymptomatic, problem-oriented practitioners may exclude the entire phorometric battery as having little relevance.

In the OEP model, in contrast, the analytical examination is viewed as a unitary procedure, a single test composed of several findings, each of which enters into case analysis regardless of the direction of the phoria or the presence or absence of symptoms. To properly obtain and analyze data in the OEP model, each of the procedures in the 21-point analytical examination must be performed.

NORMATIVE AND EXPECTED VALUES

Assessment of findings requires comparison to normative or expected values. Normative findings are measures that have been determined to be normal, or average, for a given group. Expecteds, in contrast, are findings that are theorized to be optimal for a given population.

Norms for phoria, prism vergence, and accommodative findings have been determined in a number of studies, and are summarized in Table 8-2. Shepard's data (1941) are derived from a clinical population of 2,000 adults and children. Clinical data were also used by Haines (1941), Morgan (1944a, 1944b), and Jackson and Goss (1991) to determine norms. Haines' data were obtained from his own practice, on 500 nonpathological, nonpresbyopic, comfortable, visually efficient individuals. Morgan's data were obtained from a nonselected group of 800 pre-presbyopic patients, and Jackson and Goss (1991) report data obtained from a clinical sample of 244 school-age children.

Betts and Austin (1941), Saladin and Sheedy (1978), and Griffin and Lee (1984) used nonclinical data to determine norms. Betts and Austin obtained data from a sample of 113 fifth-graders. Saladin and Sheedy's sample comprised 103 third-year optometry students, and included both asthenopic and asymptomatic individuals. Griffin and Lee studied 27 symptom-free second-year optometry students. The mean values reported for phoria, prism vergence, and relative accommodation in these various studies are similar. In addition to these studies, in which data are obtained using Risley prisms with a refractor, Wesson and Amos (1985) report norms for prism vergence measures obtained with hand-held Risley prisms and with prism bars.

In contrast with norms, which are derived statistically from clinical data, the OEP "expecteds" (Skeffington 1941–50; Lesser 1969; Hendrickson 1989) are values assumed to be the minimum required if an individual is to withstand the impact of nearpoint stress and maintain satisfactory performance. They were derived by Skeffington on the basis of clinical insight, study of many patients, and interaction with many practitioners. Despite differences in the method of derivation of the OEP expecteds and the normative data, their values are remarkably similar (see Table 8.2).

OEP CASE ANALYSIS

OEP analysis is designed to determine the optimal lens prescriptions for distance and near, and to determine whether lenses alone will provide optimal function or whether vision therapy is required. OEP analysis requires that the analytical examination findings be categorized (or checked) as high or low, based on comparison to expecteds or to one another. High and low findings are then grouped into patterns, or chains, to derive syndromes or case typings. This sequence is commonly referred to as "checking, chaining, and typing." These patterns are further analyzed to determine depth of deterioration and degree of embeddedness of the problem, and guidelines are applied to determine the indications for lens prescription and vision therapy (Skeffington 1941–50, 1945–51; Manas 1965; Emery 1968–70; Lesser 1969; Hendrickson 1989). Although few practitioners today rigidly follow the classical OEP directives for checking, chaining, and typing, many functionalists use case analysis systems derived from OEP theory.

Table 8.2 Norms and expecteds for phoria, prism vergence, and accommodative measures

	Test	Haines (1941)	Shepard (1941)	Betts and Austin (1941) (rounded figures)
#3	(habitual phoria distance)		1 exo	.1 exo
#13A	(habitual phoria near)		5 exo	2.5 exo
#8	(induced phoria distance)	ortho	1 exo	.2 exo
#9	(B.O. blur, distance)	9	9	7.4
#10	(B.O. break, recovery)	22/16	21/9	21.2/7.2
#11	(B.I. break, recovery)	9/5	9/4	7.1/3.3
#12	(vertical phoria, distance) (vertical vergences)	<1 balanced, >2	ortho 4/1.5	2.4/1.0
#13B	(induced phoria, near)	5 exo	5 exo	2.8 exo
#14A	(dissociated x-cyl)		+0.37	+1.78
#15A	(induced phoria)		6 exo	
#14B	(fused x-cyl)	+0.50 D	0	+1.44
#15B	(induced phoria)		5 exo	
#16A	(B.O. blur, near)	16	13	18.3
#16B	(B.O. break, recovery)	23	25/13	21.7/6.4
#17A	(B.I. blur, near)	15	10	18
#17B	(B.I. break, recovery)	22	20/10	21.5/12.5
#18	(vertical phoria) (vertical vergences)		ortho 5/2	3/1.4
#19	(minus lens amplitude)	4.00 D	9.0 D (age 8)	11.7
#20	(PRA)	−2.00	−2.37	−4.8
#21	(NRA)	+1.75	+1.75	+2.2

Abbreviations: B.O., base-out; x-cyl, cross-cylinder; B.I., base-in; ortho, orthophoria; exo, exophoria.

From H. Haines, Normal values of visual functions and their applications in case analysis. *Am J Optom Arch Am Acad Optom* 18(1):1–8. © The Am Acad of Optom, 1941. M.W. Morgan, Analysis of clinical data. *Am J Optom Arch Amer Acad Optom* 21(12):477–491. © The Am Acad of Optom, 1944. J.J. Saladin, J.E. Sheedy, A population study of relationships between fixation disparity, heterophorias and vergences. *Am J Optom Physiol Opt* 55(11):744–750. © The Am Acad of Optom, 1978. (Data from the above studies reprinted with permission of the American Academy of Optometry.) Data from E.A. Betts, A.S. Austin, Seeing problems of school children. XXII Summary and conclusions. *Optom Weekly* 32:369–371; J.R. Griffin, R.A. Lee, Visual skills norms in college students. *Optom Monthly* 75(2):103–104, 1984; and C.F. Shepard, The most probable "expecteds." *Optom Weekly* 32:538, 1941. (Reprinted with permission of Butterworth–

Morgan (1944a, 1944b)	Saladin and Sheedy (1978)	Griffin and Lee (1984) (rounded figures)	Jackson and Goss (1991)	OEP Expecteds
				.5 exo
				6 exo
1 exo	1 exo	1.9 exo	1 exo	.5 exo
9	15	11.8	14	7 to 9
19/10	28/20	19.7/12.4	23/6	19/10
7/4	8/5	9.6/6.5	12/4	9/5
				ortho equal
3 exo	0.5 exo	4.4 exo	3 exo	6 exo
+0.50				
17	22	16.6	21	15
21/11	30/23	24.5/15.1	27/10	21/15
14	14	14.4	15	14
21/13	19/13	21.2/14.2	21/9	22/18
				ortho equal
				5.00 D
−2.37		−3.2	−2.14	−2.25 to −2.50
+2.00		+2.3	+1.91	+1.75 to +2.00

Heinemann, Boston.) Data from T.W. Jackson, D.A. Goss, Variation and correlation of standard clinical phoropter tests of phorias, vergence ranges, and relative accommodation in a sample of school-age children. *J Am Optom Assoc* 62(7):540–547, 1991. (Reprinted with permission.) Data from S.K. Lesser, *Introduction to Modern Analytical Optometry*. Rev. ed., first publ. 1935, Santa Ana, CA: Optometric Extension Program Foundation. Reprinted with permission.

Classifying Findings as High or Low

In OEP case analysis, the first step is to classify each finding as high or low. As previously noted, variations in procedure may give rise to differences in test findings. Therefore, only findings obtained using OEP standard procedure can properly be compared with OEP expecteds and subjected to OEP analysis. The OEP expecteds are given in Table 8.1.

To classify findings as high or low, the following guidelines are applied (Skeffington 1941–50, 1945–51; Manas 1965; Emery 1968–70; Lesser 1969; Hendrickson 1989):

1. The #4 finding is high if greater in plus than the #7 finding, and low if lesser in plus.
2. The #5 finding is checked high if greater in plus than the #4 finding, and low if it is less plus. However, before the #5 finding is compared with the #4, the #5 gross finding is converted to a net finding by subtracting for an assumed lag of accommodation. The lag is obtained by dividing the #15A exophoria by 8. When the #19 is less than 5.0 D, the lag is reduced proportionately. The maximum lag to be deducted is 2.0 D.
3. The #9 finding is checked as high or low compared with its expected value of 7 to 9.
4. The #10 and #11 findings are each compared with their expecteds. If one finding is low (either a low break, or a recovery less than one half of the break), it is checked as low and so placed on the diagnostic chain. If both findings are low, they are compared with one another to determine which is lower, and the lower one is so placed on the diagnostic chain. In comparing two low vergence findings, if one has a low break finding and the other is low because of its recovery, the former is considered the lower finding, since low breaks indicate greater binocular interference. When both findings are low because of low breaks, or both low because of low recoveries, the finding that is lower in proportion to its expected is considered to be the low finding and is so placed on the chain.
5. The #16B and #17B findings are classified as high or low using the same guidelines as those given for #10 and #11. For the #16B and #17B findings, the recoveries should be at least two thirds and three quarters of the breaks, respectively.
6. The #13B near-phoria finding is checked as high and placed above the line if greater than 6△ exophoria, and as low, placed below the line, if less than 6△ exophoria.
7. The #14A gross is converted to a net finding by deducting a lag. When the #19 finding is greater than 5.0 D, the following formula is used:

$$\text{lag} = \frac{\text{\#15A exo}}{6}.$$

When the #19 finding is less than 5.0 D, the formula is

$$\text{lag} = \frac{\#15\text{A exo}}{6} \times \frac{\#19}{5}.$$

The #14A net is then compared with the subjective finding (#7). If greater in plus than #7, #14A is checked high and #15A low. If lower in plus than #7, #14A is checked low and #15A high. If the #14A is exactly the same as #7, #14A and #15A are both checked high if #15A is greater than $6^\triangle$ exophoria, and both checked low if #15A is less than $6^\triangle$ exophoria.

8. The #16A is compared to #17A, and #20 is compared with #21. For each pair, the higher is checked high, and the lower is checked low.

Diagnostic Chains and Case Typing

After the analytical examination findings are each checked as high or low, a diagnostic chain is constructed by placing high findings above and low findings below a horizontal line. A significant element of OEP case analysis is the notion that high and low findings may be grouped into patterns, or case typings, which indicate the nature of the problem and provide therapeutic implications. Four such syndromes have been described: the A, B1, B2, and C case types. The characteristic pattern of high and low findings (diagnostic chain) for each of these case types is as follows:

$$\text{A type:} \quad \frac{\phantom{4\text{-}11\text{-}13\text{B-}17\text{B}}}{4\text{-}11\text{-}13\text{B-}17\text{B}}$$

$$\text{B1 type:} \quad \frac{5}{9\text{-}11\text{-}16\text{B}}$$

$$\text{B2 type:} \quad \frac{5}{9\text{-}11\text{-}17\text{B}}$$

$$\text{C type:} \quad \frac{15\text{A}}{5\text{-}10\text{-}16\text{B}}.$$

These case types were derived, through clinical experience, in an attempt to formulate guidelines for successful lens prescription. OEP case analysis was designed to aid the practitioner in determining which cases would benefit from plus lens application, and in determining a "safe," acceptable nearpoint lens (Skeffington 1945–51; Manas 1965; Emery 1968–70; Lesser 1969; Hendrickson 1989).

The A Case Type

The A case type indicates possible toxic interference with the innervational patterns of accommodation and convergence, generating a toxic esophoria. Such cases are referred and treated medically rather than through lens application and vision training (Skeffington 1931, 1945–51).

Because of the marked similarity between the A case type, which suggests toxemia, and the B2 case type, of functional origin, differentiation on the basis of case typing alone is difficult. An excessive number of patients with functional vision disorders have been inappropriately referred for systemic medical evaluation. Clinicians are therefore advised not to refer for suspected toxicity on the basis of case typing alone but, in the presence of an A case typing, to follow the appropriate dicta for lens prescribing and other optometric care, to bear in mind the possibility of toxic interference, and to refer only those patients who demonstrate corroborating evidence of pathology in the case history and visual fields, or fail to respond to optometric care (Skeffington 1941–50; Manas 1965).

The clinician should bear in mind the potential correlation between systemic toxemia, toxic esophoria, and the analytical examination findings. Referral for medical evaluation should be made whenever the case history and other findings suggest a nonfunctional origin for a deviant analytical pattern.

Development of the B1 Case

The B pattern occurs as the individual seeks to block overconvergence by creating an inhibition or interference in the accommodative system, which in turn sets in motion a series of skews in the analytical examination findings. The interference is held to be in the accommodative mechanism, in contrast with the C type, in which the interference is primarily in the convergence mechanism. The B case types constitute those functional visual problems that will accept and benefit from plus lens application at near.

There are two types of B cases: the B1 and the B2. Skeffington (1945–51) indicates that the B1 type represents the characteristic response to nearpoint stress, and that the B2 pattern occurs as an exaggeration of the B1 when nearpoint stress is intensified (see Chapter 4).

The primary characteristic of the B1 case is that the #16B finding (base-out break and recovery at near) is low, even though the #16A finding (base-out blur at near) is high. In the earliest stage of development of the B1 case, the pattern of findings is as follows:

$$\frac{7 \quad\quad 5 \quad\quad 14A \quad\quad 16A\text{-}21 \quad\quad 19}{9\text{-}11\text{-}16B \quad\quad 15A \quad\quad 17A\text{-}20} \quad.$$

The base-out to blur at near (#16A) is high, and the base-in to blur (#17A) is low, reflecting the basic tendency for convergence to localize closer than accommodation. Similarly, the #21 finding (plus lens to blur) is high, while the #20 finding (minus to blur) is low. The #20 (PRA) finding measures the ability to shift accommodation closer than convergence, in direct opposition to the stress-induced overconvergence tendency. A low PRA finding is thus one of the earliest signs of nearpoint visual difficulty.

Although the #16A base-out blur is high, the #16B base-out break is low.

In the presence of a tendency for convergence to position closer than accommodation, single binocular vision is maintained and overconvergence is blocked by inhibiting fusional convergence.

The B2 Case

The primary difference between the B1 and B2 case types is the reversal of the #16B and #17B findings

$$\text{B1:} \quad \frac{5}{9\text{-}11\text{-}16\text{B}}.$$

$$\text{B2:} \quad \frac{5}{9\text{-}11\text{-}17\text{B}}.$$

In the B1 case, the #16B finding is low; in the B2 case, the #17B finding is low.

According to Skeffington (1945–51), the B2 pattern arises as a distortion or exaggeration of the B1, occurring as a result of intensified concentration at near. With intensification of nearpoint demand, overconvergence increases to the point where inhibition of fusional convergence is insufficient, and demands on negative fusional convergence lead to a reversal of findings—#17B decreasing below #16B. Skeffington indicates that the B2 pattern reverts to the B1 during the course of proper remediation.

OEP analysis guidelines for lens prescribing are based on the case-typing. The guideline for the B1 case is to prescribe the full-plus indicated for distance, as well as the full-plus indicated for near. However, for the B2 case, the recommendation is to prescribe full-plus for near, but to cut plus for distance (Skeffington 1945–51; Manas 1965; Emery 1968–70; Lesser 1969; Hendrickson 1989).

Flax (1984) notes the apparent incongruity that the guidelines for distance lens prescribing are, in effect, determined by the near-vergence findings. The only difference between the B1 and B2 case types is the near-vergence (#16B and #17B) findings, yet it is the guideline for distance lens acceptance that differs between the two cases; full-plus is advised for near use in both cases. Flax suggests that distance lens acceptance differs for B1 and B2 cases because these individuals use different coping strategies in response to nearpoint stress. Woolf (1963–64) and Flax (1984) propose that the B1 individual attempts to restore centering to the plane of identification, while the B2 copes by bringing identification in toward the plane of centering. Flax (1984) suggests that the B1 patient accepts full-plus for distance, because the full-plus prescription assists in the attempt to shift localization away, but that the B2 patient is bothered by full-plus for distance, because it interferes with the attempt to cope by bringing identification closer.

Flax (1984) further suggests that the B1 individual is more concerned with ambient "where is it" processing, while the B2 individual is more involved with focal vision and clarity, and is consequently more disturbed by full-plus lens prescription for distance.

Stages of Deterioration. The diagnostic chain given above as characteristic of the B1 case represents the typical initial pattern of response to nearpoint stress. When stress persists, adaptation continues. As the individual seeks to block the drive toward overconvergence, the pattern of the analytical examination findings changes. Some findings become high and others low as the individual seeks to restore equilibrium and efficient function.

These changes in the pattern of analytical findings, or stages of adaptation, tend to occur in characteristic sequence, and are referred to as the stages of deterioration of the B1 case. The seven stages are as follows:

$$1. \ \frac{7 + 5 \quad\quad 14A \quad\quad 16A\text{-}21 \quad\quad 19}{9\text{-}11\text{-}16B \quad\quad 15A \quad\quad 17A\text{-}20}.$$

$$2. \ \frac{7 + 5 \quad\quad 16A\text{-}21 \quad\quad 19}{9\text{-}11\text{-}16B \quad\quad \underline{14A}\text{-}15A \quad\quad 17A\text{-}20}.$$

At this stage, sometimes 14A-15A may be high and equal, or on the line and equal, or frequently low and equal.)

$$3. \ \frac{7 + 5 \quad\quad 15A \quad\quad 16A\text{-}21\text{-}19}{9\text{-}11\text{-}16B \quad\quad \underline{14A} \quad\quad 17A\text{-}20}.$$

$$4. \ \frac{7 + 5 \quad\quad 15A \quad\quad 16A\text{-}20\text{-}19}{9\text{-}11\text{-}16B \quad\quad 14A \quad\quad 17A\text{-}\underline{21}}.$$

$$5. \ \frac{7 + 5 \quad\quad 15A \quad\quad 16A\text{-}21}{9\text{-}11\text{-}16B \quad\quad 14A \quad\quad 17A\text{-}20\text{-}\underline{19}}.$$

$$6. \ \frac{7 + 5 \quad\quad 15A \quad\quad 16A\text{-}21}{9\text{-}\underline{10}\text{-}16B \quad\quad 14A \quad\quad 17A\text{-}20\text{-}19}.$$

$$7. \ \frac{7 \quad\quad 15A \quad\quad 16A\text{-}21}{\underline{5}\text{-}9\text{-}10\text{-}16B \quad\quad 14A \quad\quad 17A\text{-}20\text{-}19}.$$

The patterns of adaptation for B2 cases are identical to those given for the B1, except that in the B2 case the #17B finding would characteristically be low, rather than the #16B.

At each stage of deterioration, the underlined finding is that whose change from high to low is characteristic of that particular level. Following the impact of nearpoint stress, the first change in pattern is the lowering of the dissociated cross-cylinder finding (#14A); this is followed sequentially by reversal of the #20 and #21 findings; lowering of the amplitude of accommodation (#19) in the pre-presbyope; reduction of the base-out at far (#10); and finally, by lowering of the dynamic retinoscopy (#5). Although considerable variation may occur, these stages represent the typical sequence of adaptation.

The various stages of deterioration indicate progressive reduction in nearpoint plus acceptance. As the patient moves through these stages, plus lens application is progressively less likely to effect beneficial changes in performance, and vision therapy becomes more necessary to restore efficient visual function (Skeffington et al. 1945–51; Manas 1965; Emery 1968–70; Lesser 1969; Hendrickson 1989).

Embedded and Nonembedded Cases. As nearpoint stress persists and adaptation continues, the pattern of the analytical examination findings moves through the stages of deterioration. At any of these stages, the adaptation may become sufficient to allow the individual to achieve satisfactory performance. If no new stress occurs to trigger further adaptation, the adaptation will become habituated. Findings that became very low at the initial impact of the impairing task increase toward expected levels as the individual seeks, through time, to restore the best equilibrium possible. Refractive adaptations that began as distortions of visual function become embedded in structure.

This process of reorganization is known as *embedding*. It may take place at whatever stage of deterioration the adaptive changes are satisfactory for the individual. As the adaptation becomes habituated and the findings move toward expected levels, the case is considered embedded or more highly organized (Skeffington 1945–51; Manas 1965; Emery 1968–70).

As the adaptation becomes more embedded, characteristic changes occur in the analytical examination findings. The #4 distance retinoscopy finding becomes equal to or greater than the #7; the #14B net becomes equal to or greater than the #14A net; and the fusional vergence recovery findings and the #9 base-out blur each increase to expected levels.

Seven factors are considered in determining whether a pattern of findings is embedded or nonembedded (Manas 1965; Emery 1968–70).

Syndrome of the *Embedded Case*	*Syndrome of the* *Nonembedded Case*
1. #4 equal to or greater in plus than #7	1. #4 lower in plus than #7
2. #9 up to its expected value or higher	2. #9 excessively low, except in myopia, when #9 will be high
3. #10 break low (below 13) but recovery above or equal to its expected	3. #10 recovery excessively low
4. #11 break and recovery up; recovery at its expected or higher	4. #11 break and recovery excessively low
5. #14B net equal to or greater than #14A net	5. #14B net lower than #14A net
6. In B1 case, #16B break low (below 13), with recovery at or above expected. In B2 case, #17B break low (below 13), with recovery at or above expected	6. In B1 case, #16B recovery excessively low; in B2 case, #17B recovery excessively low

7. #19 and #20 are not both low; one high and the other low	7. #19 and #20 both excessively low

In determining nonembeddedness, the #9, #10, #11, and #16B findings are considered low if they are 3$^\Delta$ or more below expected values. The #19 and #20 findings are considered low if they are 0.50 D or more below expecteds.

A case is diagnosed as embedded or nonembedded when at least five of the seven factors listed are consistent with that diagnosis. When fewer than five of the factors are consistent, the status is considered indefinite.

According to Skeffington (1945–51), the visually efficient individual functions with high automaticity and little conscious effort. Stress causes interference with the effector systems involved in nearpoint activity, so that greater effort and conscious attention are required to sustain performance. Achievement and comprehension are impaired and asthenopic symptoms ensue. The embedding process does not restore optimal performance, but does allow the individual to restore the best equilibrium possible and to shift operation back to a more highly automatic level, with consequent reduction in symptoms and improved performance.

When the case has become highly organized or embedded, the patient may experience little discomfort, in contrast with the nonembedded case in which there is typically much symptomatology. If the patient is relatively symptom-free, and if performance levels are satisfactory, there may be little reason to consider treatment. If symptoms do exist, or if visual performance is inadequate, treatment should be undertaken. However, treatment is more difficult, since the embedded pattern is more resistant to change.

While embedding is advantageous in allowing function in the presence of a visual problem, the embedded pattern is more highly structured and more resistant to therapy. Therefore, depending on the degree of efficiency achieved, it may be viewed as either advantageous or disadvantageous to embed a visual problem.

In the nonembedded case, plus lens application is more readily accepted and is frequently sufficient to reverse the adaptation and restore adequate function. As the case becomes more embedded, it becomes increasingly difficult to reverse the adaptation. Both the pattern of high and low analytical findings and any structural adaptations that may have developed, including myopia, adverse high hyperopia, astigmatism, and anisometropia, become more highly organized and resistant to change. The more embedded the pattern, the less effective plus lens application will be in resolving the problem. In embedded cases, vision training is required to disembed if treatment is to be undertaken. Determination of whether the case is embedded or nonembedded thus plays an important role in determining the therapeutic approach and prognosis in OEP analysis (Skeffington 1945–51; Emery 1968–70; Lesser 1969; Hendrickson 1989).

The C Case Type
The C case type is frequently categorized as a convergence problem. The patient typically presents with high exophoria and impaired convergence func-

tion, reflected by low PRC (#16B) and receded convergence near point. The patient usually has severe nearpoint symptoms.

The pattern of findings characteristic of the C-case is

$$\frac{7 \quad 15A \quad 17A \quad 20 \quad 19}{5\text{-}10\text{-}16B \quad 14A \quad 16A \quad 21}.$$

This syndrome is usually reduced to key elements and given in shortened form as follows (Skeffington 1941–50, 1945–51; Manas 1965):

$$\frac{15A}{5\text{-}10\text{-}16B}.$$

The C case type is encountered far less frequently than the B case type. Skeffington (1945–51) and Manas (1965) indicate that approximately 95% of all functional vision problems are B cases, and the remaining 5% are C cases. According to Skeffington (1945–51), the C case represents a noncharacteristic response to nearpoint stress, occurring in individuals whose biochemical response is atypical.

A low #16B finding is characteristic of both the B1 and C case-typings. The diagnostic pattern of these cases is similar. Differentiation is often difficult, particularly in the deteriorated B1 case, since the C case-typing is virtually identical to the final stage (B1-7) of deterioration of the B1 case (Skeffington 1945–51; Manas 1965).

Manas (1965) offers guidelines for differentiating C from B1 case types. The C case does not go through stages of deterioration on continued exposure to nearpoint stress, as does the B case. The C case maintains a constant pattern. Therefore, to qualify as a true C-type case, the pattern of findings must not deviate in any respect from the full C case-type syndrome. Manas indicates that to be a true C case type, the following conditions must be present:

1. the case typing must be exactly $\dfrac{15A}{5\text{-}10\text{-}16B}$;

2. the equilibrium pattern must not vary from $\dfrac{17A\text{-}20}{16A\text{-}21}$;

3. the #9 (true adduction at far) and #19 (amplitude) findings must both be high.

The traditional label "convergence insufficiency" is commonly used to describe cases with impaired convergence. Since the B1 and C case types each show a low #16B (PRC) finding, they are often grouped together as convergence insufficiencies. Such grouping masks significant differences in etiology and prognosis postulated by the OEP model.

While most convergence insufficiency cases respond well to vision therapy, a small minority do not. The cases that respond well are probably functional in origin, arising as adaptive responses to nearpoint stress, and correspond to the

OEP case B type. In these cases, convergence usually improves rapidly with vision training. Signs of overconvergence are frequently present from the beginning, or become evident as training progresses and the case disembeds. In the nondeteriorated B case type, plus lens application at near is indicated by the analytical examination findings and is well accepted. In deteriorated B cases, in which plus is not accepted initially, plus acceptance is often demonstrated as treatment proceeds.

In the C case, in contrast, convergence is more severely impaired and more resistant to treatment. The overconvergence tendency characteristic of nearpoint stress is not demonstrable. Plus increases nearpoint exophoria, impairs convergence, and is poorly accepted. The OEP analysis guideline for lens prescribing in the C case is to cut plus at both distance and near. While the deteriorated B case may demonstrate overconvergence and increased plus acceptance as treatment proceeds, the C case does not (Skeffington 1945–51; Manas 1965; Lesser 1969; Hendrickson 1989). The C cases constitute the small minority of convergence insufficiency cases that respond poorly to treatment, and are probably organic rather than functional in origin.

Tight and Loose Cases

Some individuals are more highly structured in their spatial judgements than others. Individuals who are loosely organized in space make less accurate spatial judgements. They show greater difficulty orienting themselves in space. Spatial-computing and information-processing are less reliable. Phorias tend to be variable and unstable. Subjective judgements tend to be noncritical. Lens power changes induce little change in phoria, indicating a loose relationship between accommodation and convergence. Lenses are readily accepted by such individuals, but tend to have little impact on performance and therefore minimal patient benefit.

Individuals who are tightly organized for spatial operation are highly critical in their judgements. They have overcompensated in the effort to achieve accurate, reliable spatial judgements and dependable operation in visual space, and show restricted flexibility within and between the effector systems of accommodation and convergence. Phoria measures are precise and highly reliable, as are judgements on subjective refraction. Lens power changes cause large phoria change. Prism vergence testing often induces a report that the eyes hurt or pull. The tightly organized individual will be highly critical and accept a very narrow range of lens power, but will often benefit substantially from appropriate, judicious lens application.

The tight and loose case each indicate inefficient levels of spatial organization. The loose case lacks accuracy, reliability, and consistency in spatial judgements. The tight case makes accurate and reliable spatial judgements, but has limited flexibility. Optimal function requires that an individual be capable of accurate, reliable spatial judgements without loss of flexibility. Vision therapy is often highly effective in achieving such integration.

The terms *tight* and *loose* should not be confused with *embedded* and *nonembedded*. The tight and loose cases described above constitute syndromes of spatial organization. The degree of embeddedness indicates the degree to which the pattern of adaptive response to nearpoint stress has become habituated and ingrained. Both the loose and the tight case will embed their patterns of operation through time, although the tight case may embed more quickly. Therefore, both loose and tight cases can be found at various stages of embeddedness (Emery 1968–70).

The tight and loose syndromes of spatial organization, formulated in the early years of OEP analysis, probably relate to broader aspects of visual information-processing, central-peripheral organization, and cognitive-perceptual style described by MacDonald (1973), Forrest (1976), and Birnbaum (1978a). Tight cases are more likely to be analytical, focal, and detail-oriented in their general approach to information-processing, while loose cases are likely to be more global.

Determining the Lens Prescription

The OEP approach implicates nearpoint stress as the cause of a broad variety of functional vision disorders. Consequently, the emphasis in OEP analysis is the determination of the lens power required at near point. The goal, where possible, is to prescribe lenses that balance accommodation and convergence despite the stress-induced drive for convergence to localize closer, thereby permitting efficient function and relieving the need for adaptation.

Although the OEP approach incorporates a strong bias toward prescribing acceptable plus for near when indicated by the analytical examination findings, low-plus lenses are prescribed judiciously, in a manner consistent with the analytical findings. They are not applied indiscriminately on a shotgun basis. Plus prescribed "out of pattern," or contrary to the dictates of OEP analysis, does not create a balance between the effector systems, but rather adds to the imbalance and may exacerbate the problem.

Nearpoint lens prescriptions derived from OEP analysis are usually low in power, on the order of +0.50 to +1.00 D, and are generally similar to those determined by graphical analysis (Borish 1970; Goss 1986) or by analysis of accommodation/convergence interactions (Schor and Narayan 1982). Such low-power lenses often permit gains in reading efficiency which, to those schooled in classical case analysis, seem disproportionate to the low power of the lenses used. The effectiveness of low-power plus lenses is predicted by both the Skeffington and Schor models, not because of the small reduction in stimulus to accommodation produced by such lenses, but rather because of their effect in restoring equilibrium between vergence and accommodation (Flax 1985).

Although OEP analysis emphasizes determination of the optimal lens prescription for near, far vision is not ignored. Rather, OEP analysis is used to determine the indicated lens values for both distance and near. When these values differ, as is often the case, the lens required for near is not compromised; the indicated far and near prescriptions are issued as bifocals or as separate pairs of glasses, depending on the needs of the particular patient.

The process of determining the indicated lens prescription for distance and for near is essentially the same regardless of whether the patient is myopic, hyperopic, astigmatic, or anisometropic. These refractive deviations are viewed as outcomes of an underlying functional vision problem. OEP analysis to determine lens prescription is based on the pattern of the analytical examination findings, and is largely independent of the individual's particular refractive state.

To determine the indicated and acceptable lens prescriptions for far and near, one must

- perform the 21-point analytical sequence;
- check the findings as high or low;
- determine the limits of maximum plus prescribable (these limits are set at distance and near by the #7 subjective and the net cross-cylinder findings, respectively);
- analyze the equilibrium patterns;
- determine the case-typing;
- determine the stage of deterioration;
- determine the pattern of embeddedness;
- assess the degree of rigidity in spatial organization.

Skeffington (1945–51) was concerned with determining a lens prescription that would not only permit efficient function, but which could be safely prescribed and well accepted by the patient. He noted that lenses prescribed on the basis of traditional refractive error neutralization often created discomfort and were rejected. As a result, the OEP system is filled with checks to ensure that the prescribed lens creates minimal disruption of existing patterns of function, and is hence unlikely to be rejected.

In OEP analysis, the #7 subjective and the cross-cylinder nets set the upper limits of plus lens power that may ordinarily be considered for prescription for distance and near, respectively. To determine the safe lens prescription that will be well accepted by the patient, these maximums are further modified based on the patient's tolerance and flexibility as indicated by the blur-point findings, case-typing, embeddedness, deterioration, and spatial organization, as well as by the needs of the patient.

The #7 subjective finding, the maximum plus to a good 20/20, determines the maximum plus considered for distance. Although the #7 is used as a control through which to take the subsequent findings, it is seldom if ever given as the final distance prescription. Modification is usually made, since crowding maximum plus for far is rarely desirable (Skeffington 1945–51; Manas 1965; Emery 1968–70; Lesser 1969; Hendrickson 1989).

The Cross-Cylinder Tests

The cross-cylinder tests (#14A and #14B) indicate the patient's ability to inhibit or relax accommodation. These tests are performed under conditions that facilitate accommodative relaxation: the illumination is low, the cross-cylinder makes precise focus impossible, and plus lens power is increased as the test proceeds. Since these conditions tend to maximize accommodative relaxation, the net cross-cylinder findings are viewed as the very maximum plus lens power that can be safely prescribed for near use. These values are not necessarily optimal or desirable; rather, they indicate the upper limit of acceptable plus, based on the degree to which accommodation is relaxed during the test (Manas 1965; Emery 1968–70).

Calculation of the #14A net was given earlier. The #14B net is calculated by subtracting from the #14B gross a lag factor determined by the accommodative convergence associated with the #14B, as indicated by the #15B phoria:

$$\text{lag} = \frac{\text{\#15B exo}}{9}.$$

If the #15B is orthophoric or esophoric, no lag is subtracted. If the #19 amplitude is less than 5 D, the lag is proportionally reduced (Manas 1965).

Accommodation is inhibited more readily under dissociated conditions. Therefore, in a nonembedded case, the #14A is usually higher in plus than the #14B finding. As the case passes through successive stages of deterioration in response to sustained stress, the #14A finding usually becomes lower. The maximum prescribable nearpoint plus in any particular case is determined by the lower of the #14A and #14B nets (Manas 1965; Emery 1968–70).

Minus Projection   Minus projection exists when the patient does not accept plus on the cross-cylinder tests, but demonstrates a preference for minus. The term is defined slightly differently among authors. According to Margach (cited in Hendrickson 1989), minus projection exists when the cross-cylinder nets are more minus (or less plus) than the #7 subjective finding at far.

Manas (1965) differentiates minus projection from a condition he terms *minus-at-near*. Minus projection exists when the gross cross-cylinder finding is in plus or plano, but the exophoria through this finding is so great that the net finding is in minus. In response to overconvergence, exophoria has been built in of such magnitude that plus acceptance is lost; plus no longer restores balance between accommodation and convergence. If treatment is indicated, vision training will be required.

Manas defines minus-at-near as the situation in which not only the cross-cylinder net, but even the gross is in minus. Minus projection and minus-at-near are viewed as stages in the sequence of myopia development in which plus acceptance is progressively lost and minus is increasingly indicated at all distances.

A bias toward plus lens application at near point is inherent in OEP analysis. In the presence of minus projection or minus-at-near, arbitrary limits are placed on minus lens prescription at near. For a myope, the prescribable nearpoint lens is never more minus than the #7 subjective at far; for a hyperope or emmetrope, it is never less than plano (Manas 1965).

Equilibrium (Blur) Findings

In OEP analysis, the cross-cylinder nets determine the maximum plus lens prescribable at near. Guidelines are then applied to determine how much of this maximum plus will actually be accepted.

The relationship between the nearpoint blur findings (#16A and #17A; #20 and #21) is held to reflect the pattern of equilibrium between vergence and accommodation habituated by the patient. A lens that disrupts this pattern may create a new interference and may not be well accepted. The safe nearpoint lens is one that maintains the habitual pattern of the equilibrium findings. The prescribable near net, or maximum spherical dioptric acceptable (MSDA), is that part of the cross-cylinder net which does not reverse the habitual pattern of the #16A as compared with the #17A, or of the #20 as compared with the #21 findings.

To be certain that the lens prescribed for near use does not reverse the equilibrium pattern of the blur-point findings, the #20 and #21 findings and the #16A and #17A findings are determined with both the habitual and contemplated lens prescriptions. The pattern of high and low findings obtained with the tentative prescription should not reverse the habitual pattern; if reversal is obtained, the clinician may wish to reduce the prescribed lens power so as to preserve the habitual pattern (Manas 1965; Emery 1968–70).

Thus, if the NRA is greater than the PRA, and the PRC is greater than the NRC through the lens habitually used for near work (or through plano if no lens is habitually used), care should be taken not to prescribe so much plus that these relationships reverse.

The following example, derived from Manas (1965) and Emery (1968–70), illustrates comparison of the equilibrium patterns:

#7 O.U.: +2.25
#14A net O.U.: +3.00
#14B net O.U.: +2.75
Habitual lens Rx: O.U. +2.00 sph.
Control: #7
#16A: 26
#17A: 14
#20: −1.75
#21: +2.50.

In standard OEP practice, only one set of equilibrium findings is actually taken, through the indicated control lens. The expected value of the equilibrium findings through the habitual and tentative lens prescriptions is then calculated. For the #20 and #21 findings, this is a simple calculation: the measures are simply adjusted to reflect a different control or base lens. The #16A and #17A findings are recalculated for different lens bases assuming a 4:1 AC/A ratio. For each 0.25-D difference in control lens, a 1^Δ shift in #16A and #17A is assumed. If the findings were taken through 0.25 D more plus, the #17A finding would be expected to increase 1ᐃ, and the #16A finding to decrease 1ᐃ. The #21 would decrease 0.25 D, and the #20 would increase 0.25 D. Many practitioners prefer to actually take the phoria and prism vergence measures through habitual and various tentative nearpoint lens prescriptions, to assess the relative impact of different lenses on the findings.

In the example given, the derived equilibrium findings and patterns are as follows:

	#7 Control (+2.25)	#14A (+3.00)	#14B (+2.75)	Habitual Rx (+2.00)
#16A	26	23	24	27
#17A	14	17	16	13
#20	−1.75	−2.50	−2.25	−1.50
#21	+2.50	+1.75	+2.00	+2.75
Equilibrium	16A-21	16A-20	16A-20	16A-21
pattern	17A-20	17A-21	17A-21	17A-20

Through the habitual nearpoint correction, the #16A and #21 are respectively higher than the #17A and #20 findings. This pattern is reversed by the #14A and #14B findings, both of which reverse the #20 and #21 findings, so that #20 becomes higher. While each lens preserves the habitual equilibrium pattern of the #16A and #17A findings, +2.50 is the maximum plus that will preserve the habitual pattern of #21 being higher than #20. The prescribable near net, or MSDA, is therefore +2.50 D. This is the maximum plus that neither exceeds the net cross-cylinder findings nor reverses the habitual blur-point equilibrium pattern, and which can therefore be safely prescribed for near use without risk of creating new interference that could lead to rejection of the lens.

The maximum prescribable safe nearpoint lens balances (but does not reverse) the equilibrium findings. Given, through the habitual near correction

NRA (#21): +1.50

PRA (#20): 0,

+0.75 D sphere would be the indicated maximum nearpoint lens, providing that the lower cross-cylinder net is at least +0.75, and that +0.75 D does not reverse the habitual PRC (#16A) and NRC (#17A) findings.

Since the PRA and NRA findings are measures of flexibility between accommodation and convergence, the lens that equalizes these findings is commonly that which provides optimal balance between accommodation and convergence. The injunction not to prescribe for near use a lens that reverses the pattern of the equilibrium findings is thus similar to the middle-third criterion common in traditional graphical analysis, with the very center of the zone of clear, single binocular vision selected as the goal of the prescription. The lens that balances the NRA and PRA findings (without reversing them) also satisfies Donders' criterion (Donders 1864) that to maintain near work comfortably, the

PRA must be at least as great as the NRA. Thus, the plus lens power indicated by OEP analysis is similar to and frequently identical with that indicated by other methods of case analysis.

Influence of Case Typing

In OEP analysis, the B and C case typings differentiate those patients who will accept and benefit from plus lens application from those who will not. The B case will likely benefit from plus. However, the guidelines for prescribing differ for the B1 and B2 case types. In the B1 case, full-plus is accepted at both distance and near, while in the B2 case, the mandate is to prescribe full-plus at near, but to cut plus at distance. The lens-prescribing guideline for the C case is to cut plus for both distance and near. In the C case, plus lens application is less likely to be effective, and should be approached with caution (Skeffington 1945–51; Manas 1965; Emery 1968–70; Lesser 1969; Hendrickson 1989).

When case typing indicates that plus should be cut at far (in B2 and C type cases), the #7 subjective finding is reduced in plus. When the guidelines indicate that plus should be cut at near (in the C case), the maximum plus prescribable (that portion of the cross-cylinder net that does not reverse the habitual equilibrium findings) is accordingly reduced. When a reduction in plus at distance or near is indicated by the case typing, the usual cut is 0.25 D to 0.75 D, depending on the demand for concentrated application at distance and at near for the particular individual (Manas 1965).

Deterioration, Embedding, and Lens Acceptance

The OEP directives to neither exceed the cross-cylinder nets nor to reverse the habitual equilibrium patterns are designed to determine a lens prescription that operates within the patient's established patterns of function to reduce the stress of the task. A lens prescription that is greater in plus than indicated by these guidelines creates new stress on the patient, a demand to alter established patterns of function, and consequently has greater potential for rejection.

However, under some circumstances, lenses that exceed the guidelines for safe prescribing may serve a useful purpose. Lenses that do not operate within the patient's established pattern of function may serve as a stimulus to trigger effective restructuring and adaptation, so that the patient begins to reorganize his or her visual pattern in a more desirable direction.

However, lenses prescribed out of pattern also have greater potential for rejection. The acceptance or rejection of such lenses may be predicted, at least in part, on the basis of the degree of embedding. The more embedded the case, the greater the degree to which the patient has rigidly organized his pattern of function. In such cases, plus prescribed out-of-pattern is less likely to stimulate desirable change; it is more likely to interfere with established function, with greater likelihood of rejection.

Thus, there is greater freedom to attempt the use of out-of-pattern plus lenses as a stimulus for change when the case is nonembedded. However, even in nonembedded cases, the clinician cannot be certain that such lenses will be effective or that they will be used comfortably.

Not only is there greater freedom to exceed the guidelines in nonembedded cases, but, in general, it is in such cases that indicated plus lenses are expected to have the greatest value. In nonembedded cases, plus lenses for near are generally well accepted and have the greatest potential to increase achievement, prevent adverse adaptation, and reverse adaptation that has already occurred.

The initial impact of nearpoint stress generates interference with binocular function and substantial reduction in the vergence findings. As the patient adapts, reorganizes, and embeds the visual pattern, the findings recover in the direction of the expected values. In OEP theory, low-plus nearpoint lenses are expected to be of greatest benefit in the nonembedded cases (in which the findings are lower). Low-plus lenses resolve the effector system mismatch induced by nearpoint stress, and permit reorganization and normalization of vergence ranges. Vision therapy may not be required.

In embedded cases, although the findings may approach expected levels, nearpoint plus lenses are less well accepted and less beneficial. If treatment is desirable, vision therapy is usually required to disembed the established pattern. This is in contrast with traditional models, in which vision therapy is usually reserved for those cases in which vergence findings are more severely restricted. In OEP theory, the latter are frequently the nonembedded cases in which nearpoint lens application alone may suffice.

As B1 and B2 cases progress through the stages of deterioration, the cross-cylinder and equilibrium findings typically indicate diminished plus lens acceptance. Therefore, in both deteriorated and embedded cases, plus lens application is less likely to improve visual efficiency; vision therapy is required if change is to be achieved (Skeffington 1945–51; Manas 1965; Emery 1968–70).

As deterioration and embedding proceed, plus is less likely to be indicated on the basis of the findings. Further, as the adaptive pattern becomes more rigidly structured, the patient is less likely to accept even that plus which is indicated by the findings. Therefore, the more embedded the case, and the more advanced the syndrome of deterioration, the more caution in lens prescribing is indicated, and the clinician is cautioned to cut the plus lens prescription below that indicated by the analytical examination findings. If change is desired in embedded cases, vision therapy is required to disembed the existing pattern of function (Emery 1968–70).

Astigmatism and Anisometropia

The degree of embedding also plays a role in the determination of astigmatic and anisometropic lens prescriptions. Astigmatism and anisometropia may occur functionally in response to nearpoint stress–induced effector system mismatch or to postural skews that interfere with visual-motor integration. Such adaptations may be present functionally before they become embedded in structure, and are often transient (Skeffington 1951a; Harmon 1958; Birnbaum 1978b, 1985a).

The syndrome of embeddedness indicates the degree to which astigmatism and anisometropia have become structured and require optical compensation. When the pattern of the analytical examination findings is nonembedded, there is greater likelihood that these conditions are transient, or that stress-relieving nearpoint lenses may permit a beneficial reorganization with reduction in astigmatism and anisometropia. If low astigmatic and anisometropic components are incorporated in the prescription at this stage, they may serve to embed a deviation that had previously been nonembedded. It is advisable, therefore, in nonembedded cases, to ignore small astigmatic and anisometropic components of the lens prescription, and to reduce larger ones. However, once the pattern has been embedded, there is less potential for remedial change and greater likelihood that the patient will demand full astigmatic and anisometropic correction. It is well to avoid sudden large changes in prescription, since the embedded case may resist change (Skeffington 1945–51, 1951a; Emery 1968–70).

Lens Acceptance and Spatial Organization

Lens acceptance is also influenced by the patient's pattern of spatial organization (degree of tightness or looseness), which determines the rigidity with which one reacts to induced spatial change. The "tight" patient has restricted flexibility and is more likely to reject lenses that alter perception of space. The clinician is well advised, in the tight case, to modify the spherical, astigmatic, and anisometropic components of the indicated lens in the direction of the habitual prescription, so as not to induce excessive change in spatial perception. Spatial changes are particularly bothersome at distance, but may cause disturbance during near work as well.

Patients whose spatial organization is rigid and inflexible often demonstrate a tight relationship between accommodation and convergence. Since small changes in lens power induce larger phoria changes in such patients, the clinician may anticipate substantial benefit. However, the tight patient may reject a lens that induces a major change in phoria, since the lens may create new interference between accommodation and convergence. It is therefore advised that the lens prescription be reduced if it induces a substantial change in phoria from that obtained with the habitual lens.

Although tight patients tend to reject lenses that disturb spatial orientation, they may benefit substantially from lens changes that are within their capacity to accept. The clinician should thus be cautious in changing the tight patient's prescription, but should also recognize that such patients may benefit substantially from small but appropriate lens changes, sometimes showing dramatic improvement in comfort and visual efficiency with minimal lens change.

The "loose" patient, in contrast, is less structured with respect to spatial organization. Spatial processing is unstable and less reliable. Phoria measures are often variable. The relationship between accommodation and convergence is usually also loose, so that lens changes induce little change in phoria.

Since the AC/A is low and spatial judgements are unreliable, lens changes have little impact on the relationship between accommodation and convergence or on the patient's spatial orientation. Spatial organization is less rigid, and lens changes are well accepted. However, for the same reasons, lens changes often have little impact on performance and provide minimal patient benefit (Emery 1968–70).

Lens Prescribing in Presbyopia

In prescribing for presbyopes, assessment of the individual's task demands, working distances, and special needs assumes even greater importance than in the care of nonpresbyopes. To neglect these factors is to risk prescribing a lens that is correct by all methods of case analysis, but which nevertheless fails to satisfy the patient's needs.

With the exception of this major proviso, case analysis in presbyopia is, in OEP theory, similar to that for nonpresbyopes. In presbyopia, the #14B net (rather than the #7) is used as the control through which to take the nearpoint findings, and the lowered amplitude is taken into account in determining the #5, #14A, and #14B nets. Otherwise, the analytical sequence is performed and the findings are checked and chained in the same manner, regardless of whether the patient is presbyopic.

In determining the lens prescription for the presbyope, as for the nonpresbyope, the limits for distance and near are set by the #7 subjective and the cross-cylinder nets, respectively, and these limits are modified in accordance with the equilibrium findings, case-typing, deterioration, embedding, and spatial organization of the patient, with particular consideration given to the individual patient's special needs. Presbyopes typically show a nonembedded B pattern, since the onset of presbyopia itself serves as a disembedding factor, disrupting the patient's established pattern of organization (Emery 1968–70).

As presbyopia approaches, a decrease in accommodative amplitude exacerbates the nearpoint stress–induced tendency for accommodation to lag beyond convergence. Although standard acuity is maintained in the early stages, visual efficiency is reduced and performance suffers. Many patients experience a decrease in reading comprehension and a need to reread more frequently. Reading becomes less facile and less enjoyable, and patients often lose interest. These changes precede the more advanced symptoms of blur, eyestrain, and the need to hold reading material farther away. These early symptoms are quite subtle; although reading achievement becomes lowered, the early signs may escape notice by the patient, or be attributed to other factors.

Skeffington (1951b) advises that the practitioner, knowing of the changes about to ensue, apply increased plus at near prior to the manifestation of presbyopia, before the patient experiences difficulty, in order to prevent a loss of achievement and visual efficiency when presbyopia occurs. He states that low-plus lenses, judiciously prescribed just in advance of ensuing presbyopia, allow the patient to maintain visual function at a more nearly optimal level. Further, Skeffington implies that if such lenses are not prescribed and visual efficiency is compromised, the ensuing loss in achievement is not necessarily restored by later presbyopic lens correction. Flexibility that is lost as the patient adapts to nearpoint stress early in presbyopia does not automatically return when lenses are later provided to restore acuity.

SUMMARY

OEP case analysis is based on the assumption that it is desirable to prescribe plus lens power for near to relieve the drive for convergence to localize closer than accommodation postulated by Skeffington as intrinsic to the near-point visual tasks of society. OEP analysis is designed to determine the optimal near plus lens addition (as well as the best distance prescription) that will be well accepted and provide maximum benefit.

A 21-point analytical examination is performed and the findings are classified as high or low. High and low findings are then grouped into syndromes or case-typings, and further analyzed to determine the depth of deterioration and degree of embedding of the problem.

The #7 subjective and the cross-cylinder nets determine the maximum plus prescriptions for far and near, respectively. These maximums are modified based on the case-typing, analysis of the blur-point findings, stage of deterioration, degree of embeddedness, and pattern of spatial organization, to determine for each distance the lens prescription that can be safely prescribed.

In nonembedded cases, plus lens application has significant potential to restore visual efficiency, prevent adverse adaptation, and reverse adaptation that has already occurred. As deterioration and embedding proceed, plus lens acceptance diminishes and there is greater likelihood that vision therapy will be required to restore efficient function.

SUGGESTED READING

Emery LC (1968–70). *Optometric Case Analysis.* Optometric Extension Program Continuing Education Courses, Santa Ana, CA: Optometric Extension Program Foundation, Oct. 1968–Sept. 1970.
Hendrickson H (1989). *The Behavioral Optometry Approach to Lens Prescribing.* Rev. ed. Santa Ana, CA: Optometric Extension Program Foundation.
Lesser SK (1969). *Introduction to Modern Analytical Optometry.* Rev. ed., first publ. 1935. Santa Ana, CA: Optometric Extension Program Foundation.
Manas L (1965). *Visual Analysis.* Chicago: Professional Press.
Skeffington AM (1941–50). *An Introduction to Near Point Refraction.* Optometric Extension Continuing Education Courses, Santa Ana, CA: Optometric Extension Program Foundation, vol 1–9, Oct. 1941–Sept. 1950.
Skeffington AM, Lesser SK, Barstow R (1945–51). *Near Point Optometry.* Optometric Extension Program Continuing Education Courses, Santa Ana, CA: Optometric Extension Program Foundation, vol 1–6, Oct. 1945–Sept. 1951.

REFERENCES

Betts EA, Austin AS (1941). Seeing problems of school children. XXII. Summary and conclusions. *Optom Weekly* 32:369–371.
Birnbaum MH (1978a). Holistic aspects of visual style: A hemispheric model with implications for vision therapy. *J Am Optom Assoc* 49(10):1133–1144.

Birnbaum MH (1978b). Functional relationship between myopia, accommodative stress, and against-the-rule astigmia: A hypothesis. *J Am Optom Assoc* 49(8):911–914.

Birnbaum MH (1981). Esotropia, exotropia and cognitive/perceptual style. *J Am Optom Assoc* 52(8):635–639.

Birnbaum MH (1985a). Nearpoint visual stress. Clinical implications. *J Am Optom Assoc* 56(6):480–490.

Birnbaum MH (1985b). An esophoric shift associated with sustained fixation. *Am J Optom Physiol Opt* 62(11):732–735.

Borish IM (1970). *Clinical Refraction*. 3rd ed. Chicago: Professional Press.

Carlson NB, Kurtz D, Heath DA, et al. (1990). *Clinical Procedures for Ocular Examination*. Norwalk, CT: Appleton and Lange.

Donders FC (1864). *On the Anomalies of Accommodation and Refraction of the Eye*. Translated by W.D. Moore. London: New Sydenham Society.

Eisenberg S (1974). *Manual of Clinical Optometric Procedures*. New York: State University of New York, State College of Optometry.

Emery LC (1968–70). *Optometric Case Analysis*. Optometric Extension Program Continuing Education Courses, Santa Ana, CA: Optometric Extension Program Foundation, Oct. 1968–Sept. 1970.

Flax N (1984). A current look at the OEP B1 and B2 case typings. *J Optom Vis Dev* 15(1):19–21.

Flax N (1985). Functional case analysis: An interpretation of the Skeffington model. *Am J Optom Physiol Opt* 62(6):365–368.

Forrest E (1976). Clinical manifestations of visual information processing. *J Am Optom Assoc* 47(1):73–80; 47(4):499–507.

Getman GN (1970–71). *Vision Development and the Analytical Examination*. Optometric Extension Program Continuing Education Courses, Santa Ana, CA: Optometric Extension Program Foundation.

Getman GN, Kephart NC (1957). The Development of Ocular Fixation. In: *Developmental Vision*. Optometric Extension Program Postgraduate Courses, Santa Ana, CA: Optometric Extension Program Foundation, vol. 30, series 2, no. 3:17–23, Dec.

Goss DA (1986). *Ocular Accommodation, Convergence and Fixation Disparity: A Manual of Clinical Analysis*. New York: Professional Press.

Griffin JR, Lee RA (1984). Visual skills norms in college students. *Optom Monthly* 75(2):103–104.

Haines H (1941). Normal values of visual functions and their application in case analysis. *Am J Optom Arch Am Acad Optom* 18(1):1–8.

Harmon DB (1958). *Notes on a Dynamic Theory of Vision*. 3rd rev. ed. Austin, TX: Author.

Hendrickson H (1989). *The Behavioral Optometry Approach to Lens Prescribing*. Rev. ed. Santa Ana, CA: Optometric Extension Program Foundation.

Hirsch MJ, Bing LB (1948). The effect of testing method on values obtained for phoria at forty centimeters. *Am J Optom Arch Am Acad Optom* 25(9):407–416.

Jackson TW, Goss DA (1991). Variation and correlation of standard clinical phoropter tests of phorias, vergence ranges, and relative accommodation in a sample of school-age children. *J Am Optom Assoc* 62(7):540–547.

Kraskin RA (1968). *You Can Improve Your Vision*. Garden City, NY: Doubleday, pp. 78–81.

Kraskin RA (1981). *Lens Power in Action*. Optometric Extension Program Continuing Education Courses, Santa Ana, CA: Optometric Extension Program Foundation, vol. 54, series 1, no. 2, Nov.

Lesser SK (1969). *Introduction to Modern Analytical Optometry*. Rev. ed., first publ. 1935. Santa Ana, CA: Optometric Extension Program Foundation.

MacDonald L (1973). Presentation at annual meeting, College of Optometrists in Vision Development. Cassette recording, Insta-Tape, Pasadena, CA.

Manas L (1965). *Visual Analysis*. Chicago: Professional Press.

Margach CB (1976). Tenets of functional optometry. *Opt J Rev Optom* 113(6):38–50, 113(7):28–31.

Morgan MW (1944a). Analysis of clinical data. *Am J Optom Arch Am Acad Optom* 21(12):477–491.

Morgan MW (1944b). The clinical aspects of accommodation and convergence. *Am J Optom Arch Am Acad Optom* 21(8):301–313.

Morgan MW (1955). The reliability of clinical measurements with special reference to distance heterophoria. *Am J Optom Arch Am Acad Optom* 32(4):167–179.

Saladin JJ, Sheedy JE (1978). A population study of relationships between fixation disparity, heterophorias and vergences. *Am J Optom Physiol Opt* 55(11):744–750.

Schor CM, Narayan V (1982). Graphical analysis of prism adaptation, convergence accommodation and accommodative convergence. *Am J Optom Physiol Opt* 59:774–784.

Shepard CF (1941). The most probable "expecteds." *Optom Weekly* 32:538–541.

Skeffington AM (1928). *Procedure in Ocular Examination*. Chicago: A.J. Cox.

Skeffington AM (1928–74). Optometric Extension Program Continuing Education Courses, Santa Ana, CA: Optometric Extension Program Foundation.

Skeffington AM (1931). *Differential Diagnosis in Ocular Examination*. Chicago: A.J. Cox.

Skeffington AM (1941–50). *An Introduction to Near Point Refraction*. Optometric Extension Program Continuing Education Courses, Santa Ana, CA: Optometric Extension Program Foundation, vol 1–9, Oct. 1941–Sept. 1950.

Skeffington AM (1951a). The astigmat who required reduction in the cylinder. In: *Practical Applied Optometry*. Optometric Extension Program Continuing Education Courses, Santa Ana, CA: Optometric Extension Program Foundation, 29(9):61–70, Sept.

Skeffington AM (1951b). Lenses as preventative devices in the presbyope. In: *Practical Applied Optometry*. Optometric Extension Program Continuing Education Courses, Santa Ana, CA: Optometric Extension Program Foundation, 23(11):81–88, Nov.

Skeffington AM (1953). The phorias. In: *Practical Applied Optometry*. Optometric Extension Program Continuing Education Courses, Santa Ana, CA: Optometric Extension Program Foundation, vol. 25, Jan., Feb.

Skeffington AM (1972). *The Skeffington Colloquium Outline*. Santa Ana, CA: Optometric Extension Program Foundation.

Skeffington AM, Lesser SK, Barstow R (1945–51). *Near Point Optometry*. Optometric Extension Program Continuing Education Courses, Santa Ana, CA: Optometric Extension Program Foundation, vol. 1–6, Oct. 1945–Sept. 1951.

Smith GW (1973). If It's There, It's in the Analytical. St. Louis: Conference on Visual Training and Theoretical Optometry, transcript by Caryl Croisant, O.D., San Luis Obispo, CA.

Wesson MD, Amos JF (1985). Norms for hand-held rotary prism vergences. *Am J Optom Physiol Opt* 62(2):88–94.

Woolf D (1963–64). *Visual Function in Theory and Practice*. Optometric Extension Program Continuing Education Courses, Santa Ana, CA: Optometric Extension Program Foundation, Series 1, No. 9, June, p. 44.

9

Alternative Approaches to Lens Prescribing

PRACTICAL APPLIED CASE ANALYSIS

Formal OEP analysis is rarely performed in current practice. Similarly, few practitioners actually use a graph to formally apply graphical analysis. Most functional practitioners analyze findings informally through the use of systems derived from the Skeffington model and/or graphical methods, modified by clinical experience and insight. The following is a synthesis of this author's approach to case analysis.

In looking at the analytical findings for signs of functional vision disorder, particular consideration should be given to the refractive status, the near-phoria finding, the prism vergence measures, and the PRA finding. The expected refractive status is approximately +0.50 to +0.75 D sphere. The presence of emmetropia or low myopia is viewed as a response to nearpoint stress, and is usually accompanied by constricted phorometric findings.

The near-phoria measure is highly significant. Deviation from the expected 4 to 6$^\Delta$ exophoria suggests the presence or likely development of nearpoint stress–induced vision disorder. Low exophoria (1 to 3$^\Delta$), orthophoria, or esophoria is an early sign of nearpoint stress–induced overconvergence, since it is likely that, during sustained nearpoint application, the cumulative effect of vigilant attention, mental effort, stress, containment, and accommodation-convergence interaction is to generate greater overconvergence than is demonstrated during the analytical routine. Such overconvergence can often be demonstrated during the examination by taking consecutive near-phoria measures; many patients show a progressive shift toward esophoria as a function of intensity and time (Birnbaum 1985). Failure to initiate appropriate care is frequently followed by myopia, avoidance, or other adverse adaptation.

Exophoria greater than 6$^\Delta$ suggests that the individual has built a buffer against overconvergence so as to achieve alignment during sustained near work. Although this adaptation prevents actual overconvergence with resultant diplopia, it is less efficient than myopia. Clinically, it is noted that most high exophores avoid close work or report asthenopic symptoms.

A low PRA (#20) finding is another key sign of nearpoint stress. In nearpoint stress—induced vision disorders, the tendency is for convergence to localize closer than accommodation. Such patients have difficulty reversing this pattern to shift accommodation closer than convergence, and thus show low PRA measures.

Constricted prism vergence findings at distance or near are also viewed as signs of nearpoint stress. When accommodation and convergence are well integrated, binocular visual function is efficient and prism vergence measures approach expected levels. Effector system mismatch interferes with binocular function; this interference manifests as poor fusion ability, with low prism vergence findings. Constricted prism vergence measures can thus be viewed not as fusional reserves, to be compared with the phoria, but rather as indicators of binocular interference resulting from nearpoint stress. Which findings are low, and whether at distance, or near, or both, indicate the patterns of adaptation undertaken to cope with nearpoint stress.

Most patients show signs of functional vision disorder. However, not all such individuals require treatment. The presence of asthenopia suggests that adaptation has been inadequate to meet the needs of the patient and that treatment should be undertaken. When symptoms are absent, it may be because the patient has adapted satisfactorily, or adopted a life-style that no longer imposes near-work demands sufficient to cause difficulty. Such patients frequently do not require therapy.

However, the absence of symptoms does not mean that functional vision disorder should be ignored. Many patients with constricted phorometric findings refrain from near work and hence avoid asthenopia. Others develop or increase myopia to facilitate nearpoint function. Treatment should therefore be advised when indicated by the presence of constricted findings, even in the absence of asthenopic symptoms, if the case history shows a pattern of avoidance or disinterest in reading, or if the examination suggests the presence of ongoing adaptation (such as increasing myopia).

Treatment should also be seriously considered, even in the absence of symptoms, when a future increase in near-work demand is expected as a child progresses through school, or when an adult anticipates a vocational change that will require increased near work. When inadequate visual function is untreated, previously asymptomatic patients frequently experience severe asthenopia or demonstrate adverse adaptive change, often toward myopia, when academic or vocational demands for sustained near work increase.

Determining the Nearpoint Plus Lens Prescription

The determination as to whether plus lens application is indicated, and the amount of plus to be prescribed, is based largely on the examination findings and observation of the patient's performance with the proposed lenses. When the analytical findings suggest that nearpoint plus lens application is indicated, prescription of such lenses is viewed as desirable, rather than as something to be avoided.

During the analytical refraction, the practitioner selects a tentative nearpoint lens prescription through which to perform the prism vergence and relative accommodation findings. These findings are usually performed through the fused cross-cylinder (#14B), unless the #14B shifts the near phoria into excess exophoria. The relative convergence findings are frequently taken through both the subjective refraction and the fused cross-cylinder findings, so that the impact of plus lens application on the prism vergence measures can be determined.

After completing the analytical routine, the findings used initially by the author to assess indications for nearpoint plus prescription are the near-phoria measure (#13B), the fused cross-cylinder (#14B) and its effect on the near phoria (#15B), and the PRA and NRA (#20 and #21). Plus lens prescription is generally given (unless plus adversely lowers the NRA or prism vergence findings) under the following conditions: when the near phoria is in esophoria, orthophoria, or less than 3^Δ exophoria; when the #14B indicates plus acceptance and has a positive effect in shifting the near phoria toward a more desirable 4 to 6^Δ exophoria; and when the PRA (#20) finding is low.

If the NRA (#21) is high and the PRA (#20) is low, plus lens application is generally indicated. The #20 and #21 should not be thought of as accommodative findings, but rather as measures of the flexibility between accommodation and convergence. When the NRA is high and the PRA is low, plus is indicated to provide optimal balance, with maximum freedom of operation between vergence and accommodation. The plus lens addition usually prescribed by the author balances (or equalizes) the NRA and PRA findings. For example, if the following is obtained through the subjective refraction

$$\text{NRA: } +1.25 \text{ D}$$

$$\text{PRA: } -0.25 \text{ D,}$$

the indicated prescription would be a $+0.50$ addition for near use.

Although in most cases the plus prescribed for near is that which equalizes the NRA and PRA findings, this may be modified depending on the effect of plus on the near-phoria and prism vergence measures, the patient's subjective reaction to the indicated plus lenses, the dynamic retinoscopy findings, the case history, and probes of performance with the lenses.

In cases in which the NRA and PRA taken through the fused cross-cylinder indicate the need for additional plus, this author will generally prescribe such plus despite the OEP injunction not to exceed the cross-cylinder net, providing that the additional plus is subjectively well accepted and does not adversely affect the vergence findings. For some patients, the cross-cylinder is a less reliable finding, and more plus can be prescribed with confidence when it is indicated by the NRA and PRA findings, and subjectively preferred by the patient.

Prescribing When Near Phoria Is Esophoria or Low Exophoria

When patients demonstrate esophoria or inadequate exophoria at near, plus should be prescribed if it produces a more adequate nearpoint exophoria and is well accepted on the basis of the NRA and PRA and prism vergence findings. Following are some examples of the author's approach:

1.

> #7: plano
> #13B: 2 esophoria
> #14B: +1.00
> #15B: 3 exophoria

through O.U. +1.00 sphere:

> NRA: +1.00
> PRA: −1.00

This author would prescribe O.U. +1.00 spheres for nearpoint use.

2. Given the same findings, except through O.U. +1.00 spheres:

> NRA: +0.50
> PRA: −1.00

the author would reduce the plus lens prescription to O.U. +0.75 to balance the NRA and PRA findings.

3. If the findings are the same, except through O.U. +1.00 spheres:

> NRA: +1.00
> PRA: −0.50

the author would increase the nearpoint plus lens prescription to O.U. +1.25 to balance the NRA and PRA findings, even though such prescription exceeds the cross-cylinder net.

4. Again given the same findings, except through +1.00 spheres:

> NRA: +0.50
> PRA: −0.50

O.U. +1.00 spheres, would be prescribed for near use since it moves the near phoria toward desirable exophoria and balances the NRA and PRA findings. Although the NRA and PRA are balanced, they are quite low, indicating a lack of flexibility between vergence and accommodation. Vision therapy is advisable, in addition to nearpoint lens prescription, to develop greater flexibility.

5.

> #7: plano
> #13B: 1 exophoria
> #14B: no add
> NRA: +1.75
> PRA: −0.25
> +0.75 add gives 4 exophoria

Although the #14B suggests no plus acceptance, the NRA and PRA findings indicate that plus will be well accepted. Plus shifts the near phoria toward more desirable exophoria. I would override the #14B finding and prescribe O.U. +0.75 sphere for near use.

6.

#7: plano
#13B: 1 exophoria
#14B: no add
NRA: +0.50
PRA: −0.50

Plus lens application is not indicated on the basis of the #14B or the NRA and PRA findings. Vision therapy is indicated to develop greater plus acceptance and to develop flexibility between accommodation and convergence. Plus lens power should not be prescribed until it is better accepted.

7.

#7: plano
#13B: 1 exophoria
#14B: +0.50
#15B: 3 exophoria
through +0.50:
NRA: +0.50
PRA: −1.25

Although plus lens prescription is indicated by the favorable effect of the #14B on the near phoria, the NRA and PRA findings suggest that plus will not be well accepted. Vision therapy is indicated to develop greater flexibility between accommodation and convergence. As therapy proceeds, the examination findings frequently indicate greater plus acceptance. The development of such plus acceptance is viewed in OEP analysis as an important goal of vision therapy.

Prescribing When Near Exophoria Is High

Plus is also indicated in those cases in which the plus of the #14B reduces high exophoria toward a more desirable level. Contrary to the traditional assumption that plus always increases nearpoint exophoria, cases such as the following are sometimes encountered:

#13B: 9 exophoria
#14B: +0.75
#15B: 6 exophoria

Reduction in nearpoint exophoria with plus may occur when individuals with accommodative deficiency do not accommodate fully for near, and hence show high exophoria. Low-plus may "prime the pump" by reducing accommodative demand to more achievable levels, so that more accommodation actually comes into play, reducing the exophoria.

An alternative explanation of this phenomenon suggests that high exophoria develops as an adaptive response to buffer nearpoint stress—induced overconvergence that would otherwise manifest during near work. Low-plus lenses relieve the underlying overconvergence, and thus eliminate the need for an exophoric buffer. Reduction in exophoria may occur as an immediate adaptive response when low-plus lenses are applied.

Nearpoint plus lenses may or may not be indicated for patients who show adequate or high exophoria at near. Key indicators are the NRA and PRA findings, and the effect of plus on the near phoria:

1.
        #7: plano
        #13B: 6 exophoria
        #14B: +0.75
        #15B: 9 exophoria
        through +0.75:
        NRA: +1.50
        PRA: −2.50

This patient shows a desirable 6^Δ nearpoint exophoria through plano. The findings suggest a maximum nearpoint lens acceptance of +0.25 D. The +0.75 D of the #14B creates excessive exophoria, adversely affects the NRA/PRA balance, and is therefore not indicated. The adequate nearpoint exophoria and adequate NRA and PRA findings without lenses suggest that neither nearpoint lenses nor vision training is indicated.

2.
        #7: plano
        #13B: 5 exophoria
        #14B: +0.75
        #15B: 6 exophoria
        through +0.75:
        NRA: +0.75
        PRA: −0.75

Although the patient shows adequate exophoria at near, plus is indicated for near use. The PRA is low; if plus is not given, the PRA through plano would be 0.00 D. The appropriate prescription would be +0.75 D sphere, since the NRA and PRA are balanced through it and the #15B indicates that +0.75 will not increase the near exophoria excessively.

3.
        #7: plano
        #13B: 8 exophoria
        #14B: +0.75
        #15B: 5 exophoria
        through +0.75:
        NRA: +1.50
        PRA: −1.25

The #14B reduces excessive near exophoria, and should be prescribed. The NRA and PRA are balanced through the #14B. A nearpoint lens prescription, O.U. +0.75, should be adequate, without need for vision therapy.

4.

#7: plano
#13B: 8 exophoria
#14B: +0.75
#15B: 5 exophoria
through +0.75:
NRA: +0.50
PRA: −0.50

As in example 3, O.U. +0.75 lowers the near exophoria, balances the NRA and PRA, and should be prescribed. In addition, the severely constricted NRA and PRA findings suggest that vision therapy to expand flexibility between vergence and accommodation will be beneficial.

5.

#7: plano
#13B: 8 exophoria
#14B: +0.75
#15B: 12 exophoria
through +0.75:
NRA: +1.50
PRA: −1.25

The NRA and PRA suggest that plus is indicated, but plus increases an already high nearpoint exophoria and may not be well accepted. One course of action is to initiate vision therapy to improve binocular function, and to provide nearpoint plus lenses later. An alternative is to prescribe plus, monitor whether the exophoria reduces as adaptation takes place, and initiate vision therapy if it does not.

Indications for nearpoint plus lens prescription may develop as vision therapy proceeds in cases of convergence insufficiency. High exophoria, built in to buffer overconvergence under fused conditions, often reduces to lowered exophoria or even esophoria at near. At this stage, the #14B, the #15B induced phoria, the NRA/PRA relationship, and the shift toward esophoria at near each signal that nearpoint plus is indicated and will be well accepted.

Effect on Prism Vergences

The effect of plus lenses on the prism vergence (NRC and PRC) measures must also be considered. When plus is indicated by the #14B, NRA and PRA findings, but significantly reduces the PRC, plus may not be well accepted, and should not be prescribed until vergence ranges are expanded through vision therapy.

Mechanistic graphical analysis of the relationship between accommodation and convergence suggests that plus lens application, by reducing accommodation and hence increasing exophoria, will increase the NRC finding and decrease the PRC. This is not always the case. Often, both the NRC and PRC findings increase with plus, as plus lenses allow more effective integration of accommodation and convergence, and hence greater flexibility between systems. Plus lens prescription is strongly indicated in such cases.

Plus Lens Prescription in Presbyopia

Rules of thumb similar to Sheard's and Percival's criteria for prism prescription have been formulated to assist in the determination of the nearpoint add for presbyopes. One such rule is that the patient should not be required to sustain use of more than one half of the amplitude of accommodation. A related rule requires balancing the plus lens to blur (NRA) and minus lens to blur (PRA) findings, suggesting that the proper add is that which equalizes these findings. The near cross-cylinder test yields the lens power with which the retina is conjugate to the test target; this finding is often used to determine a tentative presbyopic add, which is then refined by testing the NRA, PRA, and range of clarity through it (Goss 1986). This author generally prescribes that plus which balances the NRA and PRA findings, since this reduces stress on accommodation and provides optimal flexibility between vergence and accommodation.

Patients who demonstrate high exophoria through indicated plus lenses may require vision therapy. However, in some cases, adaptive processes operate to reduce exophoria when plus lenses are worn, so that vision therapy is not required. When patients show high exophoria through indicated plus lenses, it may therefore be best to prescribe the plus, explain the possible need for vision therapy, and see the patient for progress evaluation in a month or two.

The clinician must differentiate those patients whose exophoria is induced by presbyopic lens correction from those whose exophoria is long-standing. Those whose exophoria is induced by plus are at significant risk for symptoms and visual inefficiency, and should either be offered vision therapy or monitored carefully. Those with long-standing exophoria frequently demonstrate patterns of suppression or avoidance that are so ingrained that there is little need for treatment.

Since presbyopes have reduced accommodative flexibility, it is important to determine the patient's typical working distance(s) and to prescribe lenses appropriate for these distances. A tape measure can be used to accurately measure simulated working distances. In addition, careful attention must be given to the selection of single vision and multifocal lens designs appropriate for the specific tasks performed by the patient.

SUPPLEMENTARY TESTS IN NEARPOINT LENS APPLICATION

The amount of plus to be prescribed may be modified on the basis of supplementary tests, including dynamic retinoscopy, the patient's subjective reaction to plus, and tests of the patient's performance through plus lenses.

Dynamic retinoscopy originated in the late 1800s, according to Pascal (1930, 1952), as a procedure to permit measurement of the amplitude of accommodation in cases in which subjective tests were not possible. Cross (1911), concerned that hyperopia masked by accommodative spasm might not be disclosed by noncycloplegic refraction, developed dynamic retinoscopic procedures to uncover latent hyperopia and thereby aid in determination of the "true" refractive state. Sheard (1920), Tait (1929), and Pascal (1930, 1952), among others, developed dynamic retinoscopy procedures designed to uncover latency, to assess the relationship between accommodation and convergence, and to determine the appropriate nearpoint lens prescription. Modern dynamic retinoscopy procedures include monocular estimate method (MEM), bell, book, and stress-point retinoscopy. Valenti (1990) has reviewed these procedures.

MEM Retinoscopy

MEM retinoscopy is a method developed by Haynes (1960, 1985) to assist in the determination of the nearpoint lens prescription. The examiner retinoscopically determines the lag of accommodation under dynamic conditions as the patient reads grade-appropriate material. The test indicates the accommodative posture (or response) under controlled conditions of reading demand with any particular tentative lens prescription.

MEM test cards are available with material suitable for preschool through adult levels. Each card has a central aperture through which the examiner observes the retinoscopic reflex. The reading material is printed adjacent to and surrounding the aperture (Figure 9.1). Error induced by off-axis oblique refraction is minimized, since retinoscopic observation takes place very close to the visual axis. The MEM card is attached to the retinoscope by means of a specially designed clip. MEM target materials and retinoscope clips are available from Dr. Jack Pierce.

Testing is usually performed either at 16 inches or the patient's Harmon distance. The patient, with both eyes open, reads the words surrounding the aperture on the MEM test card. The examiner observes the retinoscopic reflex of each eye and estimates its dioptric value. This estimate is verified by briefly interposing a neutralizing trial lens, monocularly, first before one eye and then the other (Figure 9.2). The actual or estimated lens value required to neutralize the retinoscopic reflex constitutes the MEM finding, and is an objective measure of the lag of accommodation.

It is critical that the examiner observe the motion quickly when the lens is interposed. If the lens is in place for longer than one fifth of a second (the average reaction time to an accommodative stimulus), the examiner will be observing the response to the lens, rather than the accommodative posture that existed before its interposition. If necessary, the measuring lens may be introduced repeatedly, but each interposition of the lens must be very brief.

MEM retinoscopy may be viewed as an objective correlate of the binocular cross-cylinder test, the former giving an objective and the latter a subjective measure of the lag of accommodation. The lag varies with accommodative de-

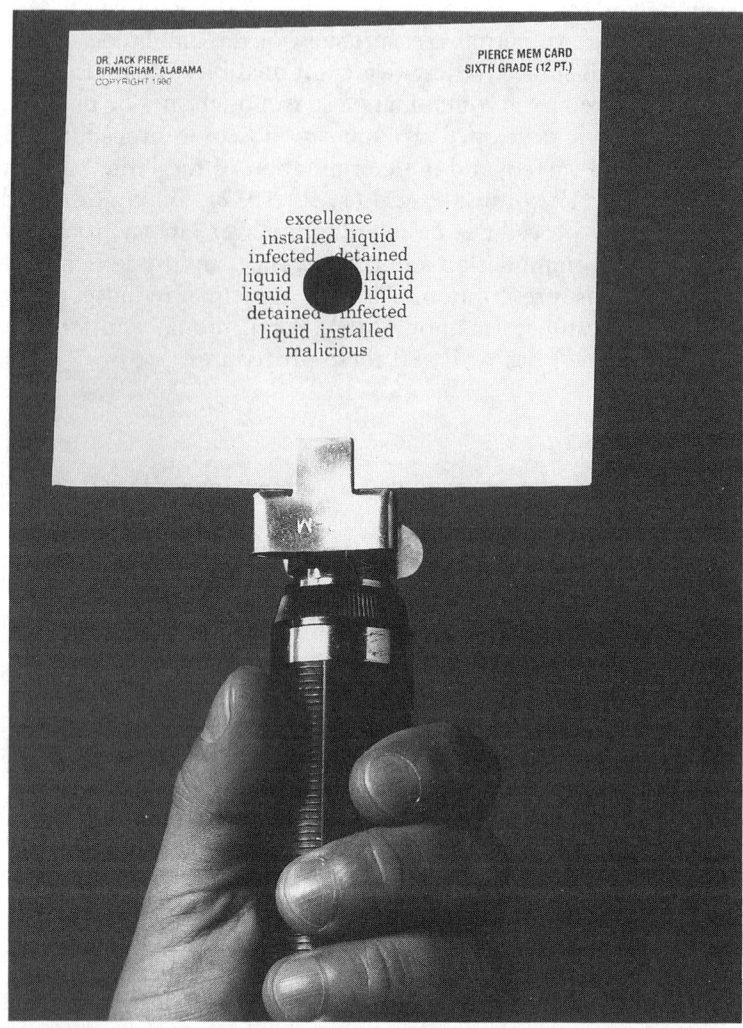

Figure 9.1 The MEM card. Reading material surrounds a central aperture through which the examiner observes the retinoscopic reflex. (Reprinted with permission of Dr. Jack Pierce.)

mand, with the size and nature of the target material, and with the level of attention and cognitive demand (Haynes 1960; Kruger 1980). The cross-cylinder grid presents less cognitive demand and requires less accommodation for identification than does the demand for reading words presenting during MEM retinoscopy. Hence, a higher lag is usually obtained on the fused cross-cylinder test. Haynes (1960) reports that when a plain white card with a vertical line target is substituted for the standard MEM card, the lag closely approximates the cross-cylinder finding, showing 0.25 to 0.50 more "with" motion than is obtained with printed words.

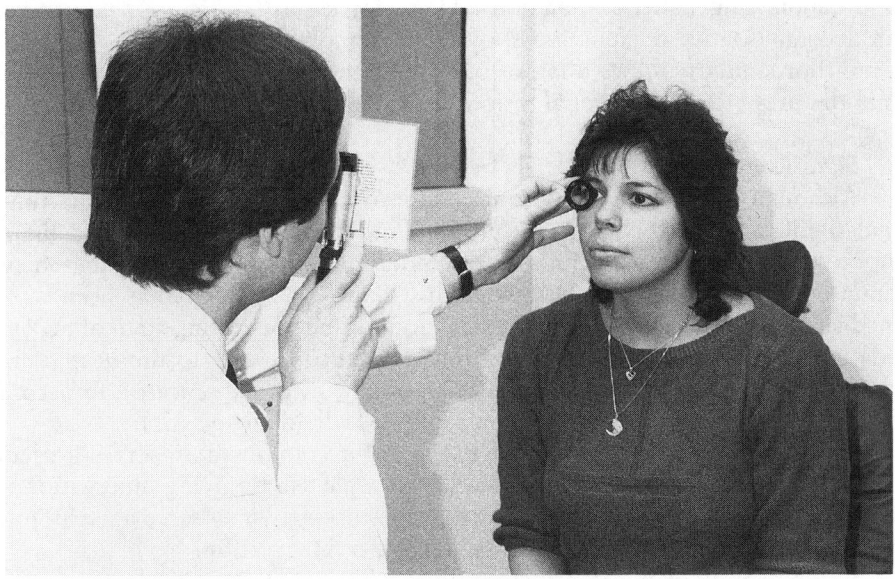

Figure 9.2 Performing MEM retinoscopy. As the patient reads the words, the examiner observes the retinoscopic reflex through the aperture of the MEM card and briefly interposes a trial lens before one eye to neutralize the motion of the reflex.

The validity of MEM retinoscopy as an objective clinical method for determining accommodative response has been documented by Rouse et al. (1982), who found a close correlation between MEM and haploscopic measures of lag of accommodation. McKee (1981) demonstrated a high degree of interexaminer reliability, two examiners agreeing with 0.25 D in 71.8% and within 0.50 D in 93% of the cases.

In any dynamic retinoscopy procedure, it is important to observe the motion in the center of the pupil. Substantial variability is obtained when observers neutralize different areas of the pupillary reflex. Greater "against" motion is usually obtained when the peripheral portion of the reflex is neutralized (Streff and Claussen 1971; Charman and Walsh 1989).

MEM Norms
Weisz (1983) reports that the normal MEM finding is usually between 0.25 and 0.50 D of "with" motion, corresponding to the normal lag of accommodation. Jackson and Goss (1991) report a mean MEM finding of +0.23 D in school-age children, and Rouse et al. (1984) obtained similar values (median, +0.25 D; range, −0.75 to +2.00 D; mean, +0.34 D; SD, ±0.34) in a sample of children age 4 to 12 years. McKee (1981) found an average MEM of +0.75 D when retinoscopy was performed at 11 inches in 5- to 10-year-old children. This relatively high lag may relate to the unusually close working distance.

Individuals with accommodative insufficiency may show excessive "with" motion, indicating a greater than normal lag. Haynes (1960) reports that patients with accommodative dysfunction show "with" motion of +0.75 to +1.75 D. This author similarly views a lag of 0.75 D or more as excessive, and likely to signal the presence of functional vision disorder.

Significance of the Lag

Although a small lag of accommodation is considered normal, the functional significance of this lag is uncertain. Traditionally, it was assumed that a lag occurs when one accommodates the minimum amount required to achieve adequate resolution at near. However, this "lazy lag" concept has been questioned since Liebowitz and Owens (1975) found that the resting state of accommodation, once assumed to be at infinity, is actually closer to the near point. Liebowitz and Owens found a mean level of TA, in the absence of an accommodative stimulus, of 1.7 D, with considerable individual variation.

Schor et al. (1986) suggest that the lag of accommodation serves a useful purpose, providing a steady-state stimulus to replenish decaying innervation to accommodation, in the same way that fixation disparity may serve a useful purpose as a stimulus to replenish decaying vergence innervation.

In the context of the Skeffington model, the normal lag of accommodation may result from a mild inhibition of accommodation that serves to reduce overconvergence associated with nearpoint stress. When this mild inhibition is not sufficient, increased inhibition of accommodation, with increased lag, is one path of adaptation. Such inhibition avoids diplopia, which would otherwise result from overconvergence, but is nevertheless maladaptive in that it contributes to visual inefficiency. In this view, excessive lag of accommodation may reflect an active inhibition, rather than a true weakness of accommodation.

Prescribing from MEM Retinoscopy

The dioptric value of the lag of accommodation measured or estimated during MEM retinoscopy constitutes the MEM finding. Once this finding is obtained, Haynes (1985) recommends that the examiner add plus lenses binocularly in 0.25-D to 0.50-D steps until the first neutral motion ("low neutral") is observed. As plus is added, the examiner makes additional MEM estimates with each change of sphere, to assess the accommodative response to plus lenses of various powers. The combined MEM/low neutral (LN) procedure thus provides an objective measure of the lag of accommodation and an indication of the accommodative response to different lens powers. Both pieces of information are used in the determination of the nearpoint lens prescription.

A high MEM finding, characterized by excessive "with" motion, indicates that accommodation is postured excessively beyond the plane of regard. A nearpoint plus lens prescription is required to bring accommodation closer to the plane of regard and permit more efficient nearpoint function.

A neutral reflex indicates that accommodation is localized at the plane of regard, with no lag, and usually with little plus acceptance.

"Against" motion indicates that accommodation is localized closer than the plane of regard. It is uncommon to obtain "against" motion when MEM is performed through the distance refraction. Such a finding is indicative of spasm of accommodation (Rutstein et al. 1988), and may be a precursor of myopia. In some cases, nearpoint plus serves to relax accommodation; more frequently, however, accommodation does not relax through plus, and MEM shows increased "against" motion, suggesting that plus lenses are unlikely to be well accepted.

When the lag of accommodation is excessive, a nearpoint plus lens addition is indicated to posture accommodation more appropriately with respect to the plane of regard. Haynes (1985) proposes two criteria for determining the nearpoint lens addition based on the MEM lag itself: (1) prescribe the average value of the MEM lag if it is 0.75 D or more; (2) prescribe the minimum plus which produces a 0.50 D "with" motion.

The amount of plus lens power required to achieve a normal lag varies with the individual patient, and is determined by adding plus spheres binocularly and repeating MEM retinoscopy. Some patients make no change in accommodative response as plus is added, and the lag reduces in direct proportion to the plus lens power added. Other patients relax accommodation as plus is added, so that more plus than predicted is necessary to reduce the lag to its normal value (Haynes 1985). This author views a lag of 0.12 to 0.50 D as normal, and typically prescribes a nearpoint lens addition that creates a lag within this range.

In addition to the two criteria listed above based on the MEM lag, Haynes (1985) proposes two criteria for nearpoint add determination based on the LN finding: (1) subtract 0.87 D from the LN finding; (2) subtract 0.37 D from the LN finding. Criterion 2 obviously yields a higher nearpoint addition than does criterion 1.

When patients show a normal lag of accommodation, but plus prescription is desirable to reduce overconvergence, the acceptance of such lenses may be predicted by adding plus lenses binocularly and observing the accommodative response to a variety of "probe lenses" or tentative prescriptions. As plus is added, some individuals with normal lag fail to relax accommodation, so that an initial 0.50-D "with" motion goes to neutral when +0.50 D spheres are added, and to "against" when plus is increased. Such individuals are unlikely to benefit from plus, since there is little physiologic effect.

Other individuals with normal lag relax accommodation as plus lens power is added, maintaining "with" motion until a point is reached where further accommodative relaxation is not possible and the retinoscopic reflex goes over to "against." When the analytical examination or other tests suggest that plus is desirable to reduce overconvergence, this demonstration of accommodative relaxation in response to plus suggests likely acceptance and benefit from such prescription. The amount of plus to be prescribed in such cases is determined by the analytical findings and by the patient's subjective response to plus, as well as by MEM retinoscopy.

When tests give differing indications as to the amount of plus lens power to prescribe, MEM retinoscopy may be used to determine the maximum plus that is likely to be accepted. This limit is determined by adding plus lens power until the high neutral (HN), the point at which additional plus power causes a shift to "against" motion, is reached. Plus greater than the HN measure causes accommodation to localize nearer than the plane of regard, and is likely to interfere with usual function.

MEM and Tonic Accommodation

Press (1990) points out that the tonic (or resting) level of accommodation is not at infinity, but considerably closer. For a patient whose TA is at 1.0 D, the demand for reflex accommodation at 40 cm 1.5 D, rather than 2.5 D as is classically conceptualized. It has been suggested that the value of low-plus lenses for near use is to reduce accommodative demand and permit accommodation to posture closer to the tonic level (Weisz 1980; Press 1990).

Weisz (1980) recommends the use of MEM retinoscopy as a means for clinical determination of TA and the optimal near prescription. She indicates that the accommodative response at near point is usually one half the dioptric difference between the resting state of accommodation and the near stimulus. This leaves a lag of accommodation, measured by MEM retinoscopy, which is equal in magnitude to this accommodative response. TA is thus determined clinically by subtracting twice the value of the MEM lag from the dioptric value of the stimulus to accommodation. The MEM lag finding is equal to the accommodative response, and is viewed as the optimal prescription to reduce accommodative demand.

Research suggests that for each individual there is a critical lens power that is associated with optimal nearpoint performance (Pierce 1966–68; Greenspan 1970, 1975; Levin et al. 1973; Sohrab-Jam 1976). This critical lens power is typically close to the MEM value. Weisz (1980) hypothesizes that the MEM finding is typically optimal for nearpoint performance because, by allowing the accommodative system to posture halfway between the resting point of accommodation and the stimulus demand level, it approximates the normal accommodative response.

Bell Retinoscopy

Bell retinoscopy (Henry 1959; Apell and Streff 1961–62; Streff 1962; Apell 1975) is a procedure to evaluate accommodative function in which the examiner observes changes in the retinoscopic reflex as the target, originally a small cat bell, but now more commonly a highly polished one-half inch chrome ball attached to a thin metal handle, is moved toward the patient. Patients are instructed to observe the reflected image of their face in the ball, and to maintain clarity as the ball is moved toward them.

The examiner scopes at a 20-inch working distance. The chrome ball target is initially held coincident with the retinoscope, just above the peephole, 20 inches from the patient. Initially, "with" motion is usually observed, since accommodation tends to lag beyond the plane of regard. As the target moves toward the patient, increased accommodation is required, and "with" motion decreases until, when accommodation is localized at the plane of the retinoscope, neutrality is obtained. Further inward movement of the target stimulates a further increase in accommodation; when accommodation localizes closer than the retinoscope, a shift into "against" motion is obtained.

The examiner notes and records the distance of the ball from the patient when neutrality is obtained or "against" motion first noted, signaling that accommodative response has crossed the plane of the retinoscope. The examiner continues to move the ball inward a few inches, then reverses direction and moves the ball slowly back toward the retinoscope, noting the distance at which the retinoscopic motion changes from "against" back to "with."

The findings are recorded in the form of a fraction. For example, a shift from "with" to "against" at 15 inches, followed by a shift back to "with" at 16 inches, is recorded as 15"/16".

A meter stick or calibrated string is used to maintain the 20-inch working distance and to determine the distance at which changes in the retinoscopic reflex are observed. The patient holds one end of the meter stick at eye level. The examiner supports the other end with the hand holding the retinoscope or with the shoulder. The experienced examiner can estimate the distance and dispense with the meter stick. When the retinoscopic reflex is basically spherical, observation is made in the horizontal meridian only. When astigmatism is observed, observation is made in the meridian in which "against" motion is first observed.

Performance is evaluated by comparing the accommodative response with the stimulus to accommodation. At the moment when neutrality of the retinoscopic reflex is obtained as the target moves toward the patient, accommodation is localized at the plane of the retinoscope. The accommodative response is thus equal to the dioptric value of the distance from retinoscope to patient, 2.0 D at the usual 20-inch working distance. The stimulus to accommodation is indicated by the dioptric value of the distance from the target to the patient. The difference between these two values is an objective measure of the lag of accommodation.

According to Apell (1975), the first "against" motion should be observed between 17 inches and 14 inches from the patient's eyes. As the ball is moved closer, increased "against" motion is observed; the ball is then moved back toward the retinoscope, and "with" motion should be observed between 15 inches and 18 inches from the patient. The shift to "with" motion as the target moves away typically occurs approximately 1 inch farther from the patient than the shift to "against" motion that occurred as the target moved toward the patient.

A typical expected response is initial "with" motion of approximately 0.50 D with the ball and retinoscope at 20 inches. As the ball approaches the patient, "neutral" or first "against" motion is expected at 15 or 16 inches. At 16 inches, the ball presents a 2.50-D stimulus to accommodation; neutral or first "against" motion indicates that accommodation is at 20 inches, the plane of the retinoscope, a 2.0-D response. The difference is the normal 0.50-D lag.

If, as the target approaches the patient, neutrality is not observed until the stimulus target is closer than normal, the indication is that lag of accommodation is excessive. If, for example, neutrality is obtained at 13 inches when the stimulus to accommodation is 3.0 D, the lag of accommodation is 1.0 D.

Excessive lag indicates the need for nearpoint plus lens application. The lens power to be prescribed may be determined by repeating bell retinoscopy with binocular plus lens additions of increasing power. The indicated plus lens prescription is that which restores a normal lag of accommodation, a finding of approximately 15″/16″.

When bell retinoscopy shows "against" motion beyond 17 inches, that is, at 18 inches or even at 20 inches where the test is started, it indicates that lag of accommodation is minimal or absent. Such a finding may suggest a myopic tendency. The effect of low-plus probe lenses should be evaluated, and such lenses should be prescribed if they relax accommodation so that "against" motion occurs closer to the patient. More commonly, plus lenses cause a shift into greater "against" motion, suggesting that plus lens power will not be accepted.

A normal bell retinoscopy finding does not necessarily contraindicate nearpoint lens application when other findings indicate the advisability of nearpoint lenses. When a normal finding is obtained (shift to "against" at 15 inches, recovery to "with" at 16 inches), bell retinoscopy allows the examiner to observe the accommodative response to plus, to determine whether low-plus lenses will reduce accommodation. A shift of neutrality toward the examiner indicates that low-plus lenses do not reduce accommodative response, and will have little value. However, if the finding remains about the same (15″/16″) with low-plus lenses, accommodation has relaxed in response to the probe lenses, since the total power of the lens/eye system has not changed with the addition of the lenses. In such cases, low-plus lenses are likely to be well accepted and may be safely prescribed if indicated on the basis of the analytical findings, performance tests, or the patient's subjective response to plus (Apell and Streff 1961–62; Apell 1975).

Astigmatism and Anisometropia

The Skeffington model predicts that nonembedded astigmatism and anisometropia, which occur adaptively in relation to nearpoint stress, or as a result of adverse posture during sustained near work, will reduce with the application of low-plus lenses that permit more appropriate posture or relieve nearpoint stress–induced effector system mismatch (Skeffington 1953). Consistent with this notion, Apell (1975) indicates that astigmatism or anisometropia may reduce with low-plus lenses. Therefore, when bell retinoscopy shows the presence of astigmatism or anisometropia, the effect of low-plus probe lenses should be evaluated. A reduction in astigmatism or anisometropia obtained with equal low-plus spheres suggests that the condition is not embedded, and that full anisometropic or astigmatic correction should not be given. Equal low-plus spheres prescribed in accordance with the analytical examination and bell retinoscopy findings may, according to Apell, lead to reduction or elimination of nonembedded astigmatism and anisometropia.

Color and Brightness

The retinoscopic reflex is normally bright and reddish-silver in color. Variations in color and brightness have been reported, and should be observed in addition to the motion of the reflex. The reflex may be described as bright, medium, or dull. In general, a bright reflex suggests attention and involvement with the task, while a dull reflex suggests lack of involvement and low interest (Apell 1975).

Stress-Point Retinoscopy

Kraskin (1965, 1981–83) uses *stress-point retinoscopy* to determine the optimal nearpoint plus lens prescription to relieve nearpoint stress, prevent nearpoint stress–induced vision disorders, and permit maximum visual efficiency. The procedure is based on Harmon's observation that, as a target moves toward an individual, a point is reached at which the person reacts to the stress of close fixation with a physiological stress response. A sharp change in color and brightness of the retinoscopic reflex is noted at this so-called stress-point; the reflex first brightens, then immediately dulls, and then returns to the previous brightness level. Flattening of the pulse pressure and observable twitch at the inner canthus occur at the same time, suggesting that, at this distance, fixation is so close as to generate a physiological stress response (Harmon 1958a).

In performing stress-point retinoscopy, the retinoscope is held at 20 inches. The patient fixates a dangled bell or chrome ball, which is held on the midline and moved toward the individual. In contrast with MEM and bell retinoscopy, the primary observation in stress-point retinoscopy is of brightness, rather than motion. It is not necessary to sweep the retinoscope beam across the pupil. The retinoscope is held stationary. The examiner observes the reflex as the target is moved toward the patient, and notes the distance at which a brightness change signals that the stress-point has been reached. Kraskin indicates that the initial brightening of the reflex is usually not observed; at the stress-point, the reflex appears to dull, followed by an immediate brightening to the original level.

It is desirable that the stress-point be closer to the individual than the habitual working distance. Harmon suggested that in children the stress-point should be approximately 4 inches closer than the near-work distance. For adults, Kraskin proposes that the stress-point should be further removed from the near-work distance, at a distance 8 to 9 inches from the face.

Stress-point retinoscopy is used to determine, for any particular individual, whether a lens prescription is required to shift the stress-point well inside the desirable near-work distance. Plus lenses allow the patient to fixate closer without stress, and therefore usually shift the stress-point closer to the patient. Minus lenses usually move the stress-point farther away. When stress-point retinoscopy shows that the stress-point is too close to the habitual near-work distance, equal plus lenses are added. The stress-point generally moves closer to the face; that plus lens power which shifts the stress-point to the desired position represents the optimal counter-stress lens formula. If too much plus is added, there is a reversal and the stress-point recedes from the face.

Kraskin (1965, 1981–83, 1985) suggests that proper plus lenses for near work can prevent the development of a visual problem. Such lenses, applied prior to the onset of the demand, reduce the stress effect of near work and eliminate the need for adverse adaptation. Kraskin uses stress-point retinoscopy to determine when a child is particularly vulnerable to the effects of nearpoint stress and likely to benefit from low-plus preventive lenses.

Kraskin advises routine evaluation of the child who does not exhibit symptoms or problems. He indicates that the stress-point recedes from the face as the child grows. When the stress-point is sufficiently receded to be within 4 inches of the child's Harmon distance, the indication is that the child is vulnerable and that preventive counter-stress lenses should be prescribed. Plus lenses are added in small increments, and the lenses that move the stress-point 4 inches closer than the Harmon distance are the indicated preventive prescription.

Book Retinoscopy

Book retinoscopy is a procedure in which nearpoint visual function is evaluated while the patient reads for comprehension. The Gray oral reading paragraphs are typically used as target material for patients who can read. The patient holds the book while the examiner aligns the retinoscope over the top of the reading material as close to the visual axis as possible (Figure 9.3). As the patient reads, the examiner observes the retinoscopic reflex, shifting from one eye to the other, noting the motion, color, and brightness of the reflex, as well as similarities and differences between the two eyes. Motion is estimated or neutralized with loose trial lenses as in MEM retinoscopy. To insure that comprehension is attempted, the patient is told that he or she will be questioned on the material. The test is begun with material that is easy, and progresses to material of increasing difficulty. No retinoscopy working lens is used, and no deduction is made for working distance. Gross amounts are recorded. In performing the test on preschoolers, a picture book or toy is substituted as a target, held by a parent if necessary (Getman 1959; Apell and Lowry 1959).

Book retinoscopy emerged from studies of child development in preschool and school-age children at the Gesell Institute. Gesell et al. (1949) and Getman and Kephart (1958) observed changes in brightness and motion of the retinoscopic reflex associated with attention, interest, and comprehension. A brightening of the reflex and a shift to "against" motion, sometimes as great as 2.0 or 3.0 D, frequently occurred when identification and comprehension took place, despite the fact that, with the retinoscope coincident with the book, neutrality of the reflex was expected.

Getman's observation that changes in color, brightness, and motion of the retinoscopic reflex are associated with cognitive demand and patient interest has been verified in the laboratory by Pheiffer (1955) and Kruger (1977, 1980).

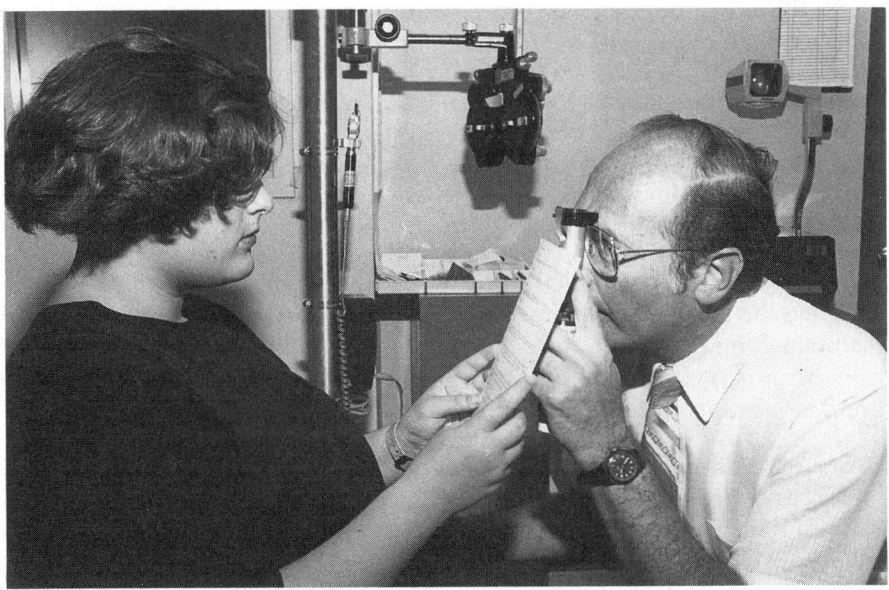

Figure 9.3 Book retinoscopy. The patient reads a book while the examiner aligns the retinoscope at the plane of the book, as close to the visual axis as possible, and observes the retinoscopic reflex.

Kruger demonstrated that these brightness and color changes result from cognitively induced changes in accommodation, and are abolished with cycloplegia.

Accommodation tends to increase, with a shift toward "against" motion, brightening of the reflex, and a color shift toward bright pink or white, when cognitive demand is great enough to require considerable mental effort, and when interest in the material is high. Accommodation tends to decrease, with a shift toward "with" motion, when interest is low or when material is so easy that good comprehension is obtained with little effort. Still greater "with" motion, accompanied by dulling of the reflex and a color shift toward dull red, occurs when material is so far beyond the patient's comprehension level that meaning cannot be obtained, so that he or she stops trying (Getman and Kephart 1958; Pheiffer 1955).

Book retinoscopy can therefore be used to determine whether reading material is easy or difficult for an individual. Further, by increasing task difficulty until "against" motion signals that substantial mental effort is required, or a dull red, high "with" reflex indicates that a frustration level has been reached, the practitioner can evaluate an individual's level of reading comprehension or capacity for problem-solving. Recognition of the potential to use this procedure to assess information-processing ability has led to use of the term *cognition retinoscopy* (Streff 1988; Getman 1990).

Four levels or stages of the retinoscopic reflex have been described, related to demand, comprehension, and interest (Gesell et al. 1949; Getman and Kephart 1958):

Stage I: Free-reading Level

In the free-reading level, the patient comprehends the material with little effort. The retinoscopic reflex is bright, whitish-pink in color, and runs from neutral to low "with" motion.

Stage II: Easy Instructional Level

When the patient reads material that is fairly easy, yet requires some effort to maintain comprehension, the reflex is bright pink and is approximately neutral, with shifts of 0.25 or 0.50 D into both "with" and "against" motion indicating momentary variations in interest and task difficulty.

Stage III: Difficult Instructional Level

When the reading material is sufficiently difficult that the patient must work hard to achieve comprehension, the reflex tends to be bright, reddish-pink in color, and demonstrates "against" motion that fluctuates from 0.25 to 1.25 D with variations in task difficulty.

Stage IV: Nonreading Stage, or Complete Frustration Level

When material is at a frustration level, far beyond the patient's capacity for comprehension, the reflex is dull, brick-red in color, and accompanied by high "with" motion. Such a reflex indicates that there is little mental effort or involvement with the task. This reflex may also occur, even when material is not too difficult, if there is a total lack of interest in the task.

Getman (Getman and Kephart 1958) found that the shift to "against" which accompanies mental effort to process information occurs not only when one reads a book or deals with visual material, but is also present when one does mental arithmetic or solves other verbally presented problems. He found that the retinoscopic shift to "against" motion coincided with the physiologic changes recorded by a lie detector, and that the shift to "against" with cognitive processing was demonstrable even in a blind individual.

These observations led Getman to emphasize the organismic aspects of the test as a probe of an individual's intellectual ability to deal with the task demand, rather than as a strictly optical phenomenon. Although the changes in motion and brightness of the reflex apparently result from changes in accommodation, it appears that these changes in accommodation are in turn induced by cognitive demand (Kruger 1977, 1980).

In observing children's perceptual responses to geometric forms, Getman and Kephart (1958) found a similar shift to "against" motion whenever interpretation or comprehension was required. In work with retarded children, retinoscopic observation was a useful tool to determine whether tasks were at an appropriate level. When, for example, a pure visual activity was accompanied by a dull red, high "with" motion indicating a lack of involvement with the task, if tactual involvement caused a shift toward "against," the implication was that training should begin with hand-eye activity.

Book retinoscopy thus serves as a developmental probe, providing information regarding attentional processes, as well as insight into the child's ability to relate to specific target material (grade-level paragraphs for the school-age child, picture books for the preschoolers, or toys for the infant). Getman (1959) and Apell and Lowry (1959) describe expected retinoscopic findings and observations at various stages of development for preschoolers and school-age children.

Apell and Lowry (1959) report that achievers and nonachievers can be differentiated on the basis of book retinoscopy observations, and that this differentiation can be made even in preschoolers. Achievers tend to shift into "against" motion as soon as the book is exposed, increase "against" the more the child participates, and release to "with" motion when requested to shift gaze to the examiner. Nonachievers tend to exhibit lack of interest, and a bright reflex that is mostly "with" or neutral, with little shift into "against." The reflex may be rigid, with little fluctuation and difficult release, or release may be excessive, with great difficulty maintaining attention on the task.

Book retinoscopy is also used to guide lens application. When excessive "with" motion is found, the effect of plus lens power in permitting greater rapport with the target material should be explored. A lens that produces some shifting into "against" motion or brightening of the reflex may facilitate performance.

Getman (1990) indicates that MEM, bell, and stress-point retinoscopy are more reliable in determining the proper lens power than is book retinoscopy. The value of book retinoscopy lies in its usefulness in predicting the effect of the lens power being considered. When the indicated lenses produce immediate brightening and stabilization of the reflexes during book retinoscopy, as compared with the reflexes through the habitual lenses or no lens, the prescribed lenses are expected to have an immediate positive effect. When increased brightness and stability are not obtained, some time may be required for visual system reorganization with the prescribed lenses.

Getman (Getman and Kephart 1958; Getman 1970–71) further views dynamic retinoscopy as a probe of *visceral binocularity*, and a means to assess the degree to which the two eyes act in synchrony. Intermittent variations in brightness, color, and stability of the reflex between the two eyes suggest inadequate binocular teaming and stability. Alternate or monocular dulling, observed through an unmoving retinoscope, suggests that one eye is "tuning out." Such variations correlate with suppressions found on visual skills tests, and suggest inadequate binocular integration.

Traditionally, optometrists have been trained to interpret retinoscopy on an optical basis, as an objective measure of refractive state. Variations and fluctuations in brightness, color, and motion are usually considered as unreliable artifacts. Practitioners trained to interpret retinoscopy as a reliable optical measure distrust observations that are fleeting and capable of various interpretations.

Consequently, retinoscopy is interpreted behaviorally by a limited number of optometrists. However, the clinical observations by Gesell, Getman, Streff, and Apell at the Gesell Institute, and subsequent documentation by Pheiffer and Kruger, suggest the potential to derive significant behavioral and developmental information from use of the retinoscope, to a much greater degree than is commonly recognized. Dynamic retinoscopic procedures such as MEM, bell, stress-point, and book retinoscopy permit assessment while the patient is actively engaged in nearpoint application. They are used to probe accommodative function, binocularity, ability to sustain, interest, attention, and information-processing ability. In addition, the tests provide valuable information regarding lens application to facilitate these processes (Streff 1988; Valenti 1990).

Performance Testing

Apell and Streff (1961–62) emphasize that, for many individuals, performance demands are primarily centered in near space. They advise that the primary lens prescription should be designed for use at near, based on performance tests at near. When the derived nearpoint lens is not satisfactory for distance performance, a bifocal lens is indicated.

They perform a number of tests to evaluate performance in near space. These tests are performed with and without contemplated nearpoint plus lens prescriptions, to determine the effect of various lens powers on performance. They are likely to prescribe the low-plus lens power, or add, that gives best nearpoint acuity, maximizes near-work distance, or permits optimal performance on tests such as pursuits, Wirt stereotest, nearpoint of convergence, bell retinoscopy, and book retinoscopy.

Apell and Streff also evaluate the effect of low-plus lenses on motor performance, observing performance on tasks such as walking rail, bilateral chalkboard circles, catching and throwing a ball, and tracking a Marsden ball. They prescribe the lenses that optimize performance.

The effect of contemplated nearpoint lenses on reading and writing performance may be evaluated directly by observing the child read and write with and without such lenses. Appropriate nearpoint lenses often produce an immediate impact on performance. Speed, fluidity, decoding, and reading comprehension may improve demonstrably. Writing may become larger, neater, better-spaced, and more legible. Posture during reading and writing may improve immediately, the patient assuming longer and more adequate working distances.

In the Harmon squares test, the child is seated at a table or desk and draws rows of squares approximating the size of his or her own handwriting. Harmon (1985b) observed that distortion of the shape or alignment of the squares tends to reflect the postural skews assumed by the child in performing the task. If, for example, the child works with head skewed so that the right eye is closer to the page, spatial projection may produce distorted squares that are smaller on the right side.

The Harmon squares test may be performed with and without contemplated low-plus lenses. Appropriate nearpoint lenses may permit more adequate posture and hence improved performance, with less distortion of the squares.

The patient's subjective response to low-plus lenses serves as a guide to prescribing. Trial lenses are held in front of the patient's eyes while viewing nearpoint material. The patient is asked to compare clarity and comfort with and without the tentative plus lens prescription. When the patient reports that the print looks clearer, that he or she feels less strain, or that it is easier to hold reading material farther away, the indicated lenses are likely to be accepted and can be prescribed with confidence.

Sometimes the lenses indicated by the analytical examination findings are subjectively rejected when held before the patient. The patient may report that the tentative nearpoint lens prescription makes the print smaller or less clear, or makes reading less comfortable. Although such responses may seem paradoxical, the experienced clinician learns to respect them as a sign that "indicated" lenses are unlikely to be worn and that prescription should be delayed. Vision training is often effective in increasing plus acceptance in such cases.

Occasionally, when the indications for nearpoint plus are uncertain, it is helpful to issue "loaner" glasses, generally +0.50, +0.75, or +1.00 D spheres, which the patient may evaluate at home for 1 to 2 weeks to assess their effect.

PRESCRIBING LENSES FOR VIDEO DISPLAY TERMINAL USE

Glasses prescribed for general use are often unsatisfactory for use at the video display terminal (VDT). The visual task demands encountered by VDT users differ in several respects from those of reading and other desk work, and frequently require lenses designed specifically for use at the terminal. In prescribing lenses for use at a VDT, the clinician must consider factors related to working distance, height of the screen, and concurrent visual demands associated with VDT use.

Working Distance

The VDT screen is generally situated at a longer working distance than that habitually used for reading and writing, typically about 18 to 22 inches. The habitual reading distance and computer working distance should be carefully determined for each patient, since prescriptions of differing power may be required for different working distances. Even small differences in working distance may be critical, especially for presbyopes. The add for VDT use can be determined by performing the NRA and PRA tests at the VDT working distance, through a tentative addition of 0.25 or 0.50 D less in plus than that obtained at 16 inches, and prescribing that lens which balances the NRA and PRA findings.

Murch (1982), using laser optometry, found that the accommodative response to a VDT screen is less than that for conventional print at the same distance. As a result, the need for nearpoint plus lens application may be greater during VDT use. Margach (1982) points out that the increased lag during VDT use suggests increasing the amount of plus prescribed, while the increased viewing distance suggests reducing it; the net result may be that the actual prescription for the VDT distance would be about the same as that determined for conventional print at 16 inches. However, presbyopes frequently prefer an add for VDT use that is slightly weaker than that required for reading at 16 inches.

Height

In contrast to conventional reading and writing in which the task demand is localized well below eye level, the VDT screen is typically located only slightly below eye level, and occasionally at or even above eye level. Consequently, a bifocal prescribed for habitual use is generally not suitable for sustained VDT application; excessive chin elevation is required to view the VDT screen through the segment, causing discomfort and neckache. If the bifocal segment is set high enough to permit comfortable viewing of the VDT screen, it interferes with habitual distance viewing. The difficulties induced by VDT use may be resolved by use of a single-vision lens prescription appropriate for the VDT screen, a high-segment occupational bifocal that provides a window for distance viewing, or a variety of intermediate/near bifocal and progressive addition lenses designed specifically for use at the VDT terminal.

Concurrent Visual Demands

The VDT operator may input data from hard copy placed to the left or right of the screen, or from other displays placed above or even across the room from the VDT screen. The console is usually just in front of the screen, but may be farther removed from it in some cases. The examiner must determine the specific visual demands and viewing distances at the patient's work station in order to design lenses appropriate for the task.

Concurrent visual demands will often require the use of multifocals with segment placement and prescription designed solely for use at the VDT work station. One such occupational lens, for example, would have a small upper window for distance viewing, a large central area with an add appropriate for the VDT screen, and a lower segment of higher power appropriate for the distance of the material being copied, which is usually located closer than the screen.

COMPENSATORY AND REMEDIAL LENSES

Lenses are prescribed to achieve a variety of goals. Apell and Streff (1961–62) conceptualize that lenses may be prescribed to compensate for refractive deviations, to remediate disorders of visual functions, to foster adequate development, and to prevent vision disorders.

Whether to prescribe a compensatory or remedial type lens depends on the visual status, needs, and desires of the patient, as well as the orientation of the doctor. The emphasis in this chapter has been the determination of the optimal nearpoint lens power for remediation and prevention. Little attention has been given to the prescription of compensatory lenses.

Compensatory lenses are frequently required and prescribed. In traditional approaches, compensatory lenses are usually designed to neutralize significant deviations from emmetropia. Such prescriptions are sometimes modified slightly to facilitate acceptance. Experienced clinicians, aware of the spatial changes induced by lenses used for everyday vision, are generally cautious about making substantial changes in lens prescription, especially in astigmatic and anisometropic prescriptions.

Although compensatory lenses are often referred to as corrective lenses, Apell and Streff (1961–62) point out that such lenses are not truly "corrective," since they neither eliminate the deviation nor influence the factors that caused it. A myope wearing minus lenses is still a myope, retaining the behavior patterns that created the myopia in the first place.

Nevertheless, a compensatory lens prescription is frequently required to permit more efficient function. Apell and Streff (1961–62) propose a functional approach to compensatory lens prescribing. They suggest that when compensatory lenses are prescribed, the primary consideration should be the individual's performance, rather than strict optical neutralization of the refractive deviation. While some patients perform best with full optical neutralization, others function most efficiently with lenses of weaker power, or with lenses modified for use at closer distances, with or without a "distance add" to provide best distance acuity.

Apell and Streff (1961–62) suggest that compensatory lens prescriptions be kept as simple as possible, especially for young children. They prescribe equal spherical lenses whenever possible, assuming that small cylindrical and anisometropic deviations may be transient adaptive changes. They suggest that neutralizing such deviations may embed them and introduce spatial distortion, which can lead to further adaptation. Small cylindrical and anisometropic prescriptions are thus given only when they actually improve performance or are demanded by the patient.

Apell and Streff (1961–62) indicate that astigmatism and anisometropia are usually less rigidly structured, with greater latitude to reduce or simplify the prescription, when a compensatory lens has not previously been used. Similarly, when small cylinders are indefinite, and one must "chase around" during the examination to pin down the cylinder, it is a sign that the astigmatism is less structured. Simplification of the prescription by eliminating or reducing cylindrical power, modifying the axis toward horizontal or vertical, and reducing anisometropic difference is more readily tolerated, and may facilitate future development in a more appropriate direction. The ability to reduce lens power and to simplify the prescription is a function of the age of the patient, the degree to which the refractive deviation is structured or embedded, and the needs of the patient in terms of acuity and performance. The goal is to provide that degree of compensation which is needed by the patient, but at the same time to give the patient room to shape refractive state in a more desirable direction.

In patients with nonembedded anisometropic tendencies, Horner (1972–

73) has had patients alternate between glasses with $+0.50$ D. O.D. and -0.50 D. O.S., and the reverse, to establish more equal plus and minus acceptance for the two eyes and develop greater flexibility to reverse anisometropic tendencies. He has also used unequal bifocal adds to attempt to reduce anisometropia. Miele (1986) reports that hyperopia and myopia can be reduced in both children and adults through the use of undercorrecting lenses. These attempts at "refractive engineering" assume that refraction is influenced by environmental interaction, and use lenses to modify the environment so as to redirect adaptive processes.

There is greater latitude to delay or modify refractive correction when the patient is receiving concurrent vision therapy. As the patient develops improved visual skills and flexibility, reduction in myopia, hyperopia, astigmatism, and/or anisometropia may occur. Low-plus lenses that relieve stress at near point may similarly effect changes in refractive state.

Yoked Prisms

Although low-plus lenses for near are the most widely prescribed remedial lenses, behavioral optometrists have explored the use of other lens combinations to disembed patterns of visual behavior and provide a stimulus to redirect visual adaptation. Several optometrists have advocated the use of yoked prisms for this purpose. *Yoked prisms* are prisms of equal power with their bases in the same direction (up, down, left, or right). Such lenses do not compensate for horizontal or vertical imbalance, since they produce no net base-up, base-down, base-in, or base-out compensatory power; their effect is rather to create spatial change (Horner 1972–73; Kaplan 1978–79; Kraskin 1981–83).

Horner (1972–73) and Kaplan (1978–79) advocate the use of vertical yoked prisms to influence spatial perception, posture, and central-peripheral organization, and hence bring about desired behavioral and performance changes. Yoked prisms are usually prescribed base-down for patients with esophoria or convergence excess, and base-up for those with exophoria or convergence insufficiency. Base-down prisms create an upward spatial shift and consequent upward gaze shift associated with divergence, expanded peripheral awareness, relaxation, outward and backwards body thrust, and increased nearpoint working distance. These expansive properties are held to make base-down yoked prisms suitable for the highly central esophoric patient.

The effects of base-down yoked prisms simulate those induced by nearpoint plus lenses. It has been reported that in cases where plus for near is desirable but is not accepted, similar effects may be achieved with base-down yoked prisms, and that use of such prisms may foster greater plus acceptance (Horner 1972–73).

Base-up yoked prisms are viewed as spatially compressive, creating decreased size, decreased distance, downward spatial shift, and downward gaze shift, associated with convergence and inward body thrust. Such prisms may facilitate awareness of figure and central visual attention in global and/or distractable individuals (Horner 1972–73; Kaplan 1978–79).

Kaplan (1978–79) suggests that low AC/A, marked differences between distance and near-phoria measures, low recovery findings, absence of blur on prism vergence tests, low accommodative amplitude, and awareness of spatial changes induced by vertical yoked prisms, are characteristic signs that patients may benefit from their use. When these characteristics are present, he recommends the use of base-up yoked prisms in cases of convergence insufficiency, and of base-down yoked prisms for convergence excess.

Kaplan suggests that vertical yoked prisms create a potential for the patient to reorganize space. He suggests that large prism powers are disruptive, while small prism powers facilitate reorganization and may be remedial. He recommends the prescription of 2^Δ base-up yoked prisms in cases of convergence insufficiency, and of 3^Δ base-down for convergence excess.

Low-power vertical yoked prisms are prescribed by Kaplan and by Horner for daily use or for specific activities. They are monitored closely, and changed as needed. These lenses are viewed as training lenses, applied to effect change, rather than as permanent lenses for long-term use. Kaplan indicates that patients using such lenses have reported reduced asthenopia, improved reading comprehension, reduced motion sickness, improved peripheral awareness, and improved sports performance. Kaplan reports positive changes in eye coordination, acuity, refractive state, AC/A, and accommodative amplitude.

There have been no controlled studies on the effectiveness of vertical yoked prisms. Clinical reports indicate that such prisms may produce positive changes in visual performance and posture (Kaplan 1978–79; Moskowitz 1981; Silver 1983; Davis et al. 1985; Garson 1986, 1987; Jacobs and Cantwell 1988; Valenti 1988). Satty (1981) reported positive changes in AC/A, convergence nearpoint, near phoria, PRA, and presenting symptoms in an uncontrolled clinical study of 10 patients.

Kraskin (1981–83) holds that vision disorders are the end result of postural skews, and advocates the use of yoked prisms to induce postural change. Kraskin relates refractive state to the tonicity of the lower back musculature. When, in coming to balance with gravity and the task at hand, an individual increases tonicity of the lower back musculature, the center of gravity shifts forward, necessitating a series of counterbalancing adjustments in the upper body that culminate in an upward, forward thrust of the chin. Myopia, according to Kraskin, is an ocular end product of these postural adjustments. Adverse high hyperopia, in contrast, is viewed by Kraskin as the ocular end result of hypotonicity of the lower back musculature that permits a backwards shift of the center of gravity.

Nearpoint lenses influence body posture during nearpoint tasks (Greenspan 1970, 1975). Kraskin indicates that the postural changes induced by lenses are accompanied by altered tonicity of the lower back musculature. Addition of plus lens power reduces lower back tonicity and, therefore, according to Kraskin, helps to counter myopia development. Minus lenses increase tonicity of the lower back musculature. When minus lenses are indicated for distance, but are inappropriately used for near, there is an increase in tonicity of the body's posturing musculature, a shifting forward of the center of gravity, and, according to Kras-kin, increased myopia.

Kraskin uses yoked prisms in those cases in which he believes it desirable to alter body posture to influence visual status. He explores the possible bene-ficial use of yoked prism in patients with myopia or adverse high hyperopia; in patients with asymmetric conditions such as anisometropia, strabismus, ambly-opia, and unequal phorias (when measures are obtained first with one eye and then the other fixating); and in patients with postural distortions, particularly of head position.

To determine whether yoked prisms may have value in these cases, Kraskin probes the effect of low power (3 to 4$^\triangle$) yoked prisms on Polaroid stereo tests such as the Wirt and the Randot. He indicates that many patients demonstrate improved stereopsis when the prisms are placed with their bases in one direction, and reduced stereopsis when prism application is reversed. Kraskin probes with vertical yoked prisms (base-up and base-down) in patients with myopia and adverse hyperopia, since he relates these conditions to lower back tonicity and compensatory postural adjustments along the vertical axis of the body. He tests with horizontal yoked prisms (base-right and base-left) in patients with lateral asymmetries such as strabismus, anisometropia, and amblyopia.

When performance is influenced positively or negatively by prisms, Kraskin advocates the use of yoked prisms to induce a postural shift and influence visual function. When there is no difference in performance with yoked prisms, such prisms are not prescribed.

When testing demonstrates that yoked prisms improve or reduce perform-ance on stereotests, Kraskin prescribes prism not in the direction that improves performance, but rather in the direction that impairs stereopsis. Such prism is prescribed to exaggerate postural stress and thus provide a stimulus for the in-dividual to rebound by organizing a postural response to counter-induced stress.

Kraskin's approach to yoked prisms frequently leads to the prescription of prism in a direction opposite to that advocated by Kaplan (1978–79). While Kaplan prescribes yoked prisms to induce spatial and postural changes favorable to a particular individual, Kraskin prescribes yoked prism in a direction that impairs performance, to induce postural stress and create a stimulus for change. Indeed, in Kraskin's method, when progress evaluation indicates that prescribed yoked prisms no longer impair performance, they are viewed as being no longer useful and are removed.

Yoked prisms cause an eye movement toward the apex of the prisms, with a shift of the hips and pelvis in the opposite direction to counterbalance. Base-down prism produces upward eye movement, accompanied by a downward pel-vic rotation and backward shift in the center of gravity. Base-up prism produces downward eye movement, pelvic tilt upward, and forward shift of the center of gravity. Base-right prisms produce an eye movement toward the left, with a compensating rotation of the pelvis toward the right. Base-left prisms produce an eye movement toward the right, and pelvic rotation toward the left.

In myopia, Kraskin conceives the postural alteration to be a pelvic tilt upward that results from increased tonicity of the musculature of the lower back, which shifts the center of gravity forward. Base-up yoked prisms exaggerate the upward pelvic tilt and provide an opportunity for the individual to rebound by reducing it.

In hyperopia, base-down yoked prisms exaggerate the downward pelvic tilt and backward shift in the center of gravity that result from hypotonicity of the lower back supportive musculature. Such prisms may, according to Kraskin, stimulate compensatory changes in body posture and lead to reduction in hyperopia.

SUMMARY

Clinical guidelines are given for practical case analysis. In prescribing near-point plus lenses, a tentative prescription is selected based on the fused cross-cylinder finding and its effect on the near phoria, and this tentative prescription is modified depending on its effect on the NRA and PRA findings and the fusional vergences at near, the patient's subjective reaction, and tests of performance through the lenses. Dynamic retinoscopy procedures such as MEM, bell, book, and stress-point retinoscopy provide additional information regarding plus lens acceptance. Some clinicians advocate the use of yoked prisms, which induce postural and spatial changes, to effect changes in visual function.

REFERENCES

Apell RJ (1975). Clinical application of bell retinoscopy. *J Am Optom Assoc* 46(10):1023–1027.

Apell RJ, Lowry RW (1959). *Preschool Vision*. St. Louis: American Optometric Association.

Apell RJ, Streff JW (1961–62). *Optometric Child Vision Care and Guidance*. Optometric Extension Program Continuing Education Courses, Santa Ana, CA: Optometric Extension Program Foundation, Oct. 1961–Sept. 1962.

Birnbaum MH (1985). An esophoric shift associated with sustained fixation. *Am J Optom Physiol Opt* 62(11):732–735.

Charman WN, Walsh G (1989). Variations in the local refractive correction of the eye across its entrance pupil. *Optom Vis Sci* 66(1):34–40.

Cross AJ (1911). *Dynamic Skiametry in Theory and Practice*. New York: Cross Optical Co.

Davis M, Glazier HS, Kotlicky MF, et al. (1985). Vision, dominance, and the use of base prisms on learning disabilities. *Invitational Skeffington Conference on Vision*, Washington, DC, Jan. 1985, transcript by Caryl Croisant.

Garson WC (1986). The use of base down prism in the treatment of the cerebral palsied patient. *Invitational Skeffington Symposium on Vision*, Washington, DC, Jan. 1986, transcript by Caryl Croisant.

Garson WC (1987). Developmental sequence as a factor in the therapeutic use of yoked prism. *Invitational Skeffington Symposium on Vision*, Washington, DC, Jan. 1987, transcript by Caryl Croisant.

Gesell A, Ilg FL, Bullis GE, Getman GN, et al. (1949). *Vision: Its Development in Infant and Child*. New York: Paul R. Hoeber, Inc. (reprinted New York: Hafner, 1967).

Getman GN (1959). *Techniques and Diagnostic Criteria for the Optometric Care of Children's Vision.* Santa Ana, CA: Optometric Extension Program Foundation.

Getman GN (1970–71). *Vision Development and the Analytical Examination.* Optometric Extension Program Continuing Education Courses, Santa Ana, CA: Optometric Extension Program Foundation.

Getman GN (1990). *Postscript* to Getman (Book) Retinoscopy, in Valenti CA: *The Full Scope of Retinoscopy.* Santa Ana, CA: Optometric Extension Program Foundation.

Getman GN, Kephart NC (1958). *Developmental Vision.* Optometric Extension Program Continuing Education Courses, Santa Ana, CA: Optometric Extension Program Foundation, vol. 30, series 2, no. 10,11; July, Aug. 1958.

Goss DA (1986). *Ocular Accommodation, Convergence and Fixation Disparity: A Manual of Clinical Analysis.* New York: Professional Press.

Greenspan SB (1970). Effects of children's nearpoint lenses upon body posture and performance. *Am J Optom Arch Am Acad Optom* 47(12):982–989.

Greenspan SB (1975). Behavioral effects of children's nearpoint lenses. *J Am Optom Assoc* 46(10):1031–1037.

Harmon DB (1958a). *Reading, Posture and Vision.* Film produced and copyright by author, Austin, TX, cited by Kraskin (1965).

Harmon DB (1958b). *Notes on a Dynamic Theory of Vision.* 3rd rev. ed. Austin, TX: author.

Haynes HM (1960). Clinical observations with dynamic retinoscopy. *Optom Weekly* 51:2243–2246, 2306–2309.

Haynes HM (1985). Clinical approaches to nearpoint lens power determination. *Am J Optom Physiol Opt* 62(6):375–385.

Henry WR (1959). Dangled Ball with Retinoscope. St. Louis: Conference on Theoretical Optometry and Visual Training, transcript by Caryl Croisant, O.D., Cayucos, CA.

Horner SH (1972–73). *The Use of Lenses and Prisms to Enhance Visual Training.* Optometric Extension Program Continuing Education Courses, Santa Ana, CA: Optometric Extension Program Foundation, vol. 45, Oct. 1972–Sept. 1973.

Jackson TW, Goss DA (1991). Variation and correlation of clinical tests of accommodative function in a sample of school-age children. *J Am Optom Assoc* 62(11):857–866.

Jacobs RR, Cantwell D (1988). Yoked prisms: A demonstration and case presentation. *Invitational Skeffington Symposium on Vision,* Washington, DC, Jan. 1988, transcript by Caryl Croisant.

Kaplan MK (1978–79). *Vertical Yoked Prisms.* Optometric Extension Program Continuing Education Courses, Santa Ana, CA: Optometric Extension Program Foundation, vol. 51, Oct. 1978–Sept. 1979.

Kraskin RA (1965). Stress point retinoscopy. *J Am Optom Assoc* 36(5):416–419.

Kraskin RA (1981–83). *Lens Power in Action.* Optometric Extension Program Continuing Education Courses, Santa Ana, CA: Optometric Extension Program Foundation, vol. 54, 55, series 1,2, Oct. 1981–Sept. 1983.

Kraskin RA (1985). Preventive vision care. *J Am Optom Assoc* 56(6):454–456.

Kruger P (1977). The role of accommodation in increasing the luminance of the fundus reflex during cognitive processing. *J Am Optom Assoc* 48(12):1493–1496.

Kruger PB (1980). The effect of cognitive demand upon accommodation. *Am J Optom Physiol Opt* 57(7):440–445.

Levin S, Ratner N, Schoenberg R (1973). *The Relationship Between M.E.M. Findings and Nearpoint Performance.* Senior Research Study, Chicago: Illinois College of Optometry.

Liebowitz HW, Owens DA (1975). Night myopia and the intermediate dark focus of accommodation. *J Optical Soc Am* 65(10):1121–1128.

McKee GW (1981). Reliability of monocular estimate method retinoscopy. *Optom Monthly* 72(12):30–31.

Margach CB (1982). Video display terminals, in *Literature and Research Review*. Optometric Extension Program Continuing Education Courses, Santa Ana, CA: Optometric Extension Program Foundation, vol. 54, series 7, no. 7, April; vol. 55, series 8, no. 1-3, Oct.-Dec.

Miele JR (1986). The range of clarity. *J Optom Vis Dev* 17(4):24–27.

Moskowitz W (1981). Studies comparing differences produced by yoked prisms and plus lenses. *Skeffington Symposium on Vision*, Washington, DC, Jan. 1981, transcript by Caryl Croisant.

Murch G (1982). How visible is your display? *Electro-Optical Systems Designs* 14(3):43–49.

Pascal JI (1930). *Modern Retinoscopy*. London: Hatton Press.

Pascal JI (1952). *Selected Studies in Visual Optics*. St. Louis: Mosby.

Pheiffer CH (1955). Book retinoscopy. *Am J Optom Arch Am Acad Optom* 32(10):540–545.

Pierce JR (1966–68). *Research Reports and Special Articles*. Optometric Extension Program Continuing Education Courses, Santa Ana, CA: Optometric Extension Program Foundation, vol. 39, 40: series 1, 2, Oct. 1966–Feb. 1968.

Press L (1990). Lenses and behavior. *J Optom Vis Dev* 21:5–17.

Rouse MW, Hutter RF, Shiftlett R (1984). A normative study of the accommodative lag in elementary school children. *Am J Optom Physiol Opt* 61(11):693–697.

Rouse MW, London R, Allen DC (1982). An evaluation of the monocular estimate method of dynamic retinoscopy. *Am J Optom Physiol Opt* 59:234–239.

Rutstein RP, Daum KM, Amos JF (1988). Accommodative spasm: A study of 17 cases. *J Am Optom Assoc* 59(7):527–538.

Satty R (1981). Effects of Vertical Yoked Prisms on Nearpoint Function: A Clinical Study. Optometric Extension Program Postgraduate Education Courses, Santa Ana, CA: Optometric Extension Program Foundation, vol. 53, *Research Reports and Special Articles*, June, pp. 1-5.

Schor CM, Kotulak JC, Tsuetaki T (1986). Adaptation of tonic accommodation reduces accommodative lag and is masked in darkness. *Invest Ophthalmol Vis Sci* 27:820–827.

Sheard C (1920). *Dynamic Skiametry*. Chicago: Cleveland Press.

Silver PA (1983). Yoked prisms: Cases in point. *Invitational Skeffington Symposium on Vision*, Washington, DC, Jan., transcript by Caryl Croisant.

Skeffington AM (1928–74). Optometric Extension Program Continuing Education Courses, Santa Ana, CA: Optometric Extension Program Foundation.

Skeffington AM (1953). *Practical Applied Optometry*. Optometric Extension Program Continuing Education Courses, Santa Ana, CA: Optometric Extension Program Foundation, vol. 25, Jan., Feb.

Sohrab-Jam G (1976). Eye movement patterns and reading performance in poor readers: Immediate effects of convex lenses indicated by book retinoscopy. *Am J Optom Physiol Opt* 53(11):720–726.

Streff JW (1962). Some early observations with a bright bell and retinoscope. *Eastern Seaboard Conference on Visual Training*, Washington, DC, transcript by Caryl Croisant, O.D., Santa Ana, CA.

Streff JW (1988). Cognitive retinoscopy. *Behav Optom* (Aust) 1(1):14–20.

Streff JW, Claussen VE (1971). Retinoscopy measurement differences as a variable of technique. *Am J Optom Arch Am Acad Optom* 48(8):671–676.

Tait EF (1929). A quantitative system of dynamic skiametry. *Am J Optom* 6(12):669–693.

Valenti CA (1988). Exploring a new technique to assess spatial localization and application of yoked prism prescriptions. *Invitational Skeffington Conference on Vision*, Washington, DC, Jan, transcript by Caryl Croisant.

Valenti CA (1990). *The Full Scope of Retinoscopy*. Rev. ed. Santa Ana, CA: Optometric Extension Program Foundation.

Weisz CL (1980). The accommodative resting state: Theoretical implications in lens prescription. *Rev Optom* 117(7):60–70; (8):62–74.

Weisz CL (1983). How to find and treat accommodative disorders. *Rev Optom* 120(1):48–53.

10

Efficacy of Low-Plus Lenses

Several research studies confirm that appropriately prescribed low-plus lenses relieve nearpoint asthenopia, improve nearpoint visual efficiency, and slow myopia progression. In addition, plus lens application has been reported to influence near-work posture, physiological activation, and electroencephalographic measures.

Low-plus lenses are commonly used in the treatment of accommodative insufficiency. Daum (1983) reported that 15 of 17 patients with accommodative insufficiency experienced at least partial relief from symptoms with plus lenses for near; nine patients reported total alleviation of symptoms.

PHYSIOLOGICAL EFFECTS OF PLUS LENS APPLICATION

Individuals involved in near-work activities at excessively close distances frequently exhibit increased muscular tension, with tightening of shoulder, jaw, and other musculature, as well as increased physiological activation as measured by indicators of sympathetic arousal. Harmon (1960) reports that use of the optimal low-plus lens power for near work is accompanied by improved posture during nearpoint visual tasks, normalization of nearpoint working distance, and reduction in physiological activation.

The effects of appropriately prescribed low-plus lenses occur because such lenses allow the individual to localize objects as being farther away in space (Skeffington 1959; MacDonald 1963; Harmon 1966; Bastien 1987; Press 1990). This property of localizing objects farther away is attributed to the geometric optics of plus lenses, which increase the convergence of light so that the observer projects the object as being farther away in space, as well as the *physical optics effect* whereby a plus lens increases the spread of light on the retina, reducing the number of photons per unit area and hence flattening the energy gradient distribution (MacDonald 1963; Harmon 1966; Press 1990). In addition, Harmon (1966) asserts that the proper low-plus lens for near acts to reduce body tonus during the near task, and that reduction in body tonus leads to an increase in perceived distance. The geometric effect of localizing the image away, the change in pattern of light distribution, and the reduction in body tonus each contribute to the interpretive effect of moving the task away from the individual, and may have positive effects on near-work posture and working distance (Press 1990).

Harmon's work was replicated and extended by Pierce (1966–68, 1970). Pierce evaluated the effect of lenses by comparing physiological activation (as measured by the electromyogram, basal resistance level of the skin, electrocardiogram, and respiration rate), posture and working distance, reading rate on a standardized reading task, and performance on an upside-down writing task, under three conditions of nearpoint lens application: (1) no lens, (2) +0.50 sphere (which was very close to the lens power determined by OEP analysis as optimal for each of the subjects in the study) and (3) +1.00 sphere (representing excessive plus lens power for these subjects).

Subjects with the +0.50-D nearpoint lens prescription demonstrated a reduction in physiological activity, improved posture and working distance, and improved reading rate and performance on the writing task, as compared with that obtained with plano or +1.00-D spheres. Pierce's data thus indicate that the optimal nearpoint lens prescription has beneficial effects on performance, physiological activation, and posture and working distance. Too little or too much plus is less effective and may have an adverse effect. Pierce assumes that the reduction in physiologic activity with the indicated nearpoint lens occurs as a result of improved posture and nearpoint working distance.

The finding that optimal plus reduces physiological activation suggests a potential general stress reduction effect. Inadequate or excessive plus may increase general stress, as indicated by increased physiological activation.

POSTURE AND PERFORMANCE EFFECTS

Greenspan (1970) evaluated the effect in children of low-plus nearpoint lenses on body posture, working distance, and performance on a timed pencil-and-paper task. For 11 subjects, 10 of whom were within 0.50 D of emmetropia, Greenspan assessed posture and performance under three different lens conditions: (1) plano lenses, (2) ametropic lens correction, and (3) arbitrary low-plus add of +0.50 to +1.00 D over the ametropic lens correction. He found statistically significant differences in nearpoint working distance and performance with the different lenses in seven of the 11 children and concluded that for many children, performance improves with use of a properly selected nearpoint lens.

Although task performance was significantly influenced by nearpoint lenses, Greenspan found that none of the three lens conditions was consistently successful in enhancing performance. Some subjects performed best with ametropic prescription, others with a lens that differed from the ametropic prescription, and still others with no lens at all. Nevertheless, for many subjects, the precise lens power to produce optimal results was critical and specific. For some children, even slight variation from this optimal nearpoint power produced significant decreases in performance and nearpoint working distance. MEM retinoscopy frequently predicted the nearpoint lens power with optimal effect.

Pierce's and Greenspan's research has been a subject of controversy. Keller and Amos (1979) criticized the research methodology and conclusions of both studies. Greenspan (1979) and Pierce (1980), as well as Flax (1980), each offered responses to these criticisms. Press (1985) reviewed both the studies and the controversy, and concluded that low-plus lenses undoubtedly enhance performance in some individuals.

Larrabee and Jones (1980) assessed the effect of indicated low-plus lenses on nearpoint working distance and performance. Eleven school-age children whose optometric examination determined that plus lenses were indicated for near use were given the motor-speed-and-precision subtest of the Detroit Test of Learning Aptitude, once with habitual correction, and once with the indicated nearpoint lens addition. Statistically significant differences in performance on the paper-and-pencil task were obtained with and without indicated nearpoint lenses. Ten of the 11 subjects showed improved performance with indicated low-plus lenses, and seven showed an increase in near working distance. Pirman and Lamb (1982) and Caden et al. (1984) similarly found that children's performance on a copy-forms test improved with nearpoint lenses determined by MEM retinoscopy, as compared with that obtained using habitual lenses.

Friedhoffer and Warren (1988) report that nearpoint visual activity produces a constriction of the central visual field, and that this constriction is reduced if low-plus spheres are worn during the near task.

Sohrab-Jam (1976) used an Eye-Trac to evaluate the effect of low-plus lenses on eye movements during reading in fourth and fifth graders. Fewer regressions, increased reading speed, and greater reading efficiency were obtained when low-plus lenses were worn by subjects for whom such lenses were appropriate, as determined by book retinoscopy. When low-plus lenses were worn by subjects for whom they were not indicated, decrement in eye movement performance was noted, with increased fixations, increased regressions, and decreased reading efficiency. In contrast, Wildsoet and Foo (1988) found no difference in eye movement recordings in subjects wearing plano lenses or their habitual low-plus prescriptions.

These several studies indicate that low-plus nearpoint lenses produce beneficial effects on performance. Some of the studies further suggest that the lens power that produces optimal effect is critical and specific. Powers that differ from the optimal by as little as 0.25 D cause alterations in posture, increased physiological activity, and decreased performance in some patients. In several of the studies, OEP case analysis and MEM retinoscopy predicted the optimal lens power.

ELECTROPHYSIOLOGICAL EFFECTS OF PLUS LENS APPLICATION

Two reports correlate plus lens application with modification in cortical electrophysiological activity. Spafford et al. (1983) reported the case of a low hyperope with inadequate accommodation who showed enhancement of the binocular visual-evoked response pattern with plus lens application. This case presents objective, neurologically based evidence that appropriate low-plus lenses may enhance binocular function.

In most individuals, amplitude of the occipital alpha rhythm is greatest when visual processing is least, and is minimal when visual activity is greatest. However, some individuals with deficient reading skills and inability to sustain attention show persistence of the alpha rhythm during attempts to process visually. Ludlam (1976) reported normalization of the alpha rhythm activation cycle, characterized by development of ability to attenuate alpha during visual processing, accompanied by improved reading performance, following successful vision training and nearpoint plus lens application.

CONTROL OF MYOPIA PROGRESSION

The use of bifocal lenses to control myopia progression has been reviewed by Birnbaum (1979), Goss (1982), Curtin (1985), and Press (1987). Both the Skeffington model and the use-abuse theory advocate plus lens application for near use. While OEP analysis generally dictates low-plus addition on the order of +0.50 to +1.00 D to achieve equilibrium between vergence and accommodation, advocates of the use-abuse theory generally prescribe high adds, on the order of +1.50 to +3.00 D, to minimize use of accommodation.

Each theory predicts that its approach to plus lens application will control myopia progression. Clinically, it appears that plus does halt or slow myopia progression in some cases. However, other cases continue to progress, leaving the clinician to wonder whether the rate of progression has been influenced by plus lens application. As a consequence, the use of bifocals to control myopia progression is controversial, and numerous studies have been undertaken to assess their effect.

These studies have produced conflicting results. A statistically significant reduction in rate of myopia progression with bifocals has been reported by Miles (1957, 1962), Roberts and Banford (1967), Oakley and Young (1975), Kelly et al. (1975), Daubs and Shotwell (1983), and Goss (1986). However, no significant effect for bifocals was found in studies by Mandell (1959), Shotwell (1981), Grosvenor et al. (1987), and Hemminki and Pärssinen (1987).

Miles (1957, 1962) reports that myopia progression is reduced in bifocal wearers as compared with single-vision controls. His data indicate that a decrease in the rate of myopia progression occurs at the beginning of bifocal wear.

Daubs and Shotwell (1983) compared the efficacy of placebo treatment, a bifocal with +1.50 D add, and a single-vision nearpoint prescription with +1.25 D add and 2$^\Delta$ base-in O.U. After 5 months, the rate of myopia progression was lower in the groups that received nearpoint lens addition than in the placebo group.

Roberts and Banford (1967) found a small but statistically significant difference in rate of myopia progression in patients wearing bifocal and single-vision lenses. Rate of progression, determined by a partial correlation technique to statistically correct for differences in age and sex distribution, was 0.31 D per year for the bifocal patients and 0.41 D for the single-vision patients. This difference is less than 0.12 D per year, but represents a rate of progression 22.8% less in the bifocal group. Bifocals were most effective in slowing myopia progression in patients with esophoria and a high AC/A ratio.

Goss (1986) similarly found that myopes wearing bifocals progress more slowly (-0.37 D/y) than myopes wearing single-vision lenses (-0.44 D/y). These differences were statistically significant for myopes with esophoria at near or a fused cross-cylinder finding of $+0.50$ D or greater, but not for those with near-point exophoria or a low-fused cross-cylinder finding. These findings suggest that bifocals are most effective in slowing myopia progression in those cases in which bifocal prescription is indicated on the basis of the nearpoint findings.

Oakley and Young (1975) found that myopes wearing bifocals progressed significantly less than those wearing single-vision lenses. In this study, the average annual rate of myopia progression was 0.50 D for single-vision lens wearers, and only 0.04 D for bifocal wearers. Oakley and Young used flat-top bifocals positioned with the segment line at the middle of the pupil in primary gaze. They suggest that this high position, insuring use of the bifocal for near, contributes significantly to the effectiveness of bifocals found in their study.

Kelly et al. (1975) treated an experimental group with bifocals and phenylephrine 5% drops at night. Refraction after 1 year showed arrest of myopia progression in 66% of the experimental group, but in only 15% of single-vision controls.

In contrast with these studies that indicate a statistically significant effect for plus lens addition in slowing myopia progression, studies by Mandell (1959), Shotwell (1981), Grosvenor et al. (1987), and Hemminki and Pärssinen (1987) report no significant effect. Given that several well-controlled studies document a positive effect for bifocals, it is possible that these negative results may have been caused by procedural differences that masked or weakened an existing positive effect. In Mandell's (1959) study for example, the bifocal wearers were significantly younger and more myopic than the single-vision group, and hence subject to greater myopic progression. Shotwell (1981) studied subjects 18 to 20 years old, over a 5-month period; both the age of the subjects and the time frame lead one to expect that myopic change will be small, and that differences between treatment groups might therefore be difficult to demonstrate. Nevertheless, Shotwell reported a rate of progression slightly lower with bifocals, although the difference was not statistically significant.

The concept that procedural differences may mask an existing positive effect is supported by a report by Goss and Grosvenor (1990). The authors point out that Roberts and Banford (1967) and Goss (1986) each found that bifocals slow childhood myopia progression for patients with nearpoint esophoria, but not for those with orthophoria or exophoria. The Houston Myopia Control Study (Grosvenor et al. 1987) found no such difference. Goss and Grosvenor (1990) noted procedural differences between the Goss (1986) and Grosvenor et al. (1987) studies, related to age of the subjects, inclusion criteria, and data analysis. To determine whether the differences in results could have been caused by these methodological differences, they reanalyzed the data of Grosvenor et al. (1987) using the methods used in the Goss (1986) study. Reanalysis produced results very similar to those obtained by Roberts and Banford (1967) and by Goss (1986): for orthophores and exophores, the rates of myopia progression with bifocal and with single-vision lenses were very similar, while for esophores, the rate of progression was less with bifocals. Further, the mean difference in rate of progression between the bifocal and single-vision lens wearers was similar for all three studies, approximately 0.20 D per year.

Issues related to compliance may further mask or weaken the effects produced by bifocals in many studies. Some bifocal wearers read through the distance prescription, rather than the bifocal segment; although they wear bifocals, they read through full minus. Many single-vision lens—wearing myopes remove their glasses for reading; although they are full minus lens wearers for the statistical analysis of the study, they actually read through a plus lens addition. These compliance factors act to statistically weaken any difference in myopia progression that in fact exists between those who actually wear full minus and reduced minus for near. Bifocals therefore may actually slow myopia progression to a degree greater than that indicated by these studies.

Random assignment of myopes to the various treatment groups further weakens the results of any research study. The inclusion, for example, of some stable myopes who would not progress regardless of the treatment method dilutes any true therapeutic effect and diminishes differences between treatment groups. Margach (1985) notes that random assignment to single-vision and bifocal treatment groups is far removed from clinical practice, and suggests that better therapeutic results should be obtained clinically when patients are appropriately selected for myopia control programs.

Another critical issue is whether high-add or low-add bifocals are more effective in slowing myopia progression. Roberts and Banford (1967), who generally used low-power lens additions of +0.75 to +1.25 D, indicate that children with weaker additions tend to progress more slowly than those with stronger bifocal adds. Oakley and Young (1975), in contrast, supplied high-add bifocals arbitrarily and indiscriminately, yet reported even more impressive results than did Roberts and Banford. Further research is needed to determine the optimal bifocal addition to minimize myopia progression.

Clinical Considerations in Prescribing Bifocals for Control of Myopia Progression

Incipient and progressing myopes typically demonstrate esophoria at near, low PRA, and greater plus acceptance on the binocular cross-cylinder test (Goss 1990, 1991). Each of the various methods of case analysis dictates that plus lens addition be prescribed for optimal nearpoint visual function in patients with such findings. In addition, studies by Roberts and Banford (1967), Goss (1986), and Goss and Grosvenor (1990) suggest that plus lens addition is most effective in slowing myopia progression in myopes who demonstrate esophoria at near. Therefore, in most cases of developing and progressing myopia, it is desirable to prescribe nearpoint plus lens addition to provide optimal nearpoint visual function, as well as for possible control of myopia progression.

When myopia has stabilized and is no longer progressing, case analysis frequently shows no further indication for nearpoint plus lens addition. Therefore, in stable myopia, a single-vision lens prescription for constant wear is often optimal.

The decision as to whether indicated plus lens addition should be prescribed in single-vision or bifocal form depends on the distance acuity through the nearpoint correction and on the nature of the tasks to be performed by the patient. Bifocals are usually preferable for school-age children, since single-vision reading glasses cannot easily be removed as the child shifts gaze from near to far in the classroom, and consequently are frequently not used as directed.

As myopia progresses, patients are sometimes advised to use their new glasses (with higher minus) for distance and to continue with the old glasses for near. In prescribing for children, this approach is usually doomed to failure, since it is virtually impossible to carry out in the classroom. Adults, too, generally find it inconvenient to switch glasses. In most cases, therefore, plus lens power for near is most effectively used when prescribed in bifocal form.

To insure that the bifocal segment is actually used for near work, many authorities use large-segment, executive-type bifocals for children, and set them considerably higher than those prescribed for adults. This author has found that most school-age children will, if properly instructed, correctly use smaller, less-visible 22-mm round and 25-mm flat-top segments set at or 1 mm above the lower lid margin. Such bifocals, if properly used, are advantageous in that they provide better cosmesis and interfere less with distance vision.

Another decision for the clinician is whether to prescribe high-add or low-add bifocals. As indicated previously, the evidence with regard to myopia progression is mixed. Roberts and Banford (1967) report less myopic progression in those with lower adds; Oakley and Young (1975) used only high adds and reported still greater effect in slowing progression. With regard to optimal nearpoint efficiency, OEP analysis, traditional graphical analysis, and graphical analysis of AC/CA interactions (Schor and Narayan 1982) each usually indicate relatively low plus addition.

In many cases, myopia continues to increase despite efforts to control progression. Patients who develop myopia at early ages, whose myopia develops rapidly, who have a family history of myopia, and who are extreme in their near-work application, intensity, and disposition toward a "myopic personality," may be least likely to respond to intervention. It is possible that even these patients may, with appropriate care, develop less myopia than would otherwise be the case.

Difficulty in the control of myopia progression is compounded by the fact that the primary stressor, near visual work, continues unabated, as do many of the behaviors and personality traits that contribute to myopia development. Intensity of near-work application and drive for achievement may be so great that plus lens application is not sufficient to halt progression.

For the clinician, the question of bifocal or single-vision distance prescription goes beyond the issue of myopia control. The myopic patient, like all patients, should be managed with the goal of providing optimal visual function. Appropriate nearpoint lenses should be prescribed when case analysis indicates their desirability, and vision training should be advised when visual skills and abilities are inadequate. When such care is provided, myopia progression will frequently slow or cease; as nearpoint visual function improves, there is less need for myopic adaptation. Even when myopia does progress, patients should be given appropriate nearpoint lens correction and vision training when indicated to permit optimal nearpoint visual efficiency.

Therapeutic Use of Cycloplegics

Several studies document the efficacy of cycloplegia in controlling myopia progression (Abraham 1966; Bedrossian 1966, 1979; Dyer 1979; Sampson 1979; Brodstein et al. 1984; Brenner 1985). This literature is thoroughly reviewed by Goss (1982). Bedrossian (1966, 1979) found that atropine instillation in one eye produced a halt in myopia progression in that eye, while the untreated eye continued to progress.

The use of cyclopegia to control myopia clinically is impractical, since prolonged cycloplegia produces adverse side effects, patient discomfort, and interference with efficient visual function (Dyer 1979; Sampson 1979; Safir 1979). Patients consequently have strong resistance to such therapy; in the study by Dyer (1979), two thirds of the subjects were dropped due to noncompliance with the regimen. However, the demonstration that cycloplegia is effective in controlling myopia progression provides strong support for theories linking myopia to near work and accommodation, and provides indirect support for the use of bifocals.

SUMMARY

Studies by Harmon, Greenspan, and Pierce suggest that for any particular individual there is an optimal low-plus lens prescription, use of which is accompanied by improved near-work posture and working distance, as well as reduction in muscular tension and general physiological activation. These and other studies report improved performance on a variety of nearpoint tasks with appropriately prescribed plus lenses. Some studies indicate that the plus lens power that produces optimal results (improved performance, improved posture, and reduced physiological activation) is critical and specific, and that even slight variation from this optimal power may reduce the effectiveness of the lens prescription. In some studies, OEP analysis and MEM retinoscopy predicted the optimal lens power. Reports indicate that use of appropriate low-plus lenses for near may also influence electrophysiologic measures.

Studies indicate that nearpoint plus lenses relieve or reduce asthenopic symptoms in patients with accommodative insufficiency, and are effective in slowing progression of myopia, particularly in myopes who demonstrate esophoria at near. Disagreement exists as to whether high- or low-addition bifocals are more effective for myopia control.

REFERENCES

Abraham S (1966). Control of myopia with tropicamide: A progress report. *J Pediatr Ophthalmol* 34(4):10–22.

Bastien AR (1987). Myopia: The Space Expanding Effect of Convex Lenses. Optometric Extension Program Postgraduate Education Courses, Santa Ana, CA: Optometric Extension Program Foundation, 59:59–69.

Bedrossian R (1966). Treatment of Progressive Myopia With Atropine. Proc XX Internat Congress of Ophthalmology, New York, NY, Excerpta Medica Foundation, pp. 612–617.

Bedrossian R (1979). The effect of atropine on myopia. *Trans Am Acad Ophthalmol* 86(5):692–694.

Birnbaum MH (1979). Management of the low myopia pediatric patient. *J Am Optom Assoc* 50(11):1281–1289.

Brenner RL (1985). Further observations on the use of atropine in the treatment of functional myopia. *Ann Ophthalmol* 17:137–140.

Brodstein RS, Brodstein DE, Olson RJ, et al. (1984). The treatment of myopia with atropine and bifocals: A long-term prospective study. *Ophthalmology* 91(11):1373–1379.

Caden BW, Lamb MW, Pirman JJ (1984). Nearpoint lenses and performance on Winter Haven Copy Forms Test. *J Optom Vision Dev* 15(3):6–8.

Curtin BJ (1985). *The Myopias: Basic Science and Clinical Management.* Philadelphia: Harper and Row.

Daubs J, Shotwell AJ (1983). Optical prophylaxis for environmental myopia: An epidemiological assessment of short-term effects. *Am J Optom Physiol Opt* 60(4):316–320.

Daum KM (1983). Accommodative insufficiency. *Am J Optom Physiol Opt* 60(5):352–359.

Dyer J (1979). Role of cycloplegics in progressive myopia. *Trans Am Acad Ophthalmol* 86(5):692–694.

Flax N (1980). Letter to the editor. *J Am Optom Assoc* 51:17.

Friedhoffer A, Warren M (1988). The effect of nearpoint visual demands upon the central visual fields and the effects of nearpoint low plus spheres upon these changes. Reprinted in Francke AW. *Introduction to Optometric Visual Training.* Optometric Extension Program Postgraduate Education Courses, Santa Ana, CA: Optometric Extension Program Foundation, vol. 60, Sept., pp. 45–53.

Goss DA (1982). Attempts to reduce the rate of increase of myopia in young people. A critical literature review. *Am J Optom Physiol Opt* 59:828–841.

Goss DA (1986). Effect of bifocal lenses on the rate of childhood myopia progression. *Am J Optom Physiol Opt* 63(8):637–640.

Goss DA (1990). Variables related to the rate of childhood myopia progression. *Optom Vis Sci* 67:631–636.

Goss DA (1991). Clinical accommodation and heterophoria findings preceding juvenile onset of myopia. *Optom Vis Sci* 68(2):110–116.

Goss DA, Grosvenor T (1990). Rates of childhood myopia progression with bifocals as a function of nearpoint phoria: Consistency of three studies. *Optom Vis Sci* 67:637–640.

Greenspan SB (1970). Effects of children's nearpoint lenses upon body posture and performance. *Am J Optom Arch Am Acad Optom* 47(12):982–989.

Greenspan SB (1979). Lenses and visual performance. *J Am Optom Assoc* 50:1381–1383.

Grosvenor T, Perrigin DM, Perrigin J, et al. (1987). Houston Myopia Control Study: A randomized clinical trial. Part II. Final report by the patient care team. *Am J Optom Physiol Opt* 64(7):482–498.

Harmon DB (1960). Nearpoint lenses and physiologic activity. Movie, produced by the author, Austin, TX.

Harmon DB (1966). *The Rationale in Developmental Training*. St. Louis: DBH Resource Center.

Hemminki E, Pärssinen O (1987). Prevention of myopia progress by glasses. Study design and the first-year results of a randomized trial among school children. *Am J Optom Physiol Opt* 64(8):611–616.

Keller JT, Amos JF (1979). Low plus lenses and visual performance: A critical review. *J Am Optom Assoc* 50(9):1005–1011.

Kelly TSB, Chatfield C, Tustin G (1975). Clinical assessment of the arrest of myopia. *Br J Ophthalmol* 59:529–538.

Larrabee PE, Jones FR (1980). Behavioral effects of low plus lenses. *Percept Mot Skills* 51:913–914.

Ludlam WM (1976). Review of the psycho-physiological factors in visual information processing as they relate to learning. In: Greenstein TN (ed), *Vision and Learning Disability*. St. Louis: American Optometric Association, pp. 179–222.

MacDonald LW (1963). *Visual Training*. Optometric Extension Program Postgraduate Education Courses, Santa Ana, CA: Optometric Extension Program Foundation, 35:45–48.

Mandell B (1959). Myopia control with bifocal correction. *Am J Optom Arch Am Acad Optom* 36:652–658.

Margach CB (1985). Research Design. In: *Literature and Research Review*. Optometric Extension Program Continuing Education Courses, Santa Ana, CA: Optometric Extension Program Foundation, vol. 58, series 11, no. 3, Dec., pp. 17–24.

Miles PW (1957). Children with increasing myopia treated with bifocal lenses. Case reports. *Missouri Med* 54:1152–1155.

Miles PW (1962). A study of heterophoria and myopia in children, some of whom wore bifocal lenses. *Am J Ophthalmol* 54:111–114.

Oakley KH, Young FA (1975). Bifocal control of myopia. *Am J Optom Physiol Opt* 52:758–764.

Pierce JR (1966–68). *Research Reports and Special Articles*. Optometric Extension Program Continuing Education Courses, Santa Ana, CA: Optometric Extension Program Foundation, vol. 39, 40, series 1, 2, Oct. 1966–Feb. 1968.

Pierce JR (1970). A study of the relation between performance and physiological activity as a function of nearpoint lenses, working distance, and posture. Ph.D. dissertation, University of Portland, OR.

Pierce JR (1980). Low plus lenses and visual performance: A critical review. *J Am Optom Assoc* 51:453–459.

Pirman JJ, Lamb MW (1982). Nearpoint lenses and performance on Winter Haven Copy Forms Test. Optometric Extension Program Postgraduate Education Courses, Santa Ana, CA: Optometric Extension Program Foundation, vol. 55. *Research Reports and Special Articles,* Oct., pp. 71–74

Press LJ (1985). Physiological effects of plus lens application. *Am J Optom Physiol Opt* 62(6):392–397.

Press LJ (1987). Myopia. *J Optom Vis Dev* 18:1–17.

Press LJ (1990). Lenses and behavior. *J Optom Vis Dev* 21(1):5–17.

Roberts WL, Banford RD (1967). Evaluation of bifocal correction technique in juvenile myopia. *Optom Weekly* 58(38):25–31; 58(39):21–30; 58(40):23–28; 58(41):27–34; 58(43):19–26.

Safir A (1979). Discussion of presentation by Dr. Robert H Bedrossian. *Ophthalmology* 86:718–719.

Sampson W (1979). Role of cycloplegia in the management of functional myopia. *Trans Am Acad Ophthalmol* 86(5):695–697.

Schor CM, Narayan V (1982). Graphical analysis of prism adaptation, convergence accommodation, and accommodative vergence. *Am J Optom Physiol Opt* 59(10):774–784.

Shotwell AJ (1981). Plus lenses, prisms, and bifocal effects on myopia progression in military students. *Am J Optom Physiol Opt* 58:349–354.

Skeffington AM (1959). The role of a convex lens. *J Am Optom Assoc* 31(5):374–378.

Sohrab-Jam G (1976). Eye movement patterns and reading performance in poor readers: Immediate effects of convex lenses indicated by book retinoscopy. *Am J Optom Physiol Opt* 53(11):720–726.

Spafford MM, Lovasik JV, Holterman JA (1983). Modification of cortical activity by low plus lenses. *Am J Optom Physiol Opt* 60(6):535–537.

Wildsoet CF, Foo KH (1988). Reading performance and low plus lenses. *Clin Exp Optom* 71(3):100–105.

PART III

Visual Skills and Abilities Testing

Routine eye examination and visual analysis generally include an eye health evaluation, refraction, cover test, tests of ocular motility and convergence near point, and a phorometric battery. These tests, often supplemented with nearpoint retinoscopy, performance tests, and assessment of the patient's reaction to the tentative lens prescription, generally yield sufficient information to determine the optimal lens prescription for distance and near, and provide considerable insight as to the adequacy of accommodative, binocular, and ocular motility functions.

In addition to this basic routine, the practitioner often finds it desirable to perform supplementary tests. Additional tests of eye movement ability, accommodative and binocular function, visual-perceptual-motor development, and spatial organization are performed as required. This additional testing is frequently referred to as the *vision training evaluation*. It generally requires that the patient return for a second visit. In some offices, when a patient or parent calling to schedule an appointment indicates that the problem is one which the receptionist knows is likely to require a vision training evaluation, a longer appointment is scheduled to permit a comprehensive one-visit evaluation.

Supplementary testing is indicated when the patient reports symptoms, achievement deficits, or other problems that are not readily explainable after the routine examination, or when the practitioner requires additional information to guide lens application, to determine the need for vision therapy, or to design a vision therapy program.

The tests performed assist the clinician in decision-making, and provide baseline data for future comparison. In addition, the tests performed in the vision therapy evaluation often serve to graphically demonstrate the problem to patients and parents so that they better understand the need for vision therapy.

This section will describe tests of eye movement and accommodative and binocular function not previously discussed. Many of these tests are performed during the initial routine examination; others are used as supplementary tests and performed as needed, often during a second visit. Tests of ocular motility are described in Chapter 11, and tests of accommodative and fusion ability in Chapter 12. Since many patients present with reading and learning difficulty as a chief concern, the significance of visual function in relation to academic achievement is discussed in Chapter 13.

11

Assessment of Eye Movement Ability

Pursuit and saccadic eye movements are routinely evaluated. Smooth pursuit movements permit continuous foveal fixation of objects moving in space. Saccades are the eye movements involved in reading and in shifting fixation from one target to another in daily life.

Eye movements are evaluated to assess the functional and structural integrity of the oculomotor system. In addition, eye movement testing provides information regarding broader aspects of behavioral and developmental maturity. Pursuits require that the individual sustain visual attention, even in the presence of distractors; that spatial organization be adequate; and, for efficient performance, that the patient be capable of moving eyes independent of head and body, a task that requires adequate motor control and organization. Saccades additionally require a high degree of central-peripheral organization if the patient is to localize a peripheral target and accurately shift fixation to it.

Leigh and Zee (1983) indicate that deficient eye movements may be caused by fatigue, aging, drugs and medications, and neurologic disease. However, in this author's experience, functional factors play a significant role in most cases. Poor eye movements commonly occur in patients who are unable to sustain attention, whose spatial organization is inadequate to predict target position, or whose fine motor development is inadequate to permit accurate tracking.

The examiner should attempt to differentiate whether inadequate eye movements are functional or organic in origin by taking a careful case history with respect to drug use, general health, and signs and symptoms of neurologic disease, as well as by looking carefully for signs of associated neuro-ophthalmic disorder. In the absence of such signs, poor eye movements are generally not the result of active treatable disease, and neurologic evaluation is not usually required.

PURSUIT EYE MOVEMENTS

Pursuits are generally tested monocularly and binocularly. Monocular pursuits are referred to as *ductions* and binocular pursuits as *versions*. Pursuit movements are typically tested by instructing the patient to follow a target that is slowly moved through the horizontal, vertical, and diagonal meridians, as well as through a circle to evaluate rotations (Figure 11.1). The patient should be seated comfortably in well-balanced posture. For the monocular phase of the test, an elastic band occluder is placed over one eye. It is best not to have the patient hold the occluder, because this may introduce postural distortion. Testing is usually performed at 16 inches or the Harmon distance. Some clinicians test as close as 6 inches to assess performance under stress.

The examiner should not move the target too rapidly. Pursuit movements are relatively slow. When target velocity is excessive, fixation is lost and pursuit movement will appear jerky. This occurs even in normal subjects, because saccadic movements, which are considerably faster than pursuits, are used to "catch-up"and regain fixation (Griffin 1984).

Typical targets include a dangled bell; a small metal sphere affixed to a

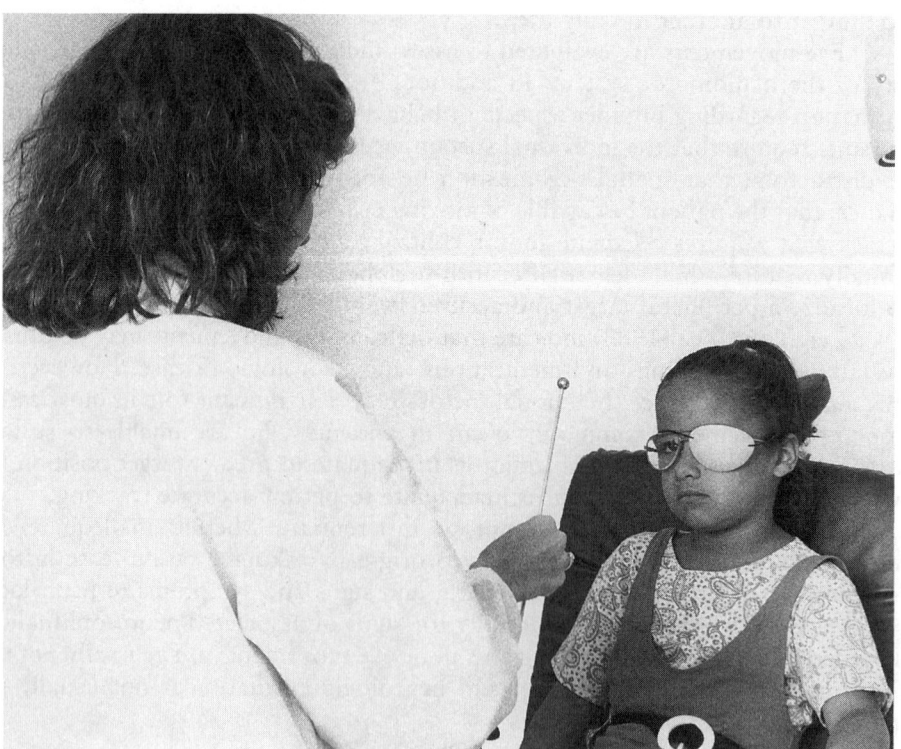

Figure 11.1 Monocular pursuits testing.

metal rod (Wolff wand); a Disney character eraser on the end of a pencil; a small picture affixed to a tongue depressor; a pen or pencil; or a small light source such as a penlight or transilluminator. The latter targets permit the examiner to observe the corneal light reflex as an aid in evaluating the quality of pursuit movements. The examiner should generally be consistent in the use of target. Routine use of the same target facilitates consistency of observation. However, use of a variety of targets may help sustain attention in preschoolers.

The performance of young children on pursuit tests differs significantly from that of adults. Since performance is influenced not only by neuromuscular integrity, but also by attention, spatial judgments, and motor organization, performance is related to age and developmental level. The experienced clinician develops the ability to evaluate eye movement skills based on observation of many patients of differing ages and developmental levels.

The presence of smooth pursuit movement has been demonstrated during the first few months of life, although such movements are inaccurate and poorly sustained (Kremenitzer et al. 1979; Aslin 1981). Pursuit movements in preschoolers are often only intermittently accurate, and are frequently accompanied by excessive head and body movement. Development is characterized by increasing accuracy, ability to sustain, and ability to inhibit head movement. Apell and Lowry (1959) describe expecteds for preschoolers of different ages. Smooth pursuit movements with minimum head movement and good ability to sustain are normally present by age 6 or 7.

In evaluating pursuit movements, the examiner should observe the following:

1. Are eye movements restricted or noncomitant?

   The clinician should be alert for signs of neurological involvement, including restricted extraocular muscle action, noncomitancy, nystagmus, and ptosis. When such conditions are present and recent in origin, medical evaluation is indicated since the causative agent may have serious health implications and may even be life-threatening (Hugonnier and Clayette-Hugonnier 1969).

2. Are ocular movements smooth, fluid, and accurate, or are they jerky or erratic?

   The examiner should observe the quality of pursuit movement as the patient tracks the moving target. Pursuits should be smooth, flowing, and well-sustained, especially in children age 8 and older (Gesell et al. 1950).

   When pursuits are inaccurate, overshooting, or (more commonly) lagging behind the target, corrective saccadic movements (which are considerably faster than pursuits) come into play to restore fixation. This phenomenon is known as *saccadic replacement*. As a consequence, inaccurate pursuits have a jerky saccadic-like appearance (Griffin, 1984).

   Pursuits are sometimes observed that are not simply jerky and inaccurate, but are actually erratic. Erratic pursuits are characterized by large random eye movements away from the target, to the examiner, to extreme gaze positions, or to other objects in the room. Erratic pursuits usually indicate that the patient is unable to sustain attention, has inadequate spatial organization, or is unduly distracted by objects in the periphery.

In assessing the quality of pursuit eye movements, the examiner should not nitpick. An occasional loss of fixation, shift from the target to the examiner, or jerk movement does not constitute grounds for failure. The examiner should consider the patient's overall performance. Are tracking movements generally smooth, accurate, and well controlled? Does the patient sustain fixation well, and not shift attention unduly? If so, quality of pursuit movements is considered to be adequate.

Differentiation between functional and organic cause for jerky pursuits is sometimes difficult. Jerky pursuit movements that smooth out even briefly when a target of greater attentional value is used, when the patient is allowed to point to or touch the target to bring in kinesthetic support, or when the patient is exhorted to look at the target more carefully, may be presumed to be functional in origin. However, differential diagnosis occasionally cannot be made until after treatment: those cases in which pursuits smooth out with training are presumed functional, and those which remain jerky are assumed be organic in origin.

3. Are pursuit movements smoother and more accurate in some directions than in others?

Observation should be made of differences in the various meridians tested. Developmentally, smooth, accurate pursuit movements are demonstrable at an earlier age in the horizontal than in the vertical or diagonal meridians. Horizontal pursuits are usually smooth and well sustained by age 6 or 7. Rotations and vertical and diagonal pursuits are more complex and mature later, generally reaching adult levels by about age 9. Even in older children and adults, vertical pursuits may exhibit a slight jerkiness that should be considered normal. Diagonal movements are the most complex, and are the last to be achieved with proficiency (Gesell et al. 1950; Apell and Lowry 1959; Kephart 1960).

4. Does head or body move as the child tracks the target?

When pursuits are tested, the child should be instructed to "follow the target as it moves." The child should not initially be told to hold the head still, since it is desirable to observe performance under habitual conditions. If head (or head and body) movement is observed, the examiner should ask the patient to follow with eyes only. The ability to inhibit head movement and track accurately with eyes alone constitutes adequate performance. If the patient is unable to inhibit head movement even when asked to, the examiner may briefly touch the child's head or cup the chin to determine whether the child is able to eliminate head movement when given this additional support (Getman 1960).

If head movement does take place, the examiner should note whether the eyes lead, with head used simply to relieve the need for extreme versions, or whether head movement is primary, occurring to take the place of eye movement. The former is often normal behavior, while the latter strongly suggests inadequate eye movement ability, so that head movement is used as a substitute. If the examiner restrains the head movement in such cases, eye movements are usually jerky and poorly controlled.

Use of head rather than eye movement is disadvantageous for several reasons. The eye muscles are so delicately controlled as compared with the neck that eye movements, when properly used, are much more accurate and efficient. In addition, head movement requires greater energy expenditure, since the mass of the head is so much greater than that of the eyes. Further, rapid head movement may cause momentary disorientation in space.

Some children tend to move the upper body along with head and eyes, so that the entire upper torso tracks the target; others exhibit significant motor overflow (nonpurposive fidgeting, wriggling, or excessive unrelated verbalization) (Getman 1960). Such behavior may reflect developmental immaturity. In infancy, any attempt at movement tends to generate activity of the entire body. Development brings increasing ability to differentiate movement patterns.

Tracking primarily with the head, or even with the entire torso, is common among young preschoolers. By age 4 or 5, head and body movement may still be used supportively, but eyes rather than head should lead the tracking activity, and the child should be capable of inhibiting head movement if so directed. The 4- or 5-year-old may demonstrate gustatory support, rolling the tongue in tandem with the eyes, as well as various forms of fidgeting and other motor and verbal overflow. These behaviors are considered immature if they persist beyond age 6 or 7.

By age 7, the child should be capable of tracking on a purely visual basis. The school-age child who moves head or body instead of eyes to track a moving object, who is unable to inhibit head movement when requested, who tracks with tongue as well as with eyes, or who shows considerable motor overflow, demonstrates immature and inefficient performance (Gesell et al. 1950; Apell and Lowry, 1959; Getman 1960). In addition to oculomotor deficit, such children may demonstrate developmental immaturity with deficient gross and fine motor abilities. Testing in these areas should be performed to determine the child's status.

5. Does the child adjust readily to the test situation?

Pursuit eye movements that are initially inaccurate, poorly sustained, and accompanied by excessive head movement and motor overflow sometimes improve considerably as the test proceeds and the child adjusts. This *adjustment difficulty*, attributable to the newness of the test situation and the surroundings, is typical in preschool children and should not mislead the examiner into believing that pursuit ability is inadequate. However, it is expected that by school age the child should adjust readily to the task. Adjustment difficulty that persists into school age is a sign of immaturity and is characteristic of nonachievers (Apell and Lowry 1959).

6. Are pursuit movements well sustained? Does performance deteriorate with time?

Pursuits are typically tested for about 30 seconds. Some clinicians advocate longer test periods to assess stamina. The ability to sustain pursuits improves as oculomotor and attentional mechanisms develop. By school age, the child should be able to sustain pursuits over the duration of the test (Apell and Lowry 1959).

7. Does kinesthetic involvement improve pursuit performance?

If pursuit performance is inadequate, the examiner should ask the child to point at or touch the target as it moves. Improved performance serves to rule out an organic basis for the pursuit deficit, and suggests that the prognosis is good for improvement with training. In such cases, it is likely that motor support will be helpful in the early stages of therapy.

8. Do the two eyes differ with regard to quality of performance on monocular pursuit testing?

Pursuit ability should be evaluated both monocularly and binocularly. When quality of performance differs for the right and left eyes, monocular training is indicated to equalize ability.

9. Is quality of performance better monocularly or binocularly?

Better monocular performance than binocular suggests the presence of binocular vision dysfunction. Under monocular test conditions, binocular perturbating factors are eliminated and performance improves. Since each ocular mechanism has achieved its own adequate motility, Getman (1964) suggests that training in such cases should emphasize binocular pursuits.

When pursuits are better under binocular than monocular test conditions, the implication is that adequate performance has not been achieved within each ocular circuit. Under binocular test conditions, one eye may reinforce the other so that binocular performance is better. Training should begin with monocular procedures, to develop more adequate performance in each ocular circuit (Getman 1964).

Pursuits may also be better under binocular than monocular conditions if pursuit ability has not developed to an adequate level of automaticity. Testing with one eye covered presents a novel situation in which the child has had little prior experience. A decrement in performance suggests that pursuit ability is fragile and easily broken down.

10. Are pursuits automatic and effortless, or do they require excessive concentration and effort? Do other demands interfere with performance?

Pursuits should be so automatic as to require minimum effort, so that the child is free to process information without concentrating on the eye movements themselves (Peachey 1991). Excessive tension, effort, and concentration during pursuit testing suggest that pursuits are not sufficiently habituated, and require concentration just to follow the target.

Reading requires accurate eye movement performance even though attention is directed toward the search for meaning, rather than toward the eye movements. Eye movements that are not fully automated and efficient may break down under these conditions, or excess attention directed toward maintaining accurate eye movement may interfere with the ability to process information.

Automaticity is demonstrated by the ability to maintain accurate eye movement in the presence of cognitive demand. To assess the degree to which pursuits are effortless and automatic, the examiner may initiate a conversation with the patient as the test proceeds (Peachey 1991). By the age of 9 or 10, a child should have habituated pursuits and be able to converse without major decrement in performance.

11. Do the eyes cross the midline smoothly?

Some patients demonstrate a small flick or jump as the target crosses the midline. A midline jump may occur under monocular or binocular test conditions, and may occur as the eyes move from left to right, from right to left, or in both directions. When a school-age child demonstrates a consistent midline jump, performance is deemed inadequate (Getman and Kephart 1957–58; Getman 1960; Kephart 1960).

Pursuit Performance Rating Scales

Several rating systems have been developed to objectively evaluate pursuit movements. One of these, developed by Heinsen and Schrock and described by Griffin (1982, 1984), uses a rating scale in which performance is graded in each of four categories, with a maximum point score of 10:

1. Degree of smoothness
   - Smooth, always on target (3 points)
   - Smooth, sometimes off target (2 points)
   - Jerky, generally on target (1 point)
2. Degree of head movement
   - Free of head movement (3 points)
   - Head movement present, but can be inhibited (2 points)
   - Slight head movement persists (1 point)
3. Degree of automaticity
   - Automated pursuits (3 points)
   - Reduced automation (2 points)
   - Much reduced automation (1 point)
4. Degree of stamina
   - Adequate stamina (1 point)

Maples and Ficklin (1988) report a somewhat similar procedure for grading pursuit performance, based on a standardized approach to testing and observation. The patient stands and follows a small test object that is moved through two clockwise and two counterclockwise rotations. Performance is graded on the basis of ability to sustain, accuracy, and degree of head and body movement. A score of one to five points is awarded in each category, as follows:

A. Can the patient sustain for two rotations in each direction?
   1. No attempt is made to follow the target.
   2. Completes one half, but not one rotation.
   3. Completes one, but not two rotations.
   4. Completes two rotations in one direction, but not the other.
   5. Completes two rotations in each direction.
B. Can the patient track accurately, with no noticeable refixation required?
   1. Makes 10 or more refixations, or makes no attempt to follow the target.
   2. Refixes four to 10 times.
   3. Refixes two to four times.
   4. Refixes two times or less.
   5. No refixations noted.
C. Can the patient maintain the pursuit without moving head and body?
   1. Gross movement of head of body.
   2. Large to moderate movement of head or body.
   3. Consistent slight movement of head or body.
   4. Intermittent slight movement of head or body.
   5. No movement of head or body.

The authors report a high degree of both interrater and test-retest reliability when this testing and scoring procedure is used by trained observers.

Groffman Tracing Test

The Groffman Tracing Test (Groffman 1966), published by Mast/Keystone, presents a series of five complex criss-crossing lines (Figure 11.2). The patient must track along each line to correctly identify the letter at the end of the line. Scoring is based on speed and accuracy; age-based norms are provided. The test is highly demanding; not only oculomotor, but also visual attention and figure-

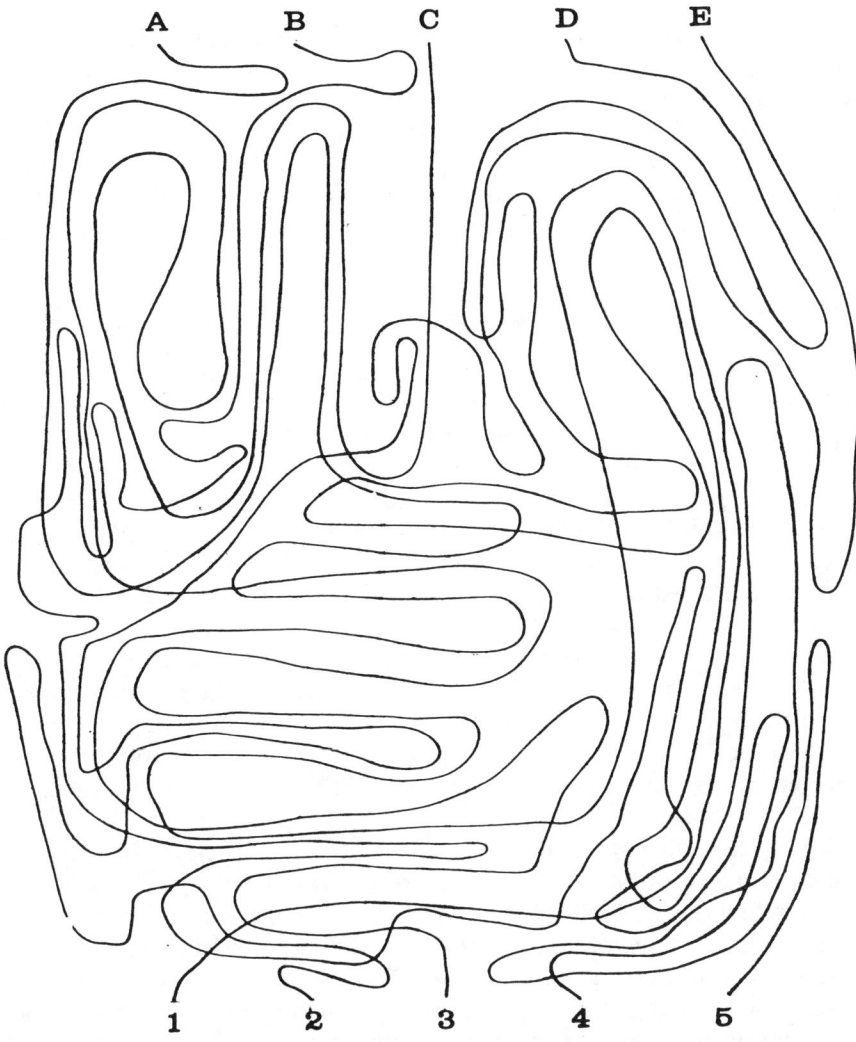

Figure 11.2   Groffman Tracing Test. (Reprinted with permission of Mast/Keystone.)

ground organization must be well developed if the patient is not to be distracted by the myriad of intersecting lines.

Pursuit Movements and Reading

Nonachievers often show jerky and erratic pursuits, a tendency to move head rather than eyes, and frequent loss of fixation (Getman 1962; Apell and Lowry 1959; Kephart 1960). In laboratory studies, Bogacz et al. (1974) and Adler-Grinberg and Stark (1978) report deficits in smooth pursuit movements in reading-disabled subjects, although Brown et al. (1983) did not find such deficits.

Although correlation between pursuit ability and academic achievement has been reported, it is saccadic eye movements and not pursuits that are involved in reading. The reported correlation may exist not because pursuits play a direct role in reading, but rather because the high level of oculomotor control and attentional ability required during pursuit testing is important for academic achievement. Further, it is possible that the ability to maintain, control, and correct pursuit movements may relate closely to the ability to make the fine saccades required in reading.

SACCADIC EYE MOVEMENTS

Saccadic eye movements occur as the individual shifts fixation from one object of interest to another. Saccades allow an individual to rapidly redirect the line of sight so as to place the image of an object of interest on the fovea.

Saccadic movements may be gross or fine. The fine saccades involved in reading consist of a series of fixations across a line of print with a return sweep at the end of each line. Larger, gross saccades are typical of daily seeing, as attention shifts from one object to another. Under natural conditions, saccades usually do not exceed 20 degrees. Saccadics of minimal amplitude measure 2 to 5 minutes of arc (Yarbus 1967).

Moving the eyes from one point of fixation to another and then sustaining fixation is achieved through a pulse-step of innervation. The *pulse* consists of a burst of neural activity to move the eyes to their new position; the *step* consists of a new tonic level of neural activity to create a steady contraction of the extraocular muscles that holds the eyes steady in their new position (Leigh and Zee 1983).

During the actual saccadic movement, vision is suppressed (or masked) to prevent the perception of blur that would result from light input being smeared across the retina during high-velocity movement. Information-processing occurs during the fixation that follows a saccadic movement (Griffin 1982; Leigh and Zee 1983). Stabilization of retinal images during fixation is prevented by head movements, by blinking, and by three types of small eye movements that occur during fixation: slow, irregular drift movements; small involuntary saccades; and tremor, a high-frequency, low-amplitude oscillating movement (Yarbus 1967).

Abnormal Saccadic Eye Movements

Saccadic eye movements may be inaccurate (or dysmetric) because the size of the rapid pulse portion of the saccade is inappropriate and the image of the target is not brought to the fovea (pulse-size dysmetria), or because the saccadic pulse and step are not appropriately matched, so that the eye drifts at the end of the saccade (pulse-step match dysmetria). Normal individuals frequently show small degrees of saccadic pulse-size dysmetria, most commonly undershooting. This undershooting (hypometria) is relatively small in degree, about 10% of the amplitude of the saccade, and is compensated by a corrective saccade. Undershooting is more pronounced with aging and with fatigue. Overshooting (hypermetria) is less common and may be a sign of neurologic disease, particularly of the cerebellum (Leigh and Zee 1983).

Abnormal saccadic eye movements include overshooting and undershooting, saccadic intrusions (inappropriate saccades that take the eyes off the target), postsaccadic drift, and a failure to sustain fixation so that the eye drifts back toward the primary position at the end of each saccade, creating gaze-evoked nystagmus. Abnormal saccades are frequently observed during routine clinical testing, but more subtle changes can be detected only by analysis of eye movement recordings (Leigh and Zee 1983).

Several studies report the existence of abnormal saccadic eye movements in children with reading disability (Lesevre 1968; Dossetor and Papaioannou 1975; Poynter et al. 1982; Jones and Stark 1983; Pavlidis 1981, 1985; Griffin et al. 1974; Goldrich and Sedgwick 1982). Other studies fail to demonstrate saccadic abnormality in the reading-disabled (Adler-Grinberg and Stark 1978; Brown et al. 1983; Stanley et al. 1983; Olson et al. 1983). These disparate findings may result from sampling differences.

Clinically, it is often found that poor eye movement ability is associated with inefficiency in reading and copying from desk or chalkboard, with frequent loss of place, need to use finger or marker to keep the place, skipping words and lines, and transposition of letters and numbers.

Evaluation of Saccadic Movements

Commonly used clinical saccadic tests evaluate gross saccadic movements, rather than the fine saccades involved in reading. In evaluating saccadic movements, the examiner typically holds two targets approximately 16 inches apart and rhythmically directs the patient to shift fixation from one to the other on command (Figure 11.3). Testing is done with the targets separated in the horizontal, vertical, and diagonal meridians, and should be performed both monocularly and binocularly.

Targets are similar to those used for pursuits. There is a trend toward using Wolff wands, small gold and silver spheres fixed to metal rods, as standard fixation targets for both pursuit and saccadic testing.

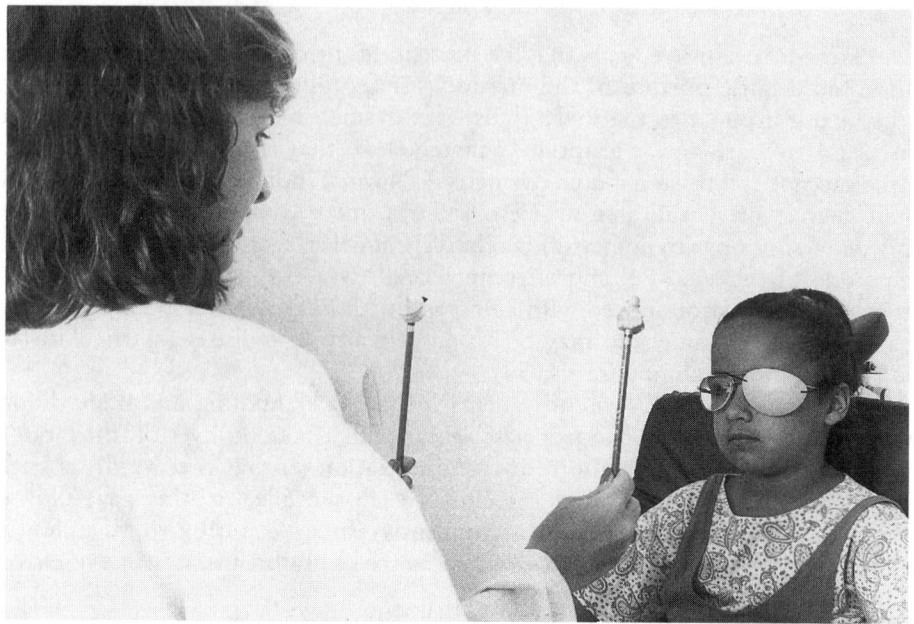

Figure 11.3 Evaluating saccadic eye movements monocularly.

Observations made by the examiner are similar to those discussed for pursuit testing. The examiner should evaluate the patient's ability to make accurate saccadic fixations; to sustain through time; to move the eyes without need for head or body support, and without random motor overflow; to perform automatically, with minimum effort, even while performing concurrent cognitive tasks; and to respond appropriately to the instructional set.

Assessment of Performance

Heinsen and Schrock designed a 10-point scale for scoring saccadic eye movement performance (Griffin 1982). The patient is given a score in each of five categories, with a maximum score of 10:

1. Head movement
   a. No head movement (3 points)
   b. Head movement, but can inhibit (2 points)
   c. Slight head movement persists (1 point)
2. Accuracy of performance
   a. Accurate (2 points)
   b. Slight inaccuracies (1 point)

3. Automaticity
   a. Highly automatic (2 points)
   b. Reduced automaticity (1 point)
4. Stability
   a. Stable saccades for 20 seconds (2 points)
   b. Stable saccades for 10 seconds (1 point)
5. Stamina
   a. Adequate stamina (1 point)

Maples and Ficklin (1988) report high interrater and test-retest reliability for a clinical test of saccadic eye movement ability. The patient stands and shifts fixation back and forth, on command, between a red and a green hatpin placed horizontally at eye level, approximately at the Harmon distance, not more than 20 cm apart. The patient is asked to perform five round trips from one target to the other, and performance is scored based on accuracy, ability to sustain, and ability to perform without head or body movement. A score of one to five points is awarded in each of three categories:

A. Can the patient sustain attention for five complete round trips?
   1. Patient can only complete one round trip, or does not attempt to perform the task.
   2. Completes two round trips.
   3. Completes three round trips.
   4. Completes four round trips.
   5. Completes five round trips.
B. Can the patient fixate accurately and consistently so that no noticeable refixation is required?
   1. Gross over- or undershooting is noted.
   2. Large to moderate over- or undershooting is noted.
   3. Constant, slight over- or undershooting is noted.
   4. Intermittent, slight over- or undershooting is noted.
   5. No over- or undershooting is noted.
C. Can the patient perform without moving head or body?
   1. Gross movement of head or body.
   2. Large to moderate movement of head or body.
   3. Consistent, slight movement of head or body.
   4. Intermittent, slight movement of head or body.
   5. No movement of head or body.

Developmental, Central-Peripheral, Spatial, and Attentional Considerations

Development and maturation bring progressive improvement on tests of saccadic performance. Preschool and young school-age children exhibit less accuracy, have greater difficulty sustaining attention, and demonstrate more head and body support, fidgeting, and motor overflow than do older children and adults. Clinically, the ability to make accurate and well-sustained saccadic movements with minimum head involvement and motor overflow is expected by age 8 or 9. As with pursuits, poor saccades may occur as a sign of neurologic disorder, but most cases are functional in origin, resulting from inadequate development of eye movement control, inability to sustain attention, inadequate central-peripheral organization, poor spatial judgements, or inability to move eyes without head and body involvement.

While normal individuals frequently show a small undershoot, about 10% of the size of the saccade, which is compensated by a corrective saccade (Leigh and Zee 1983), some patients show random errors, overshooting or undershooting extensively and erratically, or shifting gaze to the examiner, to other objects in the room, or to the extremes of gaze. These erratic, gross random errors suggest problems with oculomotor control, attention, spatial judgements, or central-peripheral organization. Saccadic fixations probe central-peripheral and spatial organization, as well as basic eye movement ability, as the patient is required to shift fixation to centrally fixate a target originally seen peripherally.

Central-peripheral organization may be further probed during saccadic testing by moving the nonfixated, peripherally viewed target to a new location. The ability to accurately shift fixation to the new target location indicates that central-peripheral organization is adequate: the patient is able to note that the target has moved and to localize it with the retinal periphery in order to initiate an accurate saccade.

Eye movement testing also reflects visual attention ability. Some patients are easily distracted by extraneous peripheral stimuli, and frequently shift fixation to the examiner, to their parents, or to other objects. Such distractibility indicates inability to sustain central attention in the presence of distractors. Vision therapy emphasizing eye movement procedures often enhances the ability to sustain visual attention.

Saccadic eye movements may also be viewed in the context of the reach-grasp-release information-processing sequence (Getman and Kephart 1957–58). Localizing the target in space and making an accurate fixation movement is a function of *reach*. The ability to sustain fixation until directed to shift to the next target relates to *grasp*, during which one inspects and derives information from an object of regard. The ability to let go and shift attention to the next target reflects the process of *release*.

The child who regularly releases too quickly demonstrates poor grasp. Such behavior is often associated with attentional deficit and impulsivity. Inability to sustain visual attention, reflected in poor grasp, is even more readily observed during pursuit testing, since pursuits are primarily involved with the grasp phase of the reach-grasp-release sequence.

Supplementary Saccadic Tests

Clinically, saccades are typically observed simply by having the patient shift fixation from one hand-held target to another. Numerous additional tests have been developed to aid in observing and quantifying saccadic performance.

A variety of opaque and transparent sequential fixation cards are used to test saccadic performance (Griffin 1982). The examiner observes as the patient sequentially fixates targets printed on the card. Targets printed on clear acetate permit the examiner to observe the patient's eye movements through the card (Figure 11.4). Tests designed by Pierce (1972), Sherman (see Treganza and Wold 1977), Vincett (1973), King and Devick (1976), and Richman and Garzia (1987) assess saccadic eye movements by determining the speed and accuracy with which the patient is able to read horizontal rows of digits or letters.

Sherman uses a distance Hart Chart, a 10 row chart with 10 letters in each row (Figure 11.5). The patient reads the first and last letter in each row. Scoring is based on time and errors. The test can be made more demanding by asking the patient to read the second and next to last letter in each row (Treganza and Wold 1977).

The Pierce Saccade Test (Pierce 1972) uses three test cards, each with a vertical column of single digit numbers at its left and right margins. The patient reads each number aloud, in horizontal rows. Difficulty increases slightly with each card. Scoring is based on time and errors, and norms are age-based. Pierce reported significant differences in performance between normal and learning-disabled children (Treganza and Wold 1977).

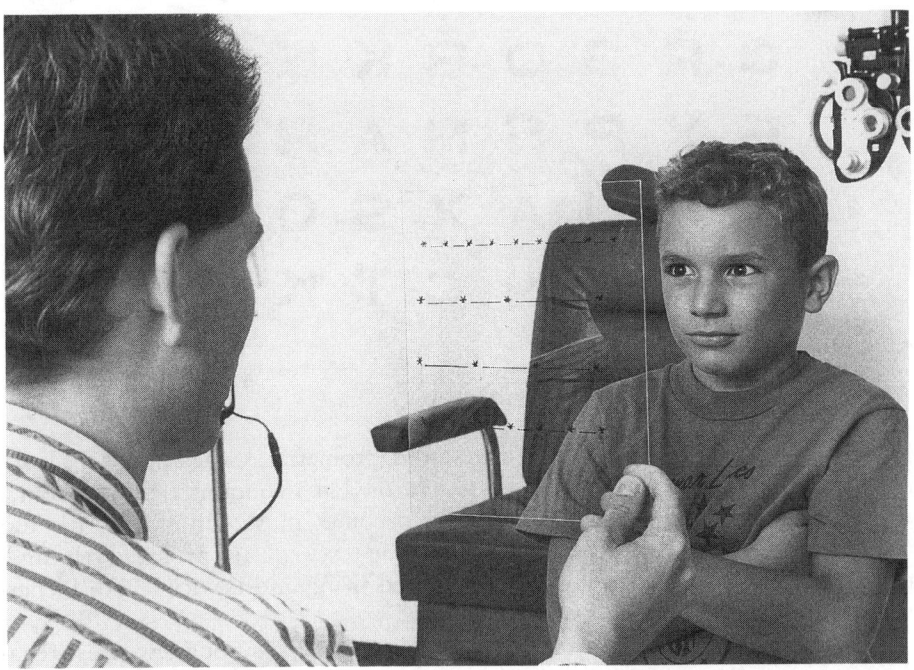

Figure 11.4 Evaluating saccadic eye movements with a sequential fixator. Use of clear acetate permits the examiner to observe the patient's eye movements through the card.

DR. HART'S REVISED VISION CHART — 100 DIGIT - 20/20 AND 10/10

20/20

		2		4		6		8		10
1	O	F	N	P	V	D	T	C	H	E
	Y	B	A	K	O	E	Z	L	R	X
3	E	T	H	W	F	M	B	K	A	P
	B	X	F	R	T	O	S	M	V	C
5	R	A	D	V	S	X	P	E	T	O
	M	P	O	E	A	N	C	B	K	F
7	C	R	G	D	B	K	E	P	M	A
	F	X	P	S	M	A	R	D	L	G
9	T	M	U	A	X	S	O	G	P	B
	H	O	S	N	C	T	K	U	Z	L

Figure 11.5 Hart chart.

The King-Devick Test (New York State Optometric Association K-D Test), published by Bernell Corp., uses three test cards. Each contains eight horizontal rows of five single-digit numbers. Spacing becomes more complex as the test proceeds from one chart to the next, so that the test requires progressively finer saccades. Norms are based on errors and speed (King and Devick 1976; Lieberman et al. 1983).

The Pierce and King-Devick saccadic tests each have poor test-retest reliability; subjects often show improved scores on retest as they become more familiar with the test. In view of this practice effect, clinicians must be cautious when using these tests to monitor the progress of therapy. Both tests may nevertheless be useful in screening for oculomotor dysfunction (Oride et al. 1986).

Another problem with the Pierce and King-Devick tests is that when a child reads the numbers slowly, the examiner cannot be certain whether failure is due to eye movement inefficiency or to inability to rapidly verbalize the names of the digits (Richman et al. 1983). The Developmental Eye Movement Test (DEM) (Richman and Garzia 1987; Garzia et al. 1990) attempts to differentiate these factors by comparing the time required to read a series of 80 vertically aligned single digits with that required to read 80 horizontal digits (Figure 11-6). If the

TEST A

3	4
7	5
5	2
9	1
8	7
2	5
5	3
7	7
4	4
6	8
1	7
4	4
7	6
6	5
3	2
7	9
9	2
3	3
9	6
2	4

Figure 11.6 Developmental Eye Movement Test (DEM). Plates A and B present 80 vertically aligned single digits; plate C presents 80 horizontal digits. (Reprinted with permission of Bernell Corp., South Bend, IN.)

TEST B

6	7
3	9
2	3
9	9
1	2
7	1
4	4
6	7
5	6
2	3
5	2
3	5
7	7
4	4
8	6
4	3
5	7
2	5
1	9
7	8

Figure 11.6 *Continued*

horizontal and vertical columns are read equally slowly, the deficit is attributed to deficient verbal response. If the horizontal rows are read more slowly than the vertical, the deficit is attributed to horizontal eye movements, since verbal response deficit would affect horizontal and vertical performance equally. Age-based norms are provided. High test-retest and interexaminer reliability have been demonstrated.

Ophthalmographic eye movement recording devices such as the Visagraph (Instructional Communications Technology) and the EDL/Biometrics Reading Eye II (Educational Developmental Laboratories) are used to objectively record saccadic eye movements while the patient reads. They provide information on

TEST C

3		7	5			9			8
2	5				7	4			6
1			4		7		6		3
7		9		3		9			2
4	5				2			1	7
5			3		7		4		8
7	4		6	5					2
9		2			3		6		4
6	3	2		9					1
7				4		6	5		2
5		3	7			4			8
4			5		2			1	7
7	9	3			9				2
1			4			7		6	3
2		5			7		4		6
3	7		5			9			8

Figure 11.6 *Continued*

the accuracy and number of fixations, the quality of the return sweep, and the number of regressions (Figure 11.7). The test may be performed with grade-appropriate cognitive or noncognitive targets. It is important not to use material that is too difficult, since the eye movement pattern during reading is influenced by the nature of the material. Material that is too difficult will produce a greater number of fixations and regressions.

SUMMARY

Pursuit and saccadic eye movements are important mechanisms for gathering information through the visual system. Tests of pursuit and saccadic eye movements are performed to evaluate the structural and functional integrity of the oculomotor system. In addition, eye movement tests provide information regarding behavioral and developmental processes such as visual attention, spa-

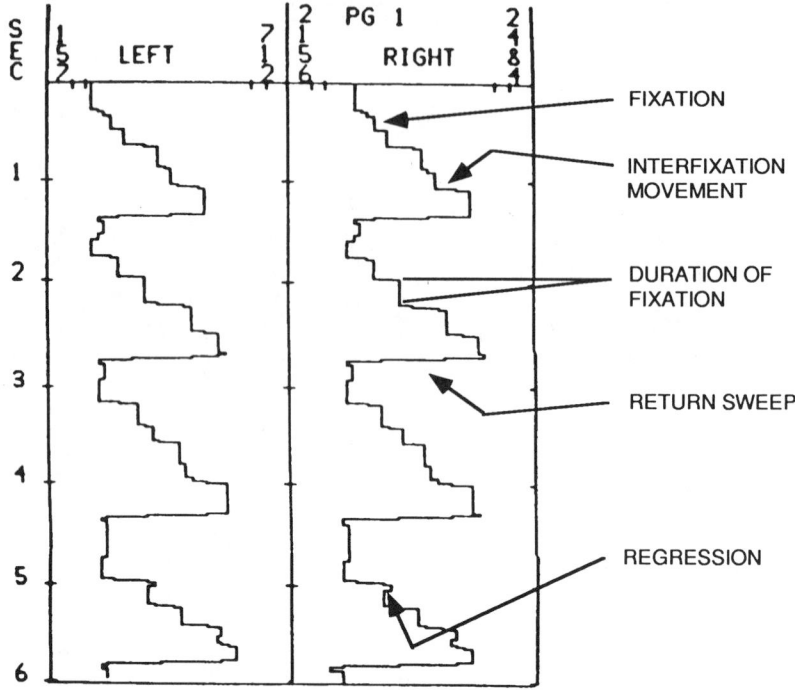

Figure 11.7 The eye movement recording provides information regarding the number of fixations, duration of fixation, number of regressions, and quality of the return sweep. (Photo reproduced with permission of Instructional Communications Technology, Inc.)

tial organization, motor control, and central-peripheral organization. Pursuits and saccades are usually tested monocularly and binocularly, and are evaluated with respect to comitancy, accuracy, ability to sustain, ability to differentiate eye movement from head movement, and automaticity. Rating scales have been developed to provide standardization. Supplementary tests include the Groffman Tracing Test, Pierce Saccadic Test, NYSOA K-D Test, Developmental Eye Movement Test, and objective eye movement recordings while reading. Some studies report abnormal eye movements in children with reading disability; other studies find no such deficits. Deficient eye movement ability is frequently remediable through vision therapy; procedures and sequences for treating deficient oculomotor function are described in Chapters 14 and 15.

SUGGESTED READING

Apell RJ, Lowry RW (1959). *Preschool Vision.* St Louis: American Optometric Association.

Getman GN (1960). *Techniques and Criteria for the Optometric Care of Children's Vision.* Santa Ana, CA: Optometric Extension Program Foundation.

Griffin JR (1982). *Binocular Anomalies: Procedures for Vision Therapy.* 2nd ed. Chicago: Professional Press.

Leigh RJ, Zee DS (1983). *The Neurology of Eye Movements.* Philadelphia: FA Davis.

REFERENCES

Adler-Grinberg D, Stark L (1978). Eye movements, scanpaths, and dyslexia. *Am J Optom Physiol Opt* 55(8):557–570.

Apell RJ, Lowry RW (1959). *Preschool Vision.* St. Louis: American Optometric Association.

Aslin RN (1981). Development of smooth pursuit in human infants. In: Fisher DF, Monty RA, Senders JW (eds), *Eye Movements: Cognition and Visual Perception.* Hillsdale, NJ: Lawrence Erlbaum Associates, pp. 31–51.

Bogacz J, Mendilaharsu C, de Mendilaharsu SA (1974). Electro-oculographic abnormalities during pursuit movements in developmental dyslexia. *EEG Clin Neurophysiol* 36:651–656.

Brown B, Haegerstrom-Portnoy G, Yingling CD, et al. (1983). Tracking eye movements are normal in dyslexic children. *Am J Optom Physiol Opt* 60(5):376–383.

Dossetor DR, Papaioannou J (1975). Dyslexia and eye movements. *Lang Speech* 18(4):312–317.

Garzia RP, Richman JE, Nicholson SB, et al. (1990). A new visual-verbal saccade test: The Developmental Eye Movement test (DEM). *J Am Optom Assoc* 61:124–135.

Gesell A, Ilg FL, Bullis GE, et al. (1950). *Vision: Its Development in Infant and Child.* New York: Paul B. Hoeber.

Getman GN (1960). *Techniques and Criteria for the Optometric Care of Children's Vision.* Santa Ana, CA: Optometric Extension Program Foundation.

Getman GN (1962). *How to Develop Your Child's Intelligence.* Santa Ana, CA: VisionExtension, Inc.

Getman GN (1964). A New Look at Ocular Motilities in Visual Development. Optometric Extension Program Continuing Education Courses, Santa Ana, CA: Optometric Extension Program Foundation, vol. 37, series 9, no. 1–3, Oct.–Dec.

Getman GN, Kephart NC (1957–58). *Developmental Vision.* Optometric Extension Program Postgraduate Courses, Santa Ana, CA: Optometric Extension Program Foundation, vol. 30, Oct.–Dec. 1958.

Goldrich SG, Sedgwick H (1982). An objective comparison of oculomotor functioning in reading disabled and normal children. *Am J Optom Physiol Optics,* 59:82P.

Griffin DC, Walton HN, Ives V (1974). Saccades as related to reading disorders. *J Learn Disabil* 7:310–316.

Griffin JR (1982). *Binocular Anomalies: Procedures for Vision Therapy.* 2nd ed. Chicago: Professional Press.

Griffin JR (1984). Visual skills—Ranking of clinical findings: Pursuit eye movements. *Optom Monthly* 75(12):499–501.

Groffman S (1966). Visual tracing. *J Am Optom Assoc* 37(2):139–141.

Hugonnier R, Clayette-Hugonnier S (1969). *Strabismus, Heterophoria, Ocular Motor Paralysis.* Translated and edited by S. Veronneau-Troutman. St. Louis: C.V. Mosby.

Jones A, Stark L (1983). Abnormal patterns of normal eye movements in specific dyslexia. In: Rayner K (ed), *Eye Movements in Reading: Perceptual and Language Processes.* New York: Academic, pp. 481–498.

Kephart NC (1960). *The Slow Learner in the Classroom.* Columbus, OH: Charles E. Merrill.

King AT, Devick S (1976). *The Proposed King-Devick Test and Its Relation to the Pierce Saccade Test and Reading Levels.* Chicago: Illinois College of Optometry, Senior Research Project.

Kremenitzer JP, Vaughan HG, Kurtzberg D, et al. (1979). Smooth-pursuit eye movements in the newborn infant. *Child Dev* 50:442–448.

Leigh RJ, Zee DS (1983). *The Neurology of Eye Movements.* Philadelphia: FA Davis.

Lesevre N (1968). Les mouvements oculaires d'exploration: etude electro-oculographique comparee des enfants normaux et des enfants dyslexiques. *Bulletin de Institut Nationale de la Sante et de la Recherche Medicale Paris* 22:467–84.

Lieberman S, Cohen AH, Rubin J (1983). NYSOA K-D test. *J Am Optom Assoc* 54(7):631–637.

Maples WC, Ficklin TW (1988). Interrater and test-retest reliability of pursuits and saccades. *J Am Optom Assoc* 59(7):549–552.

Olson RK, Kliegl R, Davidson BJ (1983). Eye movements in reading disability. In: Rayner K (ed), *Eye Movements in Reading: Perceptual and Language Processes.* New York: Academic, pp. 467–479.

Oride MKH, Marutani JK, Rouse MW, et al. (1986). Reliability study of the Pierce and King-Devick saccade tests. *J Am Optom Assoc* 63(6):419–424.

Pavlidis GTh (1981). Do eye movements hold the key to dyslexia? *Neuropsychologia* 19:57–64.

Pavlidis GTh (1985). Eye movement differences between dyslexics, normal and retarded readers while sequentially fixating digits. *Am J Optom Physiol Opt* 62(12):820–832.

Pierce J (1972). Pierce Saccade Test. Bloomington, IN: Cook.

Peachey GT (1991). Minimum attention model for understanding the development of efficient visual function. J Behav Optom 2(8):199–206.

Poynter HL, Schor C, Haynes HM, et al. (1982). Oculomotor functions in reading disability. *Am J Optom Physiol Opt* 59(2):116–127.

Richman JE, Garzia RP (1987). Developmental Eye Movement Test (DEM). South Bend, IN: Bernell Corp.

Richman JE, Walker AJ, Garzia RP (1983). The impact of automatic digit naming ability on a clinical test of eye movement functioning. *J Am Optom Assoc* 54(7):617–622.

Stanley G, Smith GA, Howell EA (1983). Eye movements and sequential tracking in dyslexic and control children. *Br J Psychol* 74:181–187.

Treganza A, Wold RM (1977). *Optometric Evaluation of Children with Academic Dysfunction.* Optometric Extension Program Continuing Education Courses, Santa Ana, CA: Optometric Extension Program Foundation, series 1, no. 9,10. June, July.

Vincett WK (1973). *Optometric Perceptual Testing and Training Manual.* PerCon Inc, 3484 Path Dr, Akron, OH 44319.

Yarbus AL (1967). *Eye Movements and Vision.* New York: Plenum Press.

12

Supplementary Tests of Accommodative and Binocular Function

Supplementary tests are performed to provide additional information regarding accommodative and binocular function. These procedures include tests of accommodative facility and both sensory and motor aspects of binocular fusion. Based on these tests, the initial evaluation, and the case history, the practitioner will determine whether functional vision disorder exists, what lens prescription is indicated, and whether vision therapy is required.

EVALUATION OF ACCOMMODATIVE FUNCTION

Because accommodation is closely related to efficient nearpoint performance, evaluation of accommodative function is an important aspect of optometric care. Relatively low correlations exist between various measures of accommodative function (amplitude, relative amplitude, lag, and facility) in school-age children (Wick and Hall 1987; Jackson and Goss 1991). Since disorder of one function may exist independently of the others, it is advisable that each function be tested to effectively evaluate accommodative status.

Previously described tests include the amplitude of accommodation, the NRA/PRA, and various near retinoscopy procedures. The following section describes the accommodative facility test and various methods of determining the amplitude of accommodation.

Amplitude of Accommodation

In the OEP 21-point analytical examination described in Chapter 8, the amplitude of accommodation (#19) test is performed as a binocular minus-to-blur procedure (Hendrickson 1989). This binocular amplitude is limited by the ability to stimulate accommodation free of convergence, and is hence a measure of flexibility between accommodation and convergence, rather than a true measure of absolute limit of accommodation.

Clinically, it is desirable to determine the monocular as well as the binocular amplitude of accommodation. When monocular amplitudes of accommodation are low or unequal, monocular accommodative training should be emphasized in the early phases of vision therapy. Monocular amplitude of accommodation usually normalizes rapidly in vision training; a failure to normalize rapidly suggests that organic factors may play a role.

Monocular and binocular amplitude of accommodation may be measured using either push-up or minus-lens-to-blur methods. In the push-up method, the patient, wearing distance refractive correction, fixates a row of nearpoint letters one or two lines larger than her best acuity, and attempts to keep the letters clear as the chart is moved toward her. The patient reports when the letters become blurry. The clinician measures the distance from the chart to the patient's spectacle plane in centimeters, and converts this linear distance into dioptric amplitude by dividing the number of centimeters into 100 (Carlson et al. 1990).

In the minus-to-blur method, the patient views a 20/30 row of letters in the phoropter at 40 cm. Minus lens power is slowly added until the patient can no longer clear the target. The minus added before the first sustained blur, plus 2.5 D (the accommodative demand for 40 cm), is the amplitude of accommodation.

The amplitude of accommodation decreases with age. Carlson et al. (1990) indicate that two systems are commonly used for determining norms by the push-up method. Hofstetter's formula states that the minimum expected amplitude should be at least 15 minus one quarter of the patient's age in years. Donders' table (Table 12.1) provides age-referenced norms. Carlson et al. (1990) indicate that the amplitude as measured by the minus-lens-to-blur method is approximately 2.0 D less than that obtained by the push-up method.

Accommodative Facility Test

Accommodative facility is the ability to make a step-change in accommodation to shift focus from one distance (or lens-induced demand level) to another. In most tests of accommodative facility, the stimulus to accommodation is altered by the interposition of lenses, and accommodative facility is quantified as the time required to clear the target material, or as the number of cycles of accommodative stimulation and relaxation that can be accomplished in a unit of time (Pierce and Greenspan 1971; Griffin 1982; Scheiman et al. 1988; Eskridge 1989). Rather than using lenses, Haynes (1979) determines the speed of response in shifting focus from a distance to a nearpoint target and back in cycles per minute.

In the procedure typically used by this author, the patient holds a nearpoint card at the Harmon distance and views a small row of letters, typically J2. The examiner interposes a +2.00/−2.00 flipper, alternately presenting the plus and minus lenses as the patient reports clearing. In older patients, lower-power lenses

Table 12.1 Donders' table for age-referenced amplitude of accommodation

Age	Amplitude
10	14.0
15	12.0
20	10.0
25	8.5
30	7.0
35	5.5
40	4.5
45	3.5
50	2.5
55	1.75
60	1.0
65	0.5
70	0.25
75	0.0

(From Carlson et al., *Clinical Procedures for Ocular Examination,* Appleton & Lange, Norwalk, CT, 1990. Reprinted with permission.)

are used in recognition of the age-expected decrease in accommodative amplitude. The test is performed monocularly with each eye, as well as binocularly.

The test is performed for 60 seconds. The patient's score is recorded as the number of cycles of alternate stimulation and relaxation achieved. In addition to recording the score, the clinician should note whether performance remains fairly consistent over the duration of the test or breaks down on repeated cycles.

If the examiner is uncertain as to whether the patient is really clearing the print, the patient is asked to read the letters or numbers aloud. The retinoscope may be used to monitor accuracy of the accommodative response (Bieber 1974; Eskridge 1989).

The Bernell #9 acuity-suppression vectogram or other Polaroid targets may be used to monitor suppression during binocular accommodative facility testing (Zellers et al. 1984; Scheiman et al. 1988).

Significance of the Accommodative Facility Test

In contrast with the monocular amplitude and the NRA/PRA tests in which the stimulus is changed gradually, the accommodative facility test probes the ability to make a step-change in accommodation in response to a sudden change in stimulus. The test is thus highly demanding; inadequate performance is a sensitive indicator of accommodative dysfunction.

The monocular accommodative facility test probes the ability to stimulate and relax accommodation with no constraints exerted by the binocular vergence system. Inadequate performance indicates a need for monocular accommodative rock training in the early phases of a vision therapy program.

The binocular accommodative facility test probes the ability to shift accommodation closer or farther than the plane of regard while maintaining binocular alignment. Inadequate performance thus indicates a lack of flexibility between vergence and accommodation.

Failure to clear the -2.00 D lens (stimulation phase) monocularly suggests a weakness of accommodation or the existence of a conditioned inhibition of accommodation. Failure to clear minus binocularly indicates an inability to shift accommodation nearer than convergence. Inability to clear minus is typically associated with nearpoint asthenopia, inability to sustain at near, avoidance and disinterest in reading, and impaired academic achievement (Pierce and Greenspan 1971; Sherman 1973; Hoffman and Rouse 1980; Levine et al. 1985).

Failure to clear the $+2.00$ D. lens (inhibition phase) suggests inadequate ability to relax accommodation. Inability to clear plus may occur when so much effort is expended in clearing the minus that accommodative relaxation ability is impaired. Failure to clear plus is often an early sign of impending myopia.

Many individuals show normal amplitude of accommodation, yet have difficulty making the step-change required by the accommodative facility test. Ability to stimulate or relax accommodation may break down, or performance may slow, as the test proceeds through several cycles. Grimacing, squinting, straining, or attempting to move the card closer or farther away also suggest difficulty.

Norms for Accommodative Facility

Studies of monocular accommodative facility in young adults typically indicate 10 to 17 cycles per minute (cpm) as normative when testing is performed with $+2.00/-2.00$ D lenses. Performance on the binocular accommodative facility test is expected to be somewhat slower, since the test requires integration between the accommodative and vergence systems, as well as a rapid shift in accommodation. Average performance for the binocular facility test is approximately 7 to 13 cpm, and is slightly less, 6 to 8 cpm, when binocular suppression control such as the acuity-suppression vectogram is incorporated (Griffin 1982; Zellers et al. 1984; Levine et al. 1985; Jackson and Goss 1991).

Scheiman et al. (1988) report lower accommodative facility rates in school-age children than those obtained for adults in the studies reported above. Children age 8 to 12 showed a mean accommodative facility of 7 cpm monocularly and 5 cpm binocularly. For 7-year-olds, the mean values were 6.5 cpm monocularly and 3.5 cpm binocularly, and for 6-year-olds monocular and binocular findings were 5.5 cpm and 3 cpm, respectively.

It is not clear whether these lower rates result from reduced accommodative facility in children, or from differences in instructional set. In the Scheiman study, children were asked to call off the numbers; this takes more time than simply saying "now" or "clear" as in the adult studies.

Reliability studies indicate that practitioners may be confident of accommodative facility findings when patients either pass the test or fail with very low scores. However, patients who fail with scores in the upper range of failure (6 to 11 cpm monocularly, 3 to 8 cpm binocularly) often show improvement due to practice effect, and subsequently pass on the next retest. A mistaken diagnosis of accommodative disorder may therefore be made if only a single test is made, particularly if the patient fails with a fairly high score. Misdiagnosis can be avoided by repeating the test or extending it for an additional minute or two for patients who fail with fairly high scores. Patients who pass the retest are considered to pass; those who again fail are considered to truly have accommodative disorder (McKenzie et al. 1987; Rouse et al. 1989, 1992).

For monocular accommodative facility, Borish (1970) proposes 6 cpm and Hoffman and Rouse (1980) 12 cpm as minimum passing values. For binocular facility, Lieberman et al. (1985) and Rosner and Rosner (1990) each suggest inability to clear 3 cycles within 30 seconds (that is, 6 cpm) as a criterion for failure. Since most studies indicate that approximately 11 cpm is normal for monocular and 8 cpm for binocular accommodative facility, this author suggests the use of 8 cpm (3 to 4 seconds per accommodative shift) and 6 cpm (5 seconds per shift) as pass-fail cut-offs for monocular and binocular testing, respectively.

EVALUATION OF FUSION AND BINOCULAR FUNCTION

Various tests are performed to evaluate sensory and motor fusion. The cover test, convergence near point, vergence facility test, Polaroid vectograms, Keystone Visual Skills test, Worth four-dot test, Stereo Optical Stereo Tests, cheiroscopic tracing, Van Orden Star, and tests of random dot stereopsis supplement the phorometric battery of the analytical examination routine and provide useful information regarding central and peripheral fusion and stereopsis, suppression, fusional stability, and fusional vergence ranges under a variety of stimulus conditions.

Although the various methods of measuring fusional vergence each have high test-retest reliability, the findings obtained by different methods differ from one another. This variation apparently relates to differences in size of the stimulus, amount of detail, method of presentation (prisms, vectograms, video display) and type of stimulus (flat fusion versus stereoscopic) (Feldman et al. 1989).

The vergence measures of the phorometric battery are particularly sensitive probes of binocular function. Whereas large targets that stimulate both peripheral and central retina constitute strong stimuli for fusional vergence (Burian 1941; Kertesz 1981), especially when they have much detail and many stereoscopic cues (Flax 1968; Feldman et al. 1989), the targets used in the phorometric battery are small and nonstereoscopic, and the periphery is excluded by the refractor. The phorometric battery is thus performed with weak stimuli for fusional vergence, and the tests are highly effective in the detection of binocular disorder.

Since patients with mild binocular disorder may show seemingly normal vergence ranges if strong stimuli are used, the use of weak stimuli increases the sensitivity of the test. Patients with even mild binocular dysfunction typically demonstrate constricted vergences when tested with weak stimuli. Moreover, mild suppression and constricted vergences demonstrable with weak stimuli in the phorometric battery may be masked, and subtle binocular disorder overlooked, if only strong fusional stimuli are used. Consequently, tests such as Polaroid vectograms, Worth four-dot, Stereo Optical Stereo Tests, and others that present strong stimuli, are used to supplement rather than to replace the analytical examination routine. Patients who demonstrate constricted vergences, suppression, or poor stereopsis even with strong stimuli have more severe binocular problems.

Convergence Near Point

The convergence near point is routinely evaluated. The target (a bell, polished sphere, pen or pencil, penlight, transilluminator, or other small object) is presented at a distance of 16 to 20 inches from the patient. The examiner observes the patient's eyes as the target is moved along the midline toward the bridge of the patient's nose (Figure 12.1). When the target doubles or the examiner notes the convergence break, the distance from the bridge of the nose is recorded as the convergence near point; the target is then moved away until the patient reports fusion or the examiner observes a fusional recovery, and the distance from the nose is noted as the recovery finding. If subjective and objective measures differ, both are recorded. The break is normally within 3 inches of the

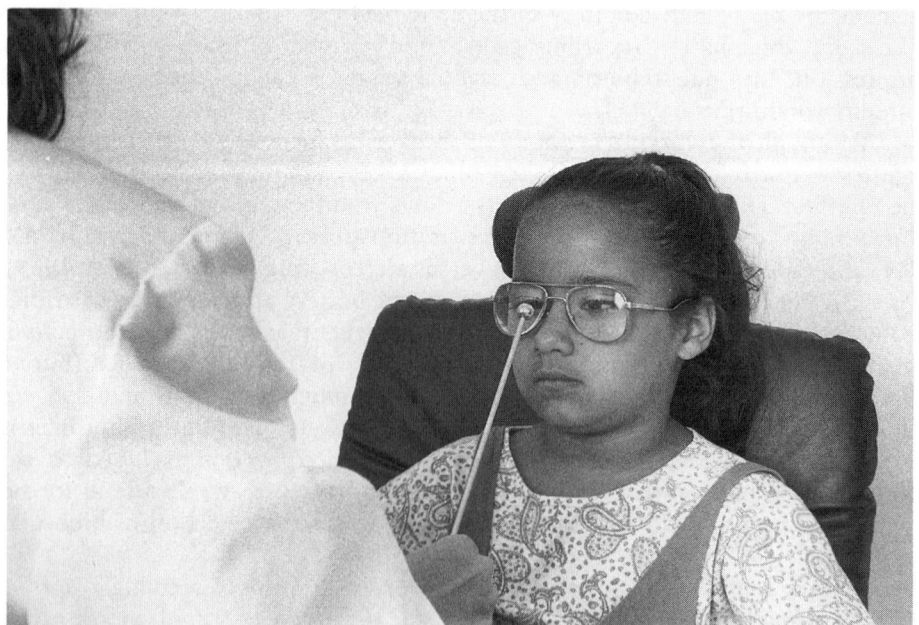

Figure 12.1 Convergence near point test.

bridge of the nose, and does not recede significantly with age. Recovery to fusion should occur not more than 3 inches beyond the break. The nonpreferred eye usually deviates at the break (Morgan 1960, 1963; Tuckman 1965; Treganza and Wold 1977; Rosner and Rosner 1990).

The examiner should not only determine the convergence nearpoint break and recovery, but should also observe the quality of the convergence movement, the effort required for performance, and any difficulty in sustaining convergence. Patients with fragile convergence often lose alignment intermittently as the target approaches the nose, demonstrating a series of breaks and recoveries. Others grimace, tense, furrow their brows, and report discomfort during testing. Some patients back away from the target to reduce convergence demand.

Sensitivity may be increased by performing the convergence nearpoint test with a red lens before one eye. In patients whose binocular function is fragile, the filter may interfere with fusion sufficiently to induce a significant recession of the convergence near point. Impairment of convergence when the test is performed with a red filter is thus a sign of binocular dysfunction (Capobianco 1952).

Patients with inadequate convergence may show a breakdown in performance when convergence nearpoint testing is repeated over several trials, or if jump convergence ability is investigated. Jump convergence is evaluated by placing the target 1 or 2 inches beyond the recovery point, and directing the patient to shift fixation back and forth from a distant object to the target. A patient with convergence difficulty may demonstrate a normal convergence near point, yet have significant difficulty achieving jump convergence (Pickwell 1989).

When a patient shows a receded convergence near point, the examiner should vary the test conditions to determine whether improved convergence is demonstrable with stronger stimuli or with increased patient involvement. A receded convergence near point may improve dramatically when the patient touches the target; when an accommodative target is used; when the test is performed through low-plus lenses, if such lenses permit more adequate integration of vergence and accommodation; or when the patient is asked to place a pointer into a straw, a task that demands both stereopsis and manual involvement (Figure 12.2). Improvement in convergence under such conditions suggests an excellent prognosis and rules out an organic basis for the impaired convergence.

Like pursuit and saccadic testing, the convergence nearpoint test permits observation of the reach-grasp-release sequence. *Reach* is observed in the patient's ability to localize and align on the target; *grasp* in the ability to sustain alignment as the target is moved toward the patient; and *release* in the patient's shift to another target when so directed (Getman and Kephart 1957–58).

Inadequate convergence is often associated with poor grasp, an inadequate ability to sustain alignment on target. Poor grasp at an oculomotor level is often characteristic of patients who are either global or impulsive in their information-processing style, and have difficulty sustaining visual attention.

Convergence ability is usually well established in the 2-year-old. The pre-

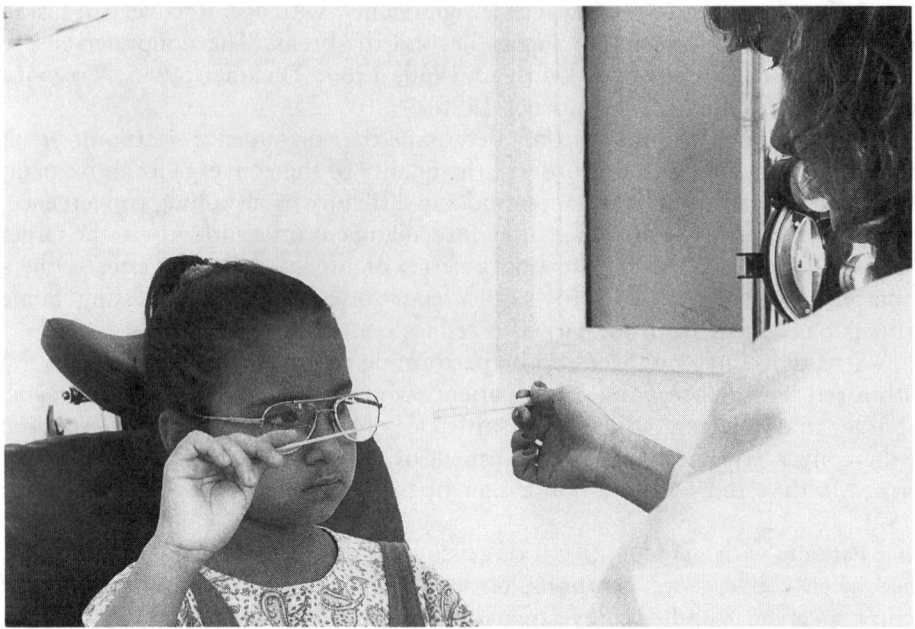

Figure 12.2 Pointer-straw test.

school years are characterized by increasing ability to sustain a smooth, well-controlled convergence movement, to release to the examiner readily, to make adequate jump convergence movements, and to touch the target, when so instructed, in an increasingly mature fashion. These abilities should be well developed by the age of 6 (Apell and Lowry 1959).

Topper Polaroid Vectogram

The Topper Polaroid vectogram (Figure 12.3) is commonly used to evaluate fusional vergence. Topper constitutes a strong stimulus for fusion, since it is large, stimulates a fairly extensive retinal area, and presents considerable variation in stereoscopic texture. Consequently, patients who show constricted phorometric vergence ranges may nevertheless demonstrate high vergence ranges with Topper. Such a finding does not imply that function is adequate or that the analytical examination measures are unreliable, but simply that vergence function, although impaired, can respond to a sufficiently strong stimulus.

The Topper vectogram is therefore used in the evaluation not so much to determine whether binocular vision disorder exists, but rather to determine the extent of impairment. The existence of constricted ranges even with a strong stimulus such as Topper suggests the presence of more severe binocular dysfunction. Because vergence ranges are generally greater with strong stimuli for fusion,

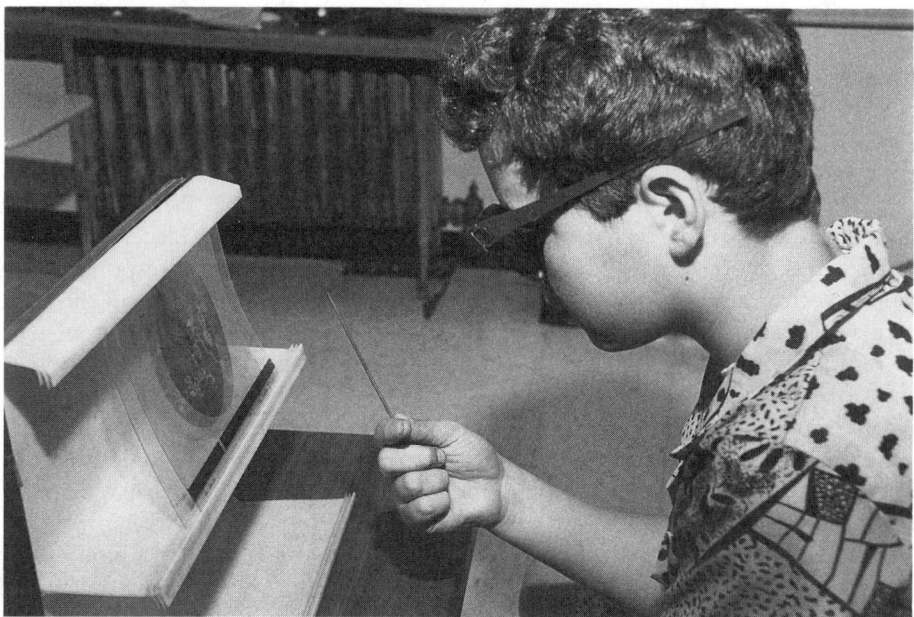

Figure 12.3   Patient viewing Topper vectogram in the polachrome orthopter.

targets such as the Topper vectogram are commonly used as target material early in vision therapy.

Differences in fusional vergence with various targets result not only from differences in stimulus strength, but also vary with the specific vergence measured. Feldman et al. (1989) found that base-out break and recovery findings are higher with Topper than with Risley prisms, as expected on the basis of greater strength of stimulus. However, base-in break and recovery are higher with Risley prisms. They suggest that base-in ranges may be lower with vectograms because, as prism base-in is added, the patients eyes must diverge beyond the plane of the vectograms. Many patients find it difficult to perceive a target beyond the plane of regard. The largest base-in ranges may thus be expected when the whole field changes, as with Risley prisms.

Testing with the Topper vectogram is usually performed at 16 inches. Testing may also be performed at distance with an overhead projector, using a transparent plastic carrier to hold the vectograms in place. Targets are disparated to determine blur, break, and recovery measures in both the base-in and base-out directions. At the standard 16-inch test distance, each number or letter on the vectogram scale corresponds to 1 prism diopter.

The Topper vectogram also provides useful information regarding the patient's ability to make spatial judgements and to localize accurately in space. As Topper is disparated base-out, the patient converges to maintain single vision.

Topper is perceived as moving closer and getting smaller, because the resulting fused retinal image, if created by a single object, would be created by one that is smaller and closer than the actual vectograms (Figure 12.4). As base-in vergence is introduced, the retinal stimulation is that which would be produced by a single object that is both larger and farther away than the actual Polaroid vectograms (Figure 12.5).

The phenomenon in which objects localized as closer or farther than their actual location are perceived as being respectively smaller or larger than their actual size is referred to as *SILO* (small-in, large-out). The SILO response to the Topper vectogram is typical of individuals who respond primarily on the basis of current visual input, since it is a response derived from and consistent with the retinal input. However, many individuals, cognizant that in real life objects that move away appear to become smaller while objects that move closer appear larger, respond to Topper with a reverse response referred to as *SOLI* (small-out, large-in). The presence of a SOLI response suggests that logic and past experience dominate current retinal input in determining the patient's spatial response to Topper.

Additional information about spatial judgements is obtained by observing the patient's ability to localize accurately with a pointer as Topper is disparated base-in and base-out, and by assessing the response to induced parallax. As the patient moves from side to side, targets that have been disparated base-out should appear to move in the same direction as the patient, and targets that have been disparated base-in should appear to move in the opposite direction.

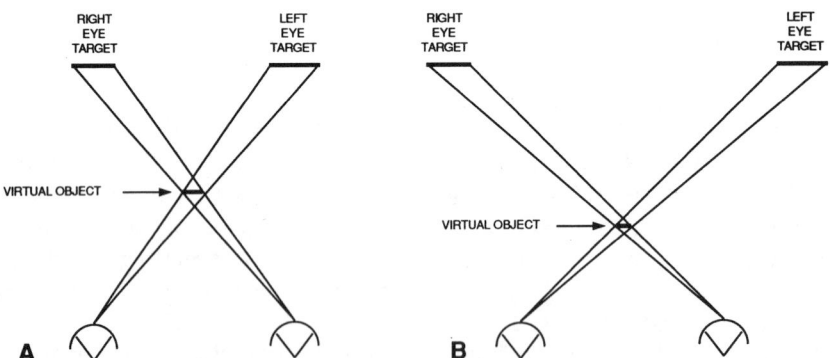

Figure 12.4 *A,* As Polaroid vectograms are disparated base-out (crossed disparity), the individual converges to maintain fusion. The fused retinal image is the same as that which would be created by a single object located in the plane for which the individual is converged. This virtual object is closer and smaller than the real object. *B,* As base-out disparity is increased, the virtual object appears to become smaller and move closer to the individual. (From a drawing by Barbara Gillam, Ph.D., and H.A. Sedgwick, Ph.D. Reprinted with permission.)

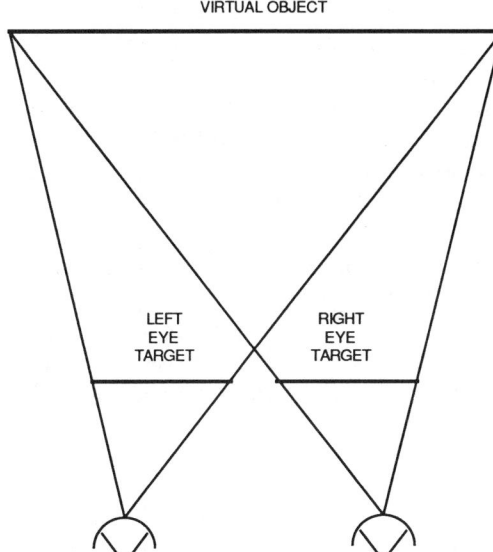

VIRTUAL OBJECT

LEFT
EYE
TARGET

RIGHT
EYE
TARGET

Figure 12.5 As Polaroid vectograms are disparated base-in (uncrossed disparity), the individual diverges to maintain fusion. The fused retinal image is the same as that which would be created by a single object located in the plane for which the patient is diverged. This virtual object is larger than the real object and is located beyond it. (From a drawing by Barbara Gillam, Ph.D., and H.A. Sedgwick, Ph.D. Reprinted with permission.)

Stereopsis

Tests of stereopsis provide information regarding the quality of binocular vision and the ability to make accurate spatial judgements. However, the correlation of performance on stereopsis tests with spatial function in the real world is uncertain, since many factors besides stereopsis contribute to depth perception and to spatial judgements.

Although a variety of nonstereoscopic cues contribute to depth perception, these cues depend on experience and learning. Stereopsis, in contrast, is an apparently innate mechanism that provides depth information which is more immediate and direct, and less dependent on context and experience. Stereopsis is therefore particularly useful in certain sports, driving, and other situations in which depth judgements must be made instantaneously, and in situations that present unusual viewing conditions, such as driving in snow or mist, where learned, experiential cues are less effective.

Stereoscopic acuity, the minimum disparity that can be perceived, has a finite limit so that stereopsis is ineffective beyond a certain critical distance. However, this distance is well beyond that at which precise spatial judgements are usually required. Von Noorden (1985) places the distance beyond which stereopsis is ineffective between 125 and 200 m; Reading (1983) indicates that when the stereothreshold is 10 arc seconds, this critical distance is approximately 0.8 miles. Stereopsis is thus involved in most of our daily spatial judgements.

The relationship between stereopsis and binocular function is complex. Patients with normal binocular vision usually perform well on clinical tests of stereopsis. However, high stereoacuity does not rule out binocular dysfunction, since patients with intermittent strabismus or nonstrabismic binocular disorder often demonstrate normal stereopsis on clinical tests.

Although occasional patients show impaired stereopsis even in the absence of clinically demonstrable binocular vision disorder (Griffin and Baldwin 1974), most patients who show reduced stereopsis do demonstrate binocular disorder. When patients demonstrate impaired stereopsis in the absence of obvious cause, the possibility of small-angle strabismus should be carefully investigated. As a general rule, normal stereopsis does not rule out binocular vision disorder, but impaired stereopsis is a strong indicator of dysfunction.

Patients with nonstrabismic binocular vision disorder usually demonstrate normal stereopsis; in some cases, however, there is central suppression and stereopsis is reduced. In such cases, measurement of stereoacuity provides a useful baseline for demonstrating improvement through vision therapy.

Clinical Stereopsis Tests
Various tests are used clinically to evaluate stereopsis. Some directly assess the ability to discriminate depth stereoscopically by determining the patient's accuracy in aligning test objects in real space. These tests include the Howard-Dolman test, the Verhoeff stereoptor, and the Diastereo test (Reading 1983).

Other tests use stereograms, vectograms, or anaglyphs in which targets are

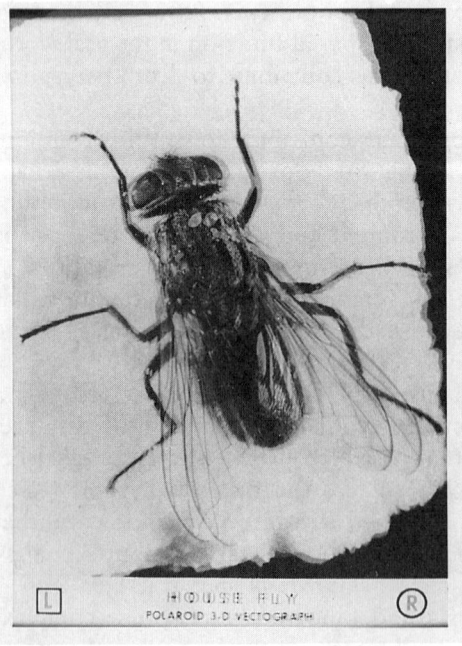 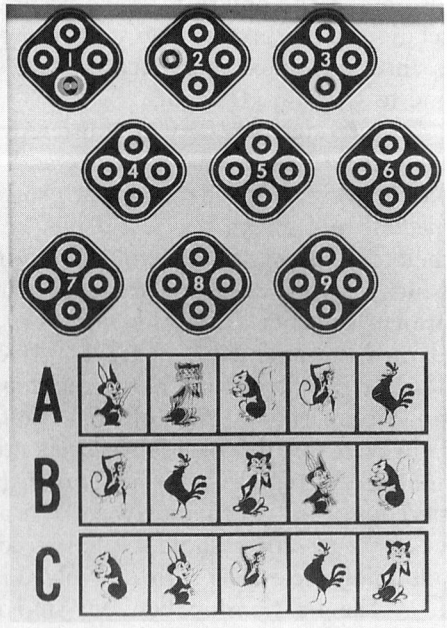

Figure 12.6 Stereo Optical Stereo Tests.

laterally displaced to create disparity and the resultant perception of depth. These artificial or "projected-depth" tests introduce a logical inconsistency, since the patient knows that the target material is really flat. Occasional patients have difficulty with such tests despite the fact that stereoscopic perception is adequate on real-depth tests (Reading 1983).

Artificial, projected-depth tests of stereopsis include the Stereo Optical Stereo Tests, the A.O. Vectographic slide (American Optical Co.), the Keystone Visual Skills Test DB-6D Stereogram (Mast/Keystone), the Stereo Reindeer Test (Stereo Optical Co., Bernell Corp.), the TNO Test (Alfred J. Poll, Inc.), the Random Dot E Stereotest (Stereo Optical Co.), the Randot Stereotests (Stereo Optical Co.), and the Frisby Stereotest (Clement Clark, Ltd.) (Griffin 1982; Reading 1983; Rosner and Rosner 1990).

Stereo Optical Stereo Tests.   Among the most commonly used projected-depth tests are the Stereo Optical Stereo Tests (Griffin 1982; Reading 1983; Rosner and Rosner 1990). It is actually one test consisting of three parts (Figure 12.6). The well-known Stereo Fly is a gross stereopsis test with approximately 3,000 arc seconds of disparity. Three rows of animal pictures present stereoscopic disparities of 400, 200, and 100 arc seconds, respectively. The most demanding portion of the test is derived from the Wirt Stereotest, and presents nine diamonds, each of which contains four circles, one of which stands out in stereoscopic depth. These circles are designed for use at 16 inches, at which distance they present stereoscopic demand as shown in Table 12.2.

The disparity range can be extended by increasing the test distance. If the circles are presented at 24 inches instead of 16 inches, diamonds 8 and 9 present stereoscopic demands of 33 and 27 arc seconds, respectively, thus increasing the sensitivity of the test (Reading 1983).

At closer working distances, the disparity presented by each target is greater, making the test less demanding. Therefore, the patient should not be permitted

Table 12.2 Stereoscopic demand presented by the diamond targets of the Stereo Optical StereoTest and the Randot Stereotest

Diamond	Binocular disparity in seconds of arc when tested at 16 inches	
	Stereo Optical Stereo Test	*Randot Stereotest*
1	800	400
2	400	200
3	200	100
4	140	70
5	100	50
6	80	40
7	60	30
8	50	20
9	40	—

to pull the test book in closer, unless the examiner desires to evaluate the response to even grosser disparities, that is, if the patient responds incorrectly with the test book at 16 inches.

Patients with poor binocularity, even with constant strabismus, sometimes correctly report the first four circles on the Wirt Stereotest, guessing on the basis of monocular displacement cues rather than true stereopsis (Simons and Reinecke 1974; Cooper and Warshowsky 1977).

Keystone DB-6D Stereogram. Another commonly used test is the Keystone Visual Skills DB-6D stereogram (Figure 12.7), designed to be viewed in the Keystone Telebinocular. This test presents 12 rows of symbols with binocular disparities that range from 1,103 arc seconds on row 1 to 82.5 arc seconds on row 12.

Random Dot Stereopsis. Random dot stereograms (Figure 12.8), developed by Julesz (1971) to study the functional hierarchy of visual processing, are widely used in the assessment of stereopsis. These computer-generated patterns are unique in that they present no monocular cues, yet a figure is perceived when the stereograms are fused. Unlike contoured stereograms, which may be correctly guessed because the monocularly perceived images are laterally displaced, random dot stereograms present no monocularly recognizable form and are hence not subject to guessing (Cooper and Warshowsky 1977; Cooper 1979).

Contoured and random dot stereograms probe different types of stereoscopic processes, referred to as local and global stereopsis, respectively, and are mediated by different neural mechanisms (Julesz 1971; Carmon and Bechtoldt 1969). In evaluating stereopsis, therefore, it is well to test with both contoured and random dot stereograms.

The Random Dot E Stereotest presents a stereoscopically perceived "E" with a disparity of 504 arc seconds at a 20-inch test distance. As the card is moved farther away from the patient, the stereoscopic disparity reduces, but the

Figure 12.7 Keystone Visual Skills DB-6D stereogram. (Reprinted with permission of Mast/Keystone.)

Figure 12.8 A random dot stereogram composed of two arrays of black and white, randomly selected cells of triangular shape. When viewed monocularly, the arrays appear as formless random textures. However, when stereoscopically fused, a large triangle is perceived in vivid depth. (Reprinted by permission of the publisher from B. Julesz, *Foundations of Cyclopean Perception,* figure 1.0-1, p. 1. Chicago: University of Chicago Press, 1971.)

target also becomes more difficult to resolve as its visual angle reduces. At a 6-foot test distance, which approaches the practical limit for resolution, the target presents a disparity of 138 arc seconds. Hence, a large range of disparities can be presented. However, because the test does not permit the measurement of threshold stereoacuity, it serves primarily as a screening instrument (Reinecke and Simons 1974; Rosner and Rosner 1990).

The original Randot Stereotest provides a more demanding test of random dot stereopsis. The test comprises three sections: a series of gross random dot forms that present disparities of 600 arc seconds at 16 inches; a series of three rows of figures that present stereoscopic disparities of 400, 200, and 100 arc seconds, respectively; and a series of eight diamonds, each of which contains four circles, one of which has crossed disparity while the other three have equal uncrossed disparity, so that one appears in front of the page and the others behind. The diamonds present progressively finer stereo demands as shown in Table 12.2.

A more recent version of the Randot Stereotest presents both random dot and contoured stereopsis targets. The test has three parts. The first, Randot Forms, presents an upper and a lower segment which contain random dot stereograms of 500 and 250 arc seconds of disparity, respectively. The second and third parts contain an Animals subtest and a Circles subtest, which are made up of contoured stimuli and are similar to those of the Stereo Optical Stereo Tests (Rosner and Rosner 1990).

Random dot stereograms are commonly used to distinguish heterophoria from small-angle strabismus, on the assumption that bifoveal fixation is required for random dot stereopsis. Random dot stereopsis cannot be perceived in most cases of microtropia (Simons and Reinecke 1974; Cooper and Feldman 1978; Griffin 1982). However, occasional small-angle strabismics do appear capable of positive responses to random dot targets (Rutstein and Eskridge 1984; Garzia and Richman 1985).

Norms For Stereopsis

Although stereoscopic acuity as low as 2 to 7 arc seconds has been demonstrated in the laboratory, a threshold of 15 to 30 seconds is considered excellent in clinical tests (von Noorden 1985). Reading (1983) suggests that stereoacuity poorer than 40 seconds of arc be considered abnormal; Rosner and Rosner (1990) suggest 50 arc seconds and Griffin (1982) proposes 67 arc seconds as cut-off values to distinguish normal from abnormal stereoacuity.

The tests commonly used in clinical practice are relatively gross and do not require extremely high levels of stereoacuity. The highest level of stereoacuity obtainable on the Stereo Optical Stereo Tests or the A.O. Vectographic slide is 40 seconds of arc, and on the Keystone Visual Skills DB-6D stereoscopic test card, only 82.5 seconds of arc. Failure to pass the entire test is thus a sign of binocular vision dysfunction.

Worth Four-Dot Test

The Worth four-dot test is commonly used to assess binocular status. The patient wears red-green anaglyph glasses and views a target that presents four lights: two green, one red, and one white. The patient who fuses will see four lights: two green, one red, and one fused in red-green lustre. The patient with central suppression will see either two lights or three, or will alternate from two to three. The patient with fragile fusion may experience diplopia and report the presence of five lights.

The Worth four-dot test is commonly performed with a flashlight designed for nearpoint use, which presents a 6-degree target at 13 inches. This target may be used at a variety of distances, becoming progressively finer as the target is moved farther from the eyes. A four-dot lantern is also available for testing at far, presenting a fine 1.25-degree target at 20 feet (Rosner and Rosner 1990).

The Worth four-dot test is relatively gross, and is most useful in the evaluation of strabismus. Nonstrabismic binocular vision disorders that cause subtle interference with fusion may not cause diplopia or suppression on a test as gross as the Worth four-dot. Failure to demonstrate fusion on the four-dot test is indicative of binocular vision dysfunction, but the presence of fusion on the Worth four-dot does not rule out binocular vision disorder.

Keystone Visual Skills Test

The Keystone Visual Skills Test (Mast/Keystone) is commonly used to screen for acuity, and binocular and color vision deficits, and is routinely administered in many optometric offices as part of an examination or pre-examination battery, providing significant information regarding binocular status.

The test battery consists of 15 target cards (10 for far point, five for near point) designed to be presented in the Keystone Telebinocular, a Brewster stereoscope with a separation of 95 mm between the optical centers of its +5.00 D lenses. The test may be administered using any Brewster-type stereoscope by adding prism to simulate the 95 mm optical center separation for which the cards are designed.

The battery includes tests of simultaneous perception (a dog is presented to one eye and a pig to the other) (Figure 12.9a); vertical imbalance (Figure 12.9b); lateral imbalance at far and near (a modified Thorington arrow and numbers test provides information as to both phoria and stability) (Figure 12.9c); fusion at far and near (Figure 12.9d); stereopsis (the DB-6D stereogram previously described); color vision; and monocular visual acuity with both eyes open at distance and near.

The tests of visual acuity at distance (Figure 12.9e) are unique in that they probe the ability to discriminate detail with each eye monocularly in a binocular field, and provide information about foveal suppression. Each stereogram presents a series of signposts that are perceived to recede into the distance. Each signpost contains five diamonds, one of which contains a small dot. The patient's task is to determine, within each signpost, which diamond contains the dot. Since the signposts, diamonds, and dots become progressively smaller, the test is a function of visual acuity.

The right eye stereogram presents the diamonds to both eyes, but the dots are presented to the right eye only. If the left eye exerts inhibitory influence on the right, right eye central vision will be suppressed and no dots will be seen. If suppression is present but less pronounced, the large dots will be visible to the right eye, but the small dots will not. When the left eye is occluded, the right eye sees the dots monocularly, free of any inhibitory influence, and will then see the small dots as well. Improvement in acuity with occlusion therefore indicates that the right eye is inhibited or suppressed under binocular conditions. The left eye stereogram is similar to that for the right eye, except that the dots are presented to the left eye. The tests for visual acuity at near (Figure 12.9f) similarly consist of targets (lines, dots, or a uniform gray field) that are presented to each eye monocularly in a binocular field.

Cheiroscopic Tracing

Cheiroscopic tracing is typically performed with the Keystone Correct-Eye-Scope or the Titmus Biopter. Each instrument consists of a Brewster stereoscope head affixed to a cheiroscopic tracing platform.

The patient is seated comfortably before the instrument with the cheiroscopic tracing sheet set at optical infinity and the test pattern on the side of the nondominant hand. The patient traces the test pattern while keeping both eyes open. Although it appears to the patient that he or she is tracing the target, the tracing is actually centered on the side of the dominant hand and is laterally displaced from the target.

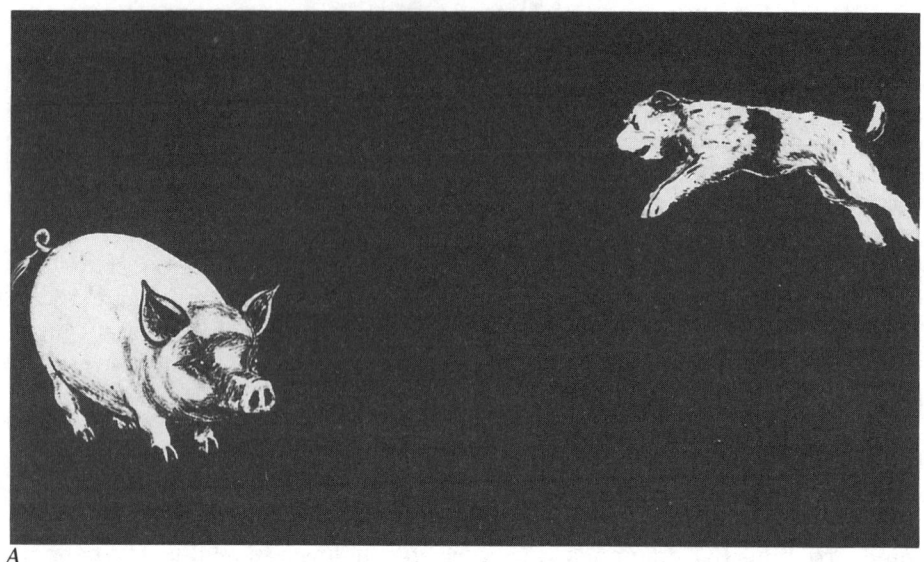

A

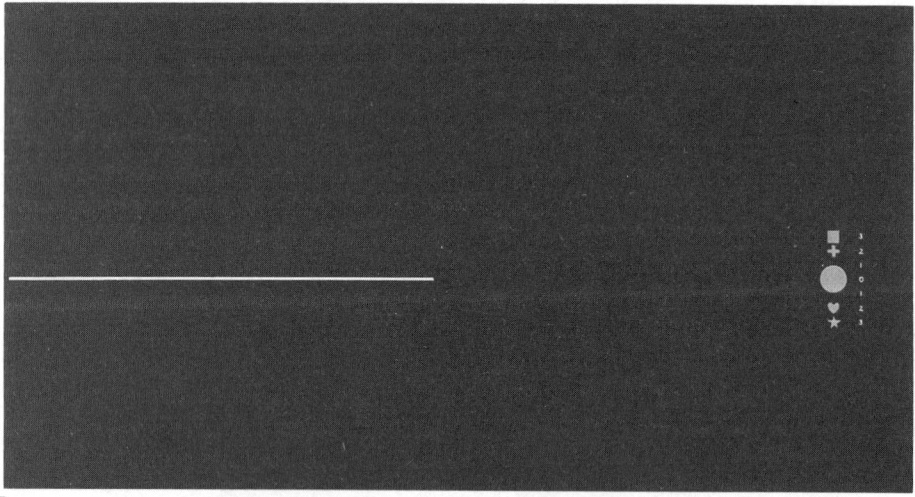

B

Figure 12.9 The Keystone Visual Skills Test (Mast/Keystone). *A,* Test 1, simultaneous perception at far. *B,* Test 2, vertical imbalance. *C,* Test 3, lateral imbalance at far (test 10, for lateral imbalance at near, is similar). *D,* Test 4, fusion at far (test 11, fusion at near, is similar). *E,* Test 6, test of usable vision, left eye, is used to assess left eye visual acuity with both eyes open. Test 5 is similar, except that the dots are presented to the right eye only. *F,* Test 13, usable vision at near, is used to assess right eye visual acuity at near with both eyes open. Test 14 is similar, except that the dots, lines, and uniform gray are presented to the left eye only.

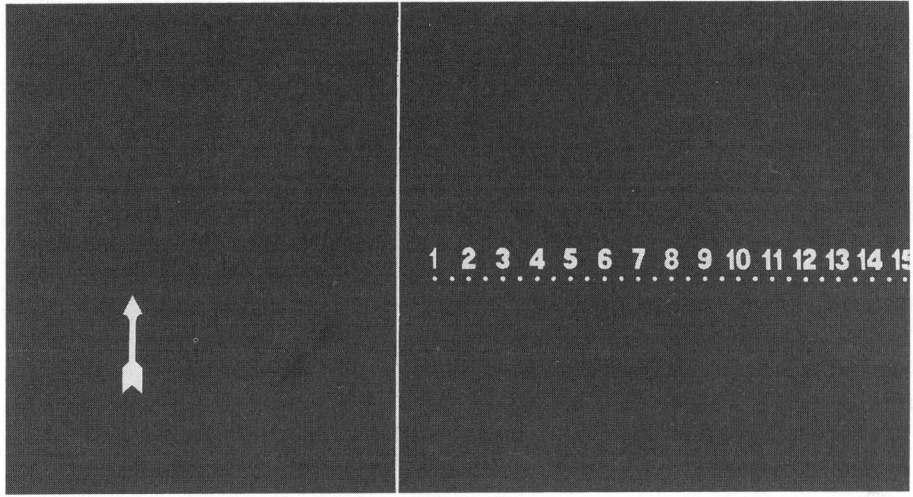

C

D

Figure 12.9 *Continued*

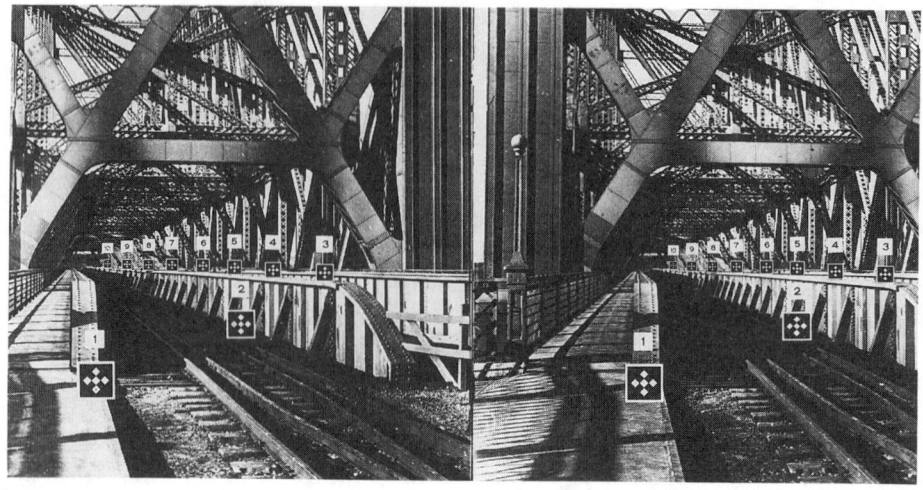

E

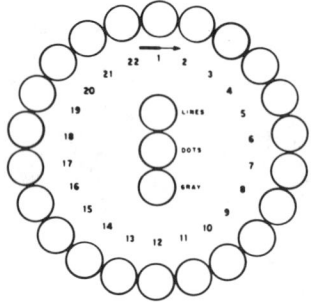
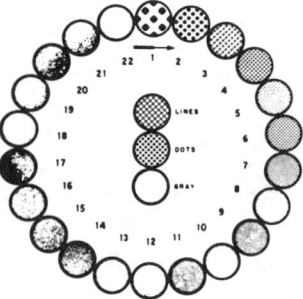

F

Figure 12.9 *Continued*

The separation of the optical centers of the lenses of the Keystone Correct-Eye-Scope is 87 mm. In orthophoria, a separation of 87 mm between corresponding points of the test pattern and the tracing is therefore expected on an optical basis. In actual practice, the involvement of the hand and the knowledge that the target is only 8 inches away usually generate proximal convergence so that the separation of test target and tracing is typically less than 87 mm. Manas (1965) suggests that an 80-mm separation be considered as *orthophoric* posture; Gruning (1981) suggests 68 mm as the orthophoric reference point. When the Correct-Eye-Scope is set for infinity, each 2-mm deviation from the expected represents 1 prism diopter.

The actual separation between the tracing and the test pattern indicates the degree of esophoric, orthophoric, or exophoric posture that exists under the conditions induced by the test. A separation greater than expected indicates exophoric posture, and a separation less than the expected value indicates esophoric posture (Figure 12.10). A tracing that is higher or lower than the target suggests the existence of vertical imbalance.

Many patients demonstrate substantial esophoric posture on a cheiroscopic tracing test. Esophoric posture may be so great that the patient's view of the pencil is blocked by the septum as she traces, so that the tracing cannot be completed. High esophoric posture suggests that the patient is particularly prone to the influence of proximal convergence, or is very intense in her performance.

In assessing performance, the practitioner should note the quality of the tracing, stability of performance, eye-hand coordination, and the existence of suppression or hyperphoria, as well as the separation between the tracing and the test pattern. Patients frequently report intermittent suppression as they trace, with either the target or the pencil briefly disappearing. Cheiroscopic tracing yields significant information regarding binocular stability.

Many patients exhibit a progressive shift, usually in an esophoric direction, as the tracing proceeds (see Figure 3.2). This progressive esophoric shift may occur regardless of whether the initial posture is esophoric, orthophoric, or exophoric. Birnbaum (1985) suggests that strong attentional involvement generates sympathetic activation, which induces a shift of accommodation toward far and creates a need for greater accommodative effort to maintain accommodation at optical infinity. Heightened accommodative effort causes a progressive esophoric shift as the test proceeds.

Cheiroscopic tracing thus provides an opportunity to observe the effect of attentional demand on oculomotor posture. The patient who shows a significant esophoric shift is likely to experience significant overconvergence in response to nearpoint tasks that present sustained demands for concentration and mental effort. A marked esophoric shift on cheiroscopic tracing thus suggests that stress

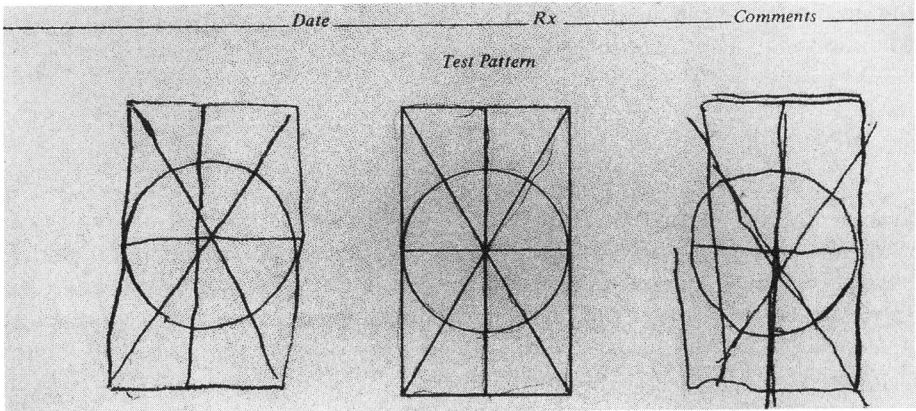

Figure 12.10 Esophoric cheiroscopic tracing.

reactivity is high and that the patient is at risk for nearpoint stress–induced vision disorder.

Van Orden Star

The Van Orden Star, like cheiroscopic tracing, is used to evaluate binocular function under conditions that demand manual involvement and sustained attention. The Van Orden Star target presents a vertical row of figures at each edge and is placed at the infinity setting of the Correct-Eye-Scope. The patient holds one pencil in each hand, and is directed to place the left-hand pencil on the top figure of the left column and the right-hand pencil on the bottom figure of the right column. The patient draws toward the center until the two pencils appear to meet. She then places the pencils at the second figure from the top on the left side and the second figure from the bottom on the right, and again draws toward the center, continuing the pattern until the star pattern is completed. Although it appears to the patient viewing through the instrument that she is completing a star pattern, the completed tracing consists of two triangles, or half-stars. The separation of the cusps or apices is determined, as in cheiroscopic tracing, by the separation of the optical centers of the instrument's lenses and by the various factors which influence oculomotor posture. Gruning (1981) suggests an expected orthophoric separation of 68 mm, comparable to his norm for cheiroscopic tracing. A greater separation indicates exophoric posture (Figure 12.11), and a smaller separation indicates esophoric posture. One apex higher than the other indicates a hyperphoric projection. Each 2 mm variation from expected is equivalent to 1 prism diopter.

The Van Orden Star provides information regarding stability and quality of binocular performance. Many patients demonstrate a progressive esophoric shift with sustained attention as the tracing proceeds. Patients may intermittently suppress one or the other pencil. When such suppression occurs, the cusp of one triangle will be missing in whole or in part, where the pencil disappeared, while the opposite cusp will be overextended (Figure 12.12). Quality of eye-hand coordination may also be observed.

Step Vergence

At times it is advantageous to use a hand-held prism bar, rather than a refractor and Risley prisms, to assess fusional vergence. The prism bar permits testing under natural conditions without the refractor in place, and permits direct observation of the eyes so that the patient's subjective responses can be objectively verified. Wesson (1982) determined normative values for step vergence ranges obtained with a prism bar in a population consisting primarily of adults. Scheiman et al. (1989) determined norms for children aged 6 to 12. Norms derived from these studies are summarized in Table 12.3.

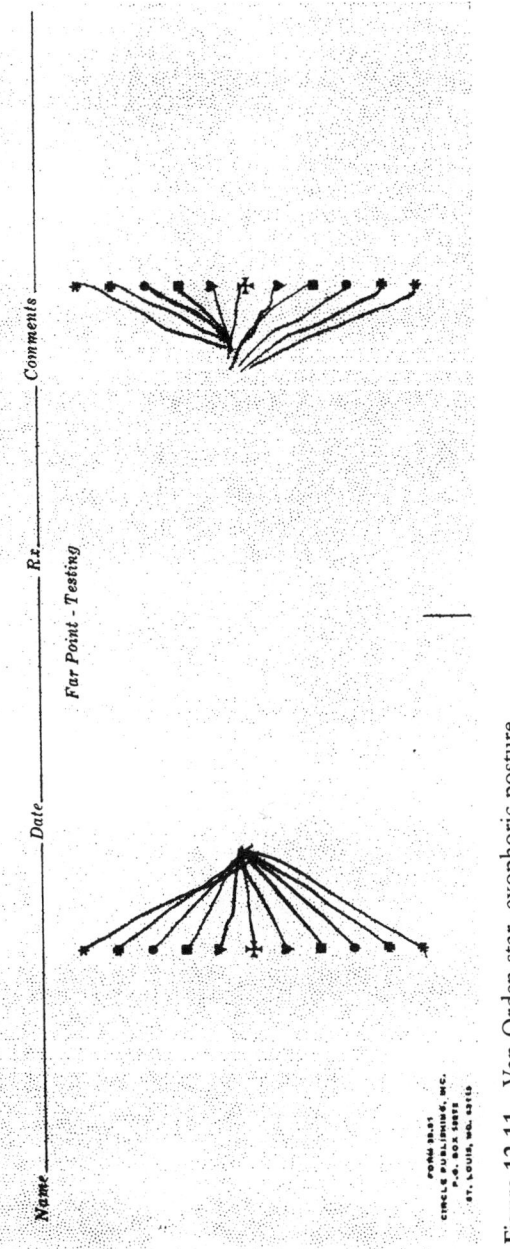

Figure 12.11 Van Orden star, exophoric posture.

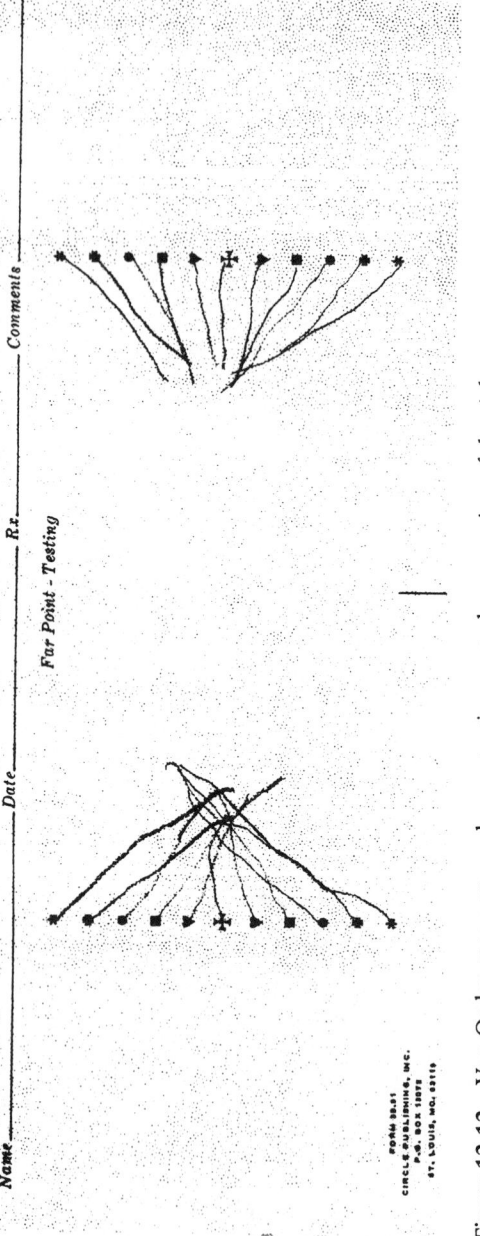

Figure 12.12 Van Orden star pattern demonstrating central suppression of the right eye.

Table 12.3 Means for step vergence ranges with prism bar in samples consisting primarily of adults (Wesson 1982) and children age 6 to 12 (Scheiman et al. 1989)

	Adults *(from Wesson 1982)*	Children age 7–12 *(from Scheiman et al. 1989)*	Children age 6
Base-out break/recovery at distance	11/7	Not determined	
Base-in break/recovery at distance	7/4	Not determined	
Base-out break/recovery at near	19/14	23/16	19/10
Base-in break/recovery at near	13/10	12/7	12/6

Vergence Facility

Vergence facility, the efficiency with which an individual can recover fusion after a step-change in vergence demand, is evaluated by observing the fusional response to interposition of loose prisms. In the reflex fusion test of vergence facility (Grisham 1983), the examiner observes the vergence response to a 6$^\Delta$ loose prism interposed in front of one eye while the patient fixates a target at 40 cm. Quality of fusion is determined on the basis of response latency, velocity, accuracy of response, and fatigue on repeated testing.

When quality of fusion is inadequate, the vergence response to the interposed prism is slow and a version movement to restore fixation is observed to precede the vergence movement which restores fusion. Amplitude of the version movement and latency of the vergence movement provide indices of the quality of fusional vergence. When vergence facility is poor, the vergence system responds slowly and a greater amplitude version movement is observed to precede it. When vergence facility is adequate, the vergence response is immediate, and the preceding version movement is small or absent. A long vergence latency implies poor quality of fusion and correlates with restricted Risley prism vergence ranges (Grisham 1983).

The reflex fusion test permits assessment of fusion without verbalization by the patient. It is therefore particularly useful in the evaluation of young children. Although the test requires judgment by the examiner as to the quality of the fusional vergence response, Grisham indicates that results correlate closely with those obtained when an infrared eye movement monitor is used to objectively identify disorders of fusional vergence dynamics.

Vergence facility can also be evaluated by using prism flippers to repeatedly change vergence demand in a manner analogous to that commonly used to assess accommodative facility. Buzzelli (1986) determined normal values for vergence facility for school-age children who viewed a target at 16 inches alternately through 16$^\Delta$ base-out and 4$^\Delta$ base-in for 1 minute. Mean vergence facility increased from approximately 7 cpm at age 5 to 11 cpm at age 13.

Computer Orthoptics

Computer programs are available to aid in both the evaluation and treatment of functional vision disorders (Cooper and Citron 1983). The Computer Orthoptics system developed by Cooper (RC Instruments, Inc.) and the OPTI-MUM system developed by Ludlam (Learning Frontiers, Inc.) each provide diagnostic programs to assess phorias, vergence ranges (with both flat fusion targets and random dot stereograms), Worth four-dot test, diplopia fields, and other visual functions.

SUMMARY

The phorometric, fixation disparity, and dynamic retinoscopy procedures described in previous chapters provide considerable information as to the adequacy of binocular and accommodative function. Supplementary tests described in this chapter include the amplitude of accommodation, accommodative facility test, convergence near point, vergence facility test, Polaroid vectograms, Keystone Visual Skills test, Worth four-dot test, Stereo Optical Stereo Tests, cheiroscopic tracing, Van Orden star, and tests of random dot stereopsis. Vision therapy is generally indicated when a patient demonstrates accommodative and/or binocular dysfunction that cannot be satisfactorily treated with lenses alone. Vision therapy sequences and procedures for the remediation of such disorders are presented in Chapters 14 and 15.

REFERENCES

Apell RJ, Lowry RW. (1959). *Preschool Vision*. St. Louis: American Optometric Association.
Bieber, JC (1974). Why nearpoint retinoscopy with children? *Optom Weekly* 65(3):54–57; 65(4):78–82.
Birnbaum MH (1985). An esophoric shift associated with sustained fixation. *Am J Optom Physiol Opt* 62(11):732–735.
Borish IM (1970). *Clinical Refraction*. 3rd ed. Chicago: Professional Press.
Burian HM (1941). Fusional movements in permanent strabismus: A study of the central and peripheral regions in the act of binocular vision in squint. *Arch Ophthalmol* 26:626–652.
Buzzelli AR (1986). Vergence facility: Developmental trends in a school age population. *Am J Optom Physiol Opt* 63(5):351–355.
Capobianco NM (1952). The subjective measurement of the nearpoint of convergence and its significance in the diagnosis of convergence insufficiency. *Am Orthopt J* 2:40–42.
Carlson NB, Kurtz D, Heath DA, et al. (1990). *Clinical Procedures for Ocular Examination*. Norwalk, CT: Appleton and Lange.
Carmon A, Bechtoldt HP (1969). Dominance of the right cerebral hemisphere for stereopsis. *Neuropsychologica* 7:29–39.
Cooper J (1979). Clinical stereopsis testing: Contour and random dot stereograms. *J Am Optom Assoc* 50(1):41–46.
Cooper J, Citron M (1983). Microcomputer produced anaglyphs for evaluation and therapy of binocular anomalies. *J Am Optom Assoc* 54(9):785–788.

Cooper J, Feldman J (1978). Random-dot stereogram performance by strabismic, amblyopic, and ocular-pathology patients in an operant-discrimination task. *Am J Optom Physiol Opt* 55(9):599–609.

Cooper J, Warshowsky J (1977). Lateral displacement as a response cue in the Titmus Stereo Test. *Amer J Optom Physiol Opt* 54:537–541.

Eskridge JB (1989). Clinical objective assessment of the accommodative response. *J Am Optom Assoc* 60(4):272–275.

Feldman JM, Cooper J, Carniglia P, et al. (1989). Comparison of fusional ranges measured by Risley prisms, vectograms, and Computer Orthopter. *Optom Vis Sci* 66(6):375–382.

Flax N (1968). *San Jose Vision Training Seminar.* Transcript by Caryl Croisant, Santa Ana, CA.

Garzia RP, Richman JE (1985). Stereopsis in an amblyopic small angle esotrope. *J Am Optom Assoc* 56(5):400–404.

Getman GN, Kephart NC (1957–58). *Developmental Vision.* Optometric Extension Program Continuing Education Courses, Santa Ana, CA: Optometric Extension Program Foundation, vol. 30, Oct. 1957–Sept. 1958.

Griffin JR (1982). *Binocular Anomalies: Procedures for Vision Therapy.* 2nd ed. Chicago: Professional Press.

Griffin JR, Baldwin RJ (1974). Absence of stereopsis during fusion. *J Calif Optom Assoc* 42(3):138–139.

Grisham JD (1983). Treatment of binocular vision dysfunctions. In: Schor CM, Ciuffreda KJ (eds), *Vergence Eye Movements: Basic and Clinical Aspects.* Boston: Butterworth–Heinemann, pp. 605–646.

Gruning C (1981). *Vision Training Laboratory Manual.* New York: State University of New York, State College of Optometry.

Haynes HM (1979). The distance rock test—A preliminary report. *J Am Optom Assoc* 50(6):707–713.

Hendrickson H (1989). *The behavioral optometry approach to lens prescribing.* Rev. ed. Santa Ana, CA: Optometric Extension Program Foundation.

Hoffman L, Rouse M (1980). Referral recommendations for binocular function and/or developmental perceptual deficiencies. *J Am Optom Assoc* 51(2):119–125.

Jackson TW, Goss DA (1991). Variation and correlation of clinical tests of accommodative function in a sample of school-age children. *J Am Optom Assoc* 62(11):857–866.

Julesz B (1971). *Foundations of Cyclopean Perception.* Chicago: University of Chicago Press.

Kertesz AE (1981). Effect of stimulus size on fusion and vergence. *J Optom Soc Am* 71:289–293.

Levine S, Ciuffreda KJ, Selenow A, et al. (1985). Clinical assessment of accommodative facility in symptomatic and asymptomatic individuals. *J Am Optom Assoc* 56(4):286–290.

Lieberman S, Cohen AH, Stolzberg M, et al. (1985). Validation study of the New York State Optometric Association (NYSOA) vision screening battery. *Am J Optom Physiol Opt* 62:165–168.

McKenzie KM, Kerr SR, Rouse MW, et al. (1987). Study of accommodative facility testing reliability. *Am J Optom Physiol Opt* 64(3):186–194.

Manas L (1965). *Visual Analysis.* 3rd ed. Chicago: Professional Press.

Morgan MW (1960). Anomalies of the visual neuromuscular system of the aging patient and their correction. In: Hirsch MJ, Wick RE (eds), *Vision of the Aging Patient.* Philadelphia: Chilton, pp. 113–145.

Morgan MW (1963). Anomalies of binocular vision. In: Hirsch M, Wick R (eds), *Vision of Children.* Philadelphia: Chilton, pp. 173–195.

Pickwell D (1989). *Binocular Vision Anomalies*. 2nd ed. London: Butterworth–Heinemann.

Pierce JR, Greenspan SB (1971). Accommodative rock procedures in V.T.—A clinical guide. *Optom Weekly* 62(33):19–23, Aug 19; 62(34):25–29, Aug 26.

Reading RW (1983). *Binocular Vision*. Boston: Butterworth–Heinemann.

Reinecke R, Simons K (1974). A new stereoscopic test for amblyopia screening. *Am J Ophthalmol* 78:714–721.

Rosner J, Rosner J (1990). *Pediatric Optometry*. 2nd ed. Boston: Butterworth–Heinemann.

Rouse MW, DeLand PN, Chous R, et al. (1989). Monocular accommodative facility testing reliability. *Optom Vis Sci* 66(2):72–77.

Rouse MW, DeLand PN, Mozayani S, et al. (1992). Binocular accommodative facility testing reliability. *Optom Vis Sci* 69(4):314–319.

Rutstein RP, Eskridge JB (1984). Stereopsis in small-angle strabismus. *Am J Optom Physiol Opt* 61(8):491–498.

Scheiman M, Herzberg H, Frantz K, et al. (1988). Normative study of accommodative facility in elementary schoolchildren. *Am J Optom Physiol Opt* 65(2):127–134.

Scheiman M, Herzberg H, Frantz K, et al. (1989). A normative study of step vergence in elementary schoolchildren. *J Am Optom Assoc* 60(4):276–280.

Sherman A (1973). Relating vision disorders to learning disability. *J Am Optom Assoc* 44:140–141.

Simons K, Reinecke RD (1974). A reconsideration of amblyopia screening and stereopsis. *Am J Ophthalmol* 78:707–713.

Treganza A, Wold RM (1977). *Optometric Evaluation of Children With Academic Dysfunction*. Optometric Extension Program Continuing Education Courses, Santa Ana, CA: Optometric Extension Program Foundation, series 1, No. 9, 10, June, July.

Tuckman H (1965). A preliminary study of the nearpoint of convergence in first grade children. *Eastern Seaboard Conference on Visual Training*, Washington, DC, transcript by Caryl Croissant, Phoenix, AZ.

von Noorden GK (1985). *Burian-von Noorden's Binocular Vision and Ocular Motility*. 3rd ed. St. Louis: C.V. Mosby.

Wesson MD (1982). Normalization of prism bar vergences. *Am J Optom Physiol Opt* 59(8):628–634.

Wick B, Hall P (1987). Relation among accommodative facility, lag, and amplitude in elementary school children. *Am J Optom Physiol Opt* 64(8):593–598.

Zellers JA, Alpert TL, Rouse MW (1984). A review of the literature and a normative study of accommodative facility. *J Am Optom Assoc* 55(1):31–37.

13

Vision and Learning

The optometrist is frequently called upon to evaluate children with reading or other academic difficulty, to determine whether vision disorder plays a significant role. Although nearpoint vision disorders do not typically cause profound interference with the process of learning to read, they often interfere significantly with reading efficiency once decoding ability has been acquired. To effectively counsel patients, the optometrist must thoroughly understand the relationships between visual function and classroom performance.

Reading and learning are complex acts involving linguistic and cognitive as well as visual processes. The role of the optometrist is to identify existing visual disorders, to determine whether visual dysfunction appears to correlate with the specific difficulties experienced by the patient, and to initiate therapy when appropriate. This requires a knowledge of the relationship between visual function and learning ability. This chapter will overview research linking vision disorders with learning difficulty, as well as clinical issues in assessing the child with learning disorder.

RESEARCH REPORTS ON VISION DISORDERS AND READING

Several studies indicate that hyperopia is frequently associated with reading problems (Eames 1932, 1935, 1948, 1955; Farris 1936; Taylor 1937; Robinson 1968; Rosner and Rosner 1987). Similar findings were obtained in a meta-analysis by Simons and Gassler (1988) and literature surveys by Grisham and Simons (1986) and Suchoff (1981). The association of reading problems with hyperopia is generally attributed to extra accommodative demand that leads to intermittent nearpoint blur, eyestrain, and avoidance of sustained nearpoint activity, and which often produces an esophoria at near that may stress the fusional vergence system (Grisham and Simons 1986). Farris (1936) and Eames (1949) report improved reading performance following refractive correction of hyperopia. Norn et al. (1969) and Helveston et al. (1985) did not find a relationship between reading and hyperopia.

Studies of the relationship of astigmatism to reading achievement have produced conflicting results. Betts (1936) reported a high incidence of astigmatism in a population of poor readers, but no such relationship was found by Eames (1932, 1948), Farris (1936), Witty and Kopel (1936a) or Norn et al. (1969).

A higher incidence of anisometropia in children with reading failure than in controls was reported by Eames (1948, 1964), but not by Norn et al. (1969). Eames (1964) found that reading ability improved following anisometropic correction.

Binocular and Accommodative Disorder

Numerous studies indicate that nonstrabismic binocular vision disorders are related to reading difficulty. Sherman (1973) and Hoffman (1980) each report that more than 85% of learning-disabled children referred for optometric evaluation demonstrate nonstrabismic binocular and accommodative disorders.

In comparison with non–learning-disabled controls, children with reading and learning problems demonstrate a higher incidence of heterophoria, especially exophoria at near (Selzer 1933; Good 1939; Robinson 1946, 1968; Park 1948; Kelly 1957; Shearer 1966; Anapolle 1967; Evans et al. 1976; Eames 1932, 1935, 1948; Park and Burri 1943a; Getz and McGraw 1980).

A greater incidence of low prism vergence ranges (Good 1939; Robinson and Huelsman 1953; Robinson 1968; Marcus, 1974; Pierce 1977; Haddad et al. 1984; Park and Burri 1943b; Stein et al. 1988); inadequate vergence facility (Buzzelli 1991); convergence insufficiency (Eames 1932, 1934; Shearer 1966; Benton 1961, 1968; Park 1948; Frankling 1961; Dunlop and Banks 1973; Dunlop 1976; Weber 1980; O'Grady 1984); fixation disparity (Sibinger and Woolf 1968; O'Grady 1984); increased lag of accommodation (Poynter et al. 1982); low PRA (Robinson 1968); and other dysfunctions relating primarily to fusion and binocular efficiency (Kephart 1953; Kephart et al. 1960; Park and Burri 1943a; Birnbaum and Birnbaum 1968; Glatt and Glatt 1956; O'Grady 1984; Witty and Kopel 1936a; Kelly 1957; Hoffman 1974; Wirt et al. 1947; King and Michael 1969; Bedwell et al. 1980; Stein et al. 1986) have been reported. In a meta-analysis of 34 studies, Simons and Gassler (1988) found exophoria at near and vertical phorias to be associated with below-average reading performance. Stolzberg et al. (1989) found that children with fusional and accommodative abnormalities made greater numbers of errors on a reading test.

In contrast with these positive studies, Clark (1935), Fendrick (1935), Swanson and Tiffin (1936), Stromberg (1937, 1938), Witty and Kopel (1936b), Dalton (1943), Spache and Tillman (1962), Park (1969), Wilson and Wold (1972), and Pierce (1977) each found no relation between reading ability and phoria. Park (1969), Blika (1982), and Helveston et al. (1985) found no relationship between reading ability and phorias, prism vergence measures, or other aspects of binocular function. Letourneau et al. (1969) found no relationship between reading disability and convergence insufficiency. A greater incidence of aniseikonia in patients with reading disability was reported by Dearborn and Anderson (1938), but not by Rosenbloom (1968).

After reviewing the literature, Simons and Grisham (1987) conclude that although there are conflicting findings, the research evidence as a whole supports the claim that binocular anomalies are involved in childhood reading problems. They note studies that indicate fewer reading problems in patients with monocular than with binocular vision (Benton et al. 1965; Norn et al. 1969; Park and Burri 1943b), and studies that report greater reading efficiency under monocular than binocular reading conditions (Birnbaum and Birnbaum 1968; Stein and Fowler 1986). These findings, together with the large number of studies reporting that disabled readers demonstrate an increased incidence of heterophoria (especially exophoria at near), lowered fusional vergence ranges, convergence insufficiency, and fixation disparity, lead them to conclude that faulty binocular function is a factor in reading problems.

Eye Movements

Smooth, accurate eye movements permit efficient, consistent chunking of the visual input and facilitate information-processing. When eye movements are irregular or erratic, the input is likely to be scrambled so that decoding is inaccurate or garbled and information-processing is impaired. As a consequence, poor eye movements are commonly held to interfere with reading efficiency (Gaarder 1975; Taylor 1966).

The relation between eye movements and reading is complex, since eye movement efficiency while reading is influenced by the reading material and by reading ability. Erratic eye movements, excessive regressions, and prolonged fixations may occur when reading material is difficult to decode or comprehend.

To determine whether poor eye movements are a cause or effect of a reading disability, it is therefore desirable to study eye movements on nonverbal materials. While deficient eye movement performance on verbal material may simply reflect cognitive difficulty, the presence of poor eye movements on nonverbal material suggests fundamental problems with oculomotor control.

Numerous studies document a correlation between poor eye movements and reading disability. Kephart et al. (1960) and Hoffman (1974) report a significant relationship between school readiness in kindergarten and performance on tests of pursuit and saccadic eye movements. Among elementary, secondary, and college-age readers, studies consistently indicate that poor readers make more fixations and regressions, have longer duration of saccadic fixation and shorter saccadic width, and consequently demonstrate considerably slower reading rates than good readers (Griffin et al. 1974).

Several studies have attempted to resolve the issue of whether poor eye movements are a perturbating factor in reading or simply reflect lack of familiarity with words and sentence structure. Lesevre (1968) and Elterman et al. (1980) report abnormal eye movements in dyslexic children during successive fixations of fixed symbols. Zangwill and Blakemore (1972) present a well-documented case of an adult dyslexic with abnormal eye movement patterns apparently unrelated to difficulty in decoding. Several studies (Griffin et al. 1974; Goldrich and Sedgwick 1982; Jones and Stark 1983; Pavlidis 1985) indicate that reading disabled individuals show less efficient saccadic eye movements than normal controls, even when eye movements are tested on nonlanguage stimuli. Maples and Ficklin (1989, 1990) found, using nonverbal stimuli, that both pursuit and saccadic eye movement were poorer in below-average readers. Griffin et al. (1974) and Goldrich and Sedgwick (1982) conclude that poor oculomotor control may contribute to reading difficulty.

Pirozzolo (1979) reports that auditory-linguistic dyslexics, like normal readers, have normal eye movements while reading easy material, but exhibit increased fixations and regressions as text difficulty increases. Visual-spatial dyslexics, in contrast, show greater numbers of fixations, regressions, and return sweep inaccuracies, and these faulty eye movements are not affected by text difficulty. Pirozzolo suggests that the faulty eye movements demonstrated by visual-spatial dyslexics while reading reflect faulty visual-spatial organization.

In contrast with studies that report abnormal saccadic eye movements in reading-impaired populations, Brown et al. (1983), Olson et al. (1983), Adler-Grinberg and Stark (1978), and Stanley et al. (1983) found that dyslexic and normal readers show no difference in saccadic characteristics on nonverbal material.

Bogacz et al. (1974) and Adler-Grinberg and Stark (1978) report that dyslexics demonstrate a greater prevalence of smooth pursuit abnormalities. This evidence supports the general notion that oculomotor dysfunction is more common among those with reading difficulty, yet raises questions about the nature of the relationship, since reading involves primarily saccadic rather than pursuit movements. Brown et al. (1983) found no difference in smooth pursuit ability between dyslexics and controls.

Poynter et al. (1982) found that the effect of oculomotor disorders on reading ability is additive, with multiple deficits increasingly predisposing toward lower reading ability. In a study of oculomotor function in fourth and sixth graders using both digits and prose, forward fixation frequency, regression frequency, and lag of accommodation each showed a small but significant relationship to reading ability. When multivariate analysis was used to examine the relationship of oculomotor functions collectively with reading ability, a much greater correlation was obtained. The combined oculomotor functions accounted for approximately 20% of the variance in reading ability, about twice the magnitude of any individual ability.

Solan (1985) reported on a sample of achieving readers with adequate interpretive skills who complained of slow and inefficient reading and showed inadequate eye movement patterns while reading. Oculomotor training produced significant improvement in reading efficiency, with increased reading rate and decrease in fixations and regressions. Rounds et al. (1991) and Taylor (1966) similarly report improved reading rate and efficiency following training to improve oculomotor function.

Visual-Perceptual-Motor Function

Although several authorities minimize the importance of visual perceptual deficit as a cause of reading disability (Larsen and Hammill 1975; Benton 1975; Fisher and Frankfurter 1977; Vellutino et al. 1977), numerous studies report that visual-perceptual-motor ability (that is, visual form perception, visual memory, visual-motor-integration) significantly correlates with reading readiness in kindergarten and with reading achievement in the early primary school grades (Silver 1961; Ayres 1969; Coleman 1968; Mattis et al. 1975; Lyon and Watson 1981; Satz and Morris 1981; Watson and Goldgar 1983; Solan et al, 1985; Solan and Mozlin 1986; Rosner and Rosner 1987; Wood et al. 1984; Robertson and Zaborske-Roy 1988; Bender and Golden 1990). Kagan (1965) reports that children in the early primary grades who respond impulsively to design-matching tests, guessing quickly with little regard for accuracy, make more word recognition errors and are poorer readers than those who are more reflective. A meta-analysis of the results of 161 studies of the relationship between visual perception and reading achievement concludes that visual perceptual skills are important correlates of reading achievement, especially at the preschool and primary level (Kavale 1982). In the later primary grades, a reduced but still significant relationship between visual perceptual function and reading achievement has been reported (Solan 1987a; Solan and Ficarra 1990).

These findings suggest that visual perceptual deficits interfere most in the early stages of learning to read, when visual form perception plays an important role in the acquisition of letter and word recognition skills. In the later primary grades, reading becomes more dependent on language and cognitive abilities, and perceptual function plays a diminished role.

Gross and Rothenberg (1979) cite numerous studies that report significant differences in visual perceptual function in dyslexic and normal readers when visual perceptual abilities are assessed by psychophysical methods. Differences in information storage and short-term visual memory have also been reported (Stanley, 1975; Lovegrove and Brown 1978; Stanley and Hall 1973a, 1973b). Differences in visual-evoked potentials between dyslexics and controls suggestive of differences in visual processing have been reported by Preston (1979), Andriola (1983), Mecacci et al. (1983), Cohen (1980), Solan et al. (1990), and Symann-Lovett (1977).

Transient System Processing Deficits

Experimental evidence suggests the existence of two parallel visual subsystems, the sustained and transient systems, which operate from the retina to the visual cortex (Livingstone and Hubel 1987). The sustained system predominates in central vision and is primarily a high-acuity pattern detection system that is most sensitive to stationary stimuli and transmits information about detail. The transient system predominates peripherally and transmits general information about stimulus change. It is primarily a flicker or motion detection system and is most sensitive to low spatial and high temporal frequencies (Garzia and Nicholson 1990).

Abnormal spatiotemporal processing attributable to transient system dysfunction is present in more than 75% of individuals with specific reading disability. This transient system dysfunction is inferred from experiments demonstrating differences in visual persistence, contrast sensitivity, and flicker masking effects between disabled readers and controls. The deficit in transient system function precedes the development of reading disorder (Lovegrove et al. 1990; Garzia and Nicholson 1990).

The sustained system responds throughout the duration of stimulus presentation, and its activity persists after removal of the stimulus. The transient system responds very briefly at the onset or cessation of a stimulus, and operates to reduce persistence of activity in the sustained channels. When reading a line of print in the presence of a transient system deficit, activity in the sustained channel from the previous fixation persists and interferes with input during the current fixation, resulting in garbled input and confused reading (Breitmeyer, 1983; Lovegrove et al. 1986, 1990; Garzia and Nicholson 1990; Williams and LeCluyse 1990).

Consistent with this model, Williams and LeCluyse (1990) report that when passages of text are displayed line by line as compared with single-word presentation, reading comprehension is reduced in disabled readers, but not in controls. This finding suggests that it is the demand for eye movements in the reading task that acts to reduce comprehension in disabled readers, apparently due to transient system deficit.

Garzia et al. (1990) and Lovegrove et al. (1990) suggest that transient system dysfunction may contribute to reading disability through interference with the process whereby peripheral visual mechanisms, mediated by the transient system, are involved in the selection of appropriate locations for fixation as one reads along a line of print. Several studies report differences in peripheral processing between normal and disabled readers (Geiger and Lettvin 1987; Grosser and Spafford 1989, 1990; Dautrich 1990; Spafford and Grosser 1991), leading Grosser and Spafford to hypothesize that photopic vision extends farther into the retinal periphery in dyslexic than in normal readers.

The performance of disabled readers on various perceptual tests is consistent with transient system dysfunction. As compared with controls, disabled readers exhibit perceptual grouping deficits and relative inability to selectively attend; require more time to make accurate temporal judgements, and to locate letters in an array of distractors; have slower processing rates for both simple and word-like stimuli; require longer integration time; and tend to be overly restricted to global processing at the expense of local detail processing (Garzia and Nicholson 1990; Williams and LeCluyse 1990).

Noting studies which indicate that most dyslexics demonstrate language disorder, but only a small percentage have primary visual-spatial perceptual deficits, Lovegrove et al. (1990) point out that most of the visual perceptual tests used in these studies involve the sustained rather than the transient visual system. Since the sustained system functions normally in individuals with specific reading disability, this finding does not conflict with Lovegrove's finding that a high percentage (>75%) of dyslexics have transient visual system deficits. Lovegrove et al. (1990) consider it likely that dyslexics have both language and transient visual-processing disorder. They suggest that transient visual system deficit that renders the appearance of graphemes unstable may interfere with learning grapheme-to-phoneme rules, and that this effect may partially explain the frequent association of language and transient system deficit in dyslexia.

CLINICAL MODELS RELATING VISION AND READING

Flax (1968, 1970a, 1970b) points out that the visual requirements for reading vary with the nature and level of the reading demand. The visual functions involved in learning to read are quite different from those required to read long passages with efficiency and comprehension at the high school and college levels. Flax suggests that visual perceptual deficits may contribute to inability to recognize words in learning to read, but that such deficits interfere less once word recognition skills have been acquired. Subtle binocular integration and accommodative disorders are unlikely to be the primary cause of early severe reading disability, but commonly interfere with reading efficiency as demands increase for sustained reading with comprehension.

Problems in Learning to Read

Developmental Immaturity

Birch (1962) suggests that dyslexia may result from inability to analyze and synthesize visual information, from deficient auditory-visual integration, and from inadequate hierarchial development of sensory systems whereby the auditory and visual systems fail to assume a dominant role. The act of reading requires that the child gather and process information through the visual system without tactile or auditory corroboration or support. The child whose development is abnormal or immature may be unable to perform at a visual level without kinesthetic or verbal support, and may therefore have considerable difficulty learning to read. Such a child may also exhibit hyperactivity, distractability, and/or attentional deficit if he is unable to inhibit movement and perform visually (Flax 1968, 1970a).

Phonics and Sight Reading

Learning to read involves both phonetic and eidetic processes (Christenson et al. 1990). Phonetic analysis involves sounding-out grapheme by grapheme. Eidetic or whole-word decoding is a more global process in which words are recognized based on their shape and configuration. In the earliest stages of reading, phonetic decoding predominates; as one becomes proficient, sight recognition is increasingly used. Visual perceptual deficits that interfere with the consistent recognition of graphemes may interfere with each of these processes.

Sight recognition is dependent on adequate visual form perception and visual memory. When these skills are inadequate, children may confuse the letters of the alphabet and confuse similar looking words. Children with inadequate visual form perception may become overly dependent on phonics, laboriously decoding one phoneme at a time with inadequate fluency and comprehension.

Dyslexia and Its Subtypes

Research suggests the existence of several subtypes of dyslexia, notably those in which auditory-language disorder is primary and those characterized chiefly by the presence of visual-spatial perceptual disorders. The auditory-linguistic form is the most common, outnumbering the visual perceptual by at least four or five to one (Pirozzolo 1979; McKinney 1984; Thomson 1984; Solan 1986).

Auditory-linguistic dyslexics typically demonstrate delays in language development, expressive speech defects, and verbal IQ that is low in relation to performance IQ. They have difficulty with phonetic analysis, and may have a store of sight words, but are unable to phonetically decipher words not in their sight vocabulary. They often make guesses from minimal cues, such as the first and last letter, substituting words that are similar in meaning, but dissimilar phonetically. Eye movements are usually normal and visual-spatial abilities relatively intact (Pirozzolo 1979).

The visual-spatial dyslexic has deficiencies in visual perception. Visual-spatial dyslexia is characterized by a performance IQ that is low in relation to the verbal, left-right disorientation, excessive reversals, transposition of letters and syllables, spatial difficulty, and faulty eye movements during reading.

Visual dyslexics have difficulty building a sight vocabulary and perceiving whole words. They make errors involving visual aspects of the text, confusing letter shapes, omitting and reversing letters and words, and guessing at words from shapes so that similar looking words are confused and miscalled.

Visual dyslexics generally have good linguistic ability. They tend to read and spell phonetically, sounding out words through auditory analysis. As a consequence, reading is slow and labored, and they have great difficulty reading and spelling irregular, nonphonetic words (Pirozzolo 1979).

Children with deficits in both auditory and visual modes have difficulty both with whole words and with phonetic analysis. As a consequence, they are virtually nonreaders.

Visual Perceptual Deficits

The fundamental visual problem in learning to read, according to Flax (1968, 1970a, 1970b), is the ability to appreciate and differentiate the shape and directional orientation of visual symbols, and to transform them into verbal symbols. The beginning reader must pay considerably greater attention to the internal detail of words than does the more advanced reader. Visual perceptual deficits that interfere with this aspect of visual function may cause confusion of similar looking words. The visual functions most important in the early stages of the reading process include visual form perception, visual memory, visual appreciation of directional differences, and visual-motor organization.

At this stage of the reading process, Flax indicates that end-organ visual function such as refractive state, visual acuity, fusion, convergence, and accommodation play a lesser role, since print is generally large, words are well isolated on the page or chalkboard, and the child is required to sustain visual attention for only brief moments. Accommodative and binocular fusion disorders, unless very severe, are therefore not usually the primary factors in severe reading disability in the early grades. However, accommodative and binocular disorders may cause asthenopia and disinterest in reading, and hence contribute to a child's failure to respond to proper teaching.

Problems in Reading Efficiency

Once basic decoding and sight recognition skills are established, perceptual organization plays a less significant role in reading proficiency. By third or fourth grade, there is a transition from "learning to read" to "reading to learn," using reading skills to acquire information. This transition is accompanied by a change in the visual abilities required for reading achievement. Efficient eye movement, and accommodative and binocular function become increasingly important as the child progresses through school and reading assignments become lengthier, demands for speed and comprehension become greater, print size becomes smaller, and spacing decreases between letters, words, and lines (Flax 1970a, 1970b).

Skeffington (1946–50) indicates that even subtle interference with visual efficiency detracts from the automaticity of the visual process. Increased effort required for visual function interferes with efficient information-processing and leads to decreased comprehension. Mild accommodative and binocular disorders contribute significantly to lowered achievement in the upper grades, causing asthenopia, blur, reduced comprehension, inability to sustain, disinterest, and avoidance.

CLINICAL ASSESSMENT OF THE READING-DISABLED CHILD

When examining a child with reading difficulty, the optometrist should perform a comprehensive vision evaluation to assess function in each of the areas that may potentially influence reading ability. Tests of eye movements and binocular and accommodative function have been described earlier (Chapters 11 and 12). Visual-perceptual-motor function should also be evaluated in the child with reading difficulty, particularly when the reading problem stems from the early grades when visual form perception and visual memory play an important role in the acquisition of word recognition skills.

Tests commonly used to evaluate visual-perceptual-motor function include tests of visual form perception and visual memory such as the Gardner Test of Visual Perceptual Skills (nonmotor), Motor-Free Visual Perception Test, Monroe Visual Tests, Frostig Developmental Test of Visual Perception, circus puzzle, SUNY pegboard test, tachistoscope, Rosner Test of Visual Analysis Skills, divided formboard, Visual Aural Digit Span Test, and the WISC-R block design and coding subtests; tests of visual-motor integration such as the Beery-Buktenica, Bender, and the Winter Haven Copy Forms test; tests of gross motor ability and bilateral integration; and the Birch-Belmont Auditory-Visual Integration Test. A full description of these perceptual tests is beyond the scope of this text; information on administration and scoring is provided by Apell and Lowry (1959), Getman (1960), Solan (1969, 1987b), Solan et al. (1985), Lowry (1970), Ilg and Ames (1972), Suchoff (1975), Rosner and Rosner (1990), and Treganza and Wold (1978–79).

Assessment of the Reading Problem

In examining a child with reading difficulty, the clinician must determine not only the presence of vision disorder, but also the nature of the reading problem, in order to determine the degree to which existing vision disorder may contribute to the specific reading difficulty. Information regarding the reading problem may be obtained from the parents during the case history and through telephone conferences with the classroom teacher and the resource room or remedial reading teacher.

The optometrist should determine whether psychoeducational evaluation has been performed at school. Such evaluation provides information regarding the child's academic difficulty and any intellectual and emotional factors that may contribute to it. When such testing has been performed, the optometrist should request a report of the results and recommendations. When psychoeducational evaluation has not been performed, the optometrist should consider recommending such testing.

The optometrist may obtain useful information regarding the specifics of the reading problem by listening to the child read. This author typically administers a shortened version of the Gates-McKillop Oral Reading Test (Lowry 1970). The test consists of seven paragraphs of increasing difficulty. It is quickly administered, easily scored, and correlates well with more extensive reading tests. The test provides the optometrist with an opportunity to assess the nature of the reading difficulty, and also provides a grade-level estimate of oral reading ability. The Gray Oral Reading Paragraphs or other suitable reading material may also be used for this purpose.

Inadequate Phonics and Sight Recognition

To be a good reader, the child must achieve proficiency in both phonics and sight recognition. Phonetic decoding permits one to sound out unfamiliar words. Sight recognition permits rapid recognition of familiar words. If either ability is poor, reading ability suffers.

The child with poor phonics may recognize familiar words, but is unable to decode unfamiliar and multisyllabic words. Poor phonetic decoding may result from auditory and language deficits, or from inadequate instruction. Inadequate phonics ability generally requires educational rather than optometric remediation.

The child with poor sight recognition is able to sound out words, but has difficulty recognizing familiar words. Reading may be slow and laborious as the child phonetically decodes each word. Because the child reads one word at a time, reading comprehension is impaired.

Poor sight recognition often correlates with inadequate visual form perception skills. The child who is unable to visually match shapes and forms will have difficulty recognizing words, since these are highly complex forms. The child with inadequate visual form perception and sight recognition skills frequently confuses similar looking words such as "look-like," "where-there," "was-saw."

Poor sight recognition is not always caused by deficits in visual form perception. Dyseidetic dyslexia, a genetic condition characterized by difficulty matching auditory and visual whole-word gestalts, is attributed to deficits in the angular gyrus of the left hemisphere (Christenson et al. 1990) and appears unrelated to visual perceptual deficit (Birch et al. 1991).

The clinician should evaluate visual perceptual skills whenever a child is overly phonetic in reading, or when excessive word confusion errors are noted. When visual form perception is inadequate, it may be assumed that dyslexia is of the visual-spatial variety, and appropriate vision therapy should be initiated. Patients who show poor sight recognition secondary to visual form perception deficit frequently demonstrate significant improvement in reading ability when visual perceptual deficits are treated.

The child who demonstrates both language and visual perceptual deficits so that phonics and sight recognition are each poor has no mechanism available for effective decoding, and typically suffers with severe reading disability. Such a child struggles unsuccessfully with most words, recognizing only the easiest and most familiar, unable to sound out the others. Even after years of educational exposure, the child may be a virtual nonreader. Although visual perceptual training is not sufficient to resolve such a disability, remediation of visual form perception and visual memory deficits may permit more adequate sight recognition and thereby be of value.

Small Word Errors

Some children make frequent small word errors, miscalling simple words like "the," "a," and "and." These errors frequently result from a global style, a tendency to perceive broadly, rather than to look carefully and note differences in detail. In contrast with word confusions, which result from poor visual form perception, these tend to be careless errors in that, if the word is pointed to and the child asked to read it again, it is usually read correctly.

Careless small word errors are commonly encountered in patients with vergence and accommodative disorders, who may scan globally as a result of their difficulty in integrating accommodation and convergence. Vision therapy is often highly effective in improving reading accuracy in such cases. Since these small words are connectors that significantly influence meaning, reading comprehension frequently improves as these errors drop out. Careless small word errors may also result from visual form perception and ocular motility deficits.

Reversal Errors

Reversal errors occur normally in preschool children and in the early primary grades, and should not be considered abnormal unless they are excessive. In normal readers, reversals usually disappear by the end of second grade as perceptual development permits more accurate and reliable directional differentiation (Gibson et al. 1962; Gardner 1978). Reading disabled children frequently make greater numbers of reversal errors in the early primary grades than do normals, and these reversals may persist long after such errors have dropped out in normally developing children (Bryant 1964; Mann 1969; Ginsberg and Hartwick 1971).

When a child presents with reversal errors, the clinician must determine whether they are normal reversals of development or abnormal reversals associated with learning disability. The Jordan Left-Right Reversal Test (Academic Therapy Publications) and the Gardner Reversal Frequency Test (Creative Therapeutics) are each useful for this purpose, providing information as to whether the frequency of reversal errors is excessive for the patient's age. However, clinicians should be aware that these tests show only low agreement with each other and with teachers' observations of reversal frequency (Cotter et al. 1987).

Persistent or excessive reversals have been attributed to rivalry in hemispheric dominance (Orton 1925), lags in visual-perceptual-motor development (Satz and Sparrow, 1973), and directional confusion and problems in left-right orientation (Kephart 1960). In many children, reversals result from inadequate visual form perception, rather than from directional confusion. When visual form perception is inadequate, children may reverse look-alikes such as "b-d" and "was-saw" as a result of difficulty in distinguishing similar shapes.

Inaccurate eye movements may also contribute to reversals, if fixations are irregular so that visual input is inconsistent. Reversals may occur when fixation lands at the end of a word or phrase, rather than at the beginning.

Inaccurate Eye Movement

Clinical tests of pursuit and saccadic eye movements generally use nonverbal target material. Patients who demonstrate inaccurate eye movements with nonverbal material may be presumed to have true oculomotor deficits, and are often inefficient readers. They frequently lose their place when reading, use a finger or marker to keep place, omit words and letters, skip and reread lines, and make small word errors. Reversals, inversions and transpositions, errors in copying from the chalkboard, and difficulty in organizing columns of numbers have also been attributed to eye movement inaccuracy. Children with accommodation/convergence dysfunction may similarly lose place frequently, skip words and lines, and use a finger to aid concentration. Significant improvement is usually obtained when vision therapy is performed to improve oculomotor function.

Children with reading problems unrelated to vision disorders may make similar errors as a result of their difficulty with the decoding process and their lack of familiarity with language. It is therefore important that the clinician evaluate the eye movements with nonverbal materials to differentiate whether the symptoms result from oculomotor dysfunction or from poor reading ability.

Evaluating the Older Disabled Reader

When the older child with reading problems is examined, it is helpful to determine when the reading difficulty began. Barring major psychological or educational interference, reading problems that began in first and second grade are usually related to inadequate phonics and/or sight recognition skills. If sight recognition skills are still poor and visual form perception ability is inadequate, appropriate visual-perceptual-motor training may provide a better foundation for the acquisition of reading skills. Appropriate educational instruction should be more effective once visual perceptual deficits have been resolved.

When examining the older child whose reading difficulty began in first or second grade, accommodation/convergence disorders are commonly found. Such disorders are usually not the primary factors causing early reading failure, but may cause asthenopia, inability to sustain, and disinterest in reading. Existing accommodative and vergence disorder should be treated to remove barriers to reading efficiency.

When reading difficulty develops in third grade or beyond, after adequate decoding skills have been acquired, visual inefficiency caused by subtle accommodative and binocular disorders is often a major factor. Some patients with such disorders make frequent small word errors. Others read accurately, yet experience discomfort, blur, and inability to read for prolonged periods. Such patients require excessive effort to maintain clear single vision. Reading is often slow and laborious, with frequent loss of concentration and need to reread. Reading comprehension is often impaired. Many patients consequently dislike and avoid reading.

Inadequate Reading Comprehension

By third or fourth grade, the good reader not only reads fluently and efficiently, but reads for meaning as well. Skeffington (1946–50) indicates that near-point stress–induced interference with vergence and accommodation causes visual inefficiency when reading, and that increased effort and attention devoted to visual function interferes with reading comprehension. This concept finds support in studies that document decreases in reading comprehension (Garzia et al.

1989) and performance on a standard intelligence test (Walton et al. 1978) when minus lenses are used to induce binocular stress or simulate uncorrected hyperopia.

Forrest (1981) points out that reading comprehension may be impaired when visual imagery or visualization abilities are inadequate or underused. Visualization skills, derived from prior experience and intersensory integration, play a major role in the acquisition of information through the visual process. The child sees an object such as an apple and is able to experience the smoothness, roundness, and hardness of its surface; its taste; and the crunch of biting into it through the process of visualization. Reading comprehension may suffer in cases in which failure in intersensory matching restricts the ability to integrate and synthesize input through the visualization process.

Many factors may contribute to poor reading comprehension. The child who has difficulty decoding will struggle with each word and likely fail to understand the reading material. The child with an intellectual or emotional disorder may similarly fail to comprehend. However, when reading comprehension is poor in a child who is a fluid reader with no language, intellectual, emotional, or attentional problem, the optometrist should consider whether inefficient vergence and accommodative function or inadequate or underused visualization ability may be a contributing factor.

Prognosis and Management

In cases in which vision disorder interferes with academic achievement, classroom performance will frequently improve when visual dysfunction is eliminated. When visual skills (oculomotor, accommodation, or vergence) disorder or visual-perceptual-motor dysfunction correlates closely with reading difficulty, vision therapy is clearly indicated. When, for example, a patient shows accommodative and/or vergence disorder and reports nearpoint asthenopic symptoms, inability to sustain, and poor reading comprehension, treatment is indicated to eliminate visual dysfunction as a barrier to reading achievement. Similarly, if a patient has poor visual form perception and inadequate sight recognition ability, or has poor eye movement ability and frequently omits small words and loses place when reading, visual dysfunction should be treated to eliminate barriers to effective reading.

In some cases, reading ability improves dramatically on remediation of underlying vision dysfunction. Immediate improvement is likely when vision disorder is the primary cause of reading difficulty, especially in those cases which are uncomplicated and in which the reading deficit is not too great. Severe reading deficit may persist after remediation of visual deficit, even if such deficit is a primary causative factor, unless appropriate educational remediation is provided. Elimination of visual deficits may permit the child to more readily benefit from educational instruction geared to the appropriate level.

In many cases, a variety of etiologic factors contribute to reading difficulty. Intellectual, verbal-linguistic, emotional, and socioeconomic factors may contribute, as well as the quality of the child's educational experience. Visual factors may play a role in such cases, and should be remediated since adequate reading ability is unlikely to be achieved in the presence of interfering vision disorder. However, the clinician should exercise caution predicting educational gains in such cases, since the continued presence of interfering psychoeducational and intellectual factors will continue to limit academic achievement.

The optometrist should be alert to the existence of other interfering factors and consider referral to other professionals when indicated. When several therapies are indicated, the clinician must determine whether they can be conducted simultaneously, whether vision therapy should be initiated prior to other therapies, or whether vision therapy should be delayed. In some cases, psychologic problems are so severe as to preclude effective vision therapy, which must therefore be delayed. In other cases, remediation of vision disorder eliminates a significant roadblock to effective classroom performance and is therefore a priority, since it may permit the patient to benefit more fully from subsequent remedial education.

Many children with reading difficulty demonstrate vision disorders that do not correlate closely with their reading problem. For example, a child with severe inability to phonetically decode may demonstrate mild accommodation/vergence disorder that is unlikely to be a significant factor in his reading problem. Such visual problems should not be ignored, since the clinician's responsibility is to properly care for the visual system. If such disorders are not treated, the patient may develop symptoms, patterns of avoidance, or adverse adaptation as reading demands increase. Appropriate vision care should not be denied simply because visual dysfunction is not the root cause of the reading difficulty. However, in such cases, the clinician must be careful to explain that vision therapy is undertaken to remediate visual dysfunction, but is unlikely to improve academic ability. Further, the priorities for such treatment must be weighed in relation to the child's need for other forms of therapy.

Although remediation of underlying vision disorder frequently leads to improved academic achievement, Hoffman and Rouse (1987) emphasize that vision therapy is a regimen for treating visual deficiencies, not learning disability. Vision disorders that are unrelated to learning difficulty should not go untreated, nor should the efficacy of vision therapy be judged on the basis of improved learning ability. However, it is important that the clinician be cognizant of the relationships between vision disorders and academic achievement in order to effectively counsel patients and prioritize recommendations for care.

VISION AND OTHER ASPECTS OF CLASSROOM PERFORMANCE

Arithmetic

In written arithmetic, children with visual perceptual, spatial, and eye movement deficits often copy inaccurately, space numbers improperly, and fail to properly align columns of numbers. Difficulties in organizing responses on a page and in keeping place interfere with ability to solve written arithmetic problems. Spatial and visual perceptual deficits interfere with mental arithmetic, which requires visualization of the spatial arrangement of the numbers, and with higher mathematical functions which require visualization of geometric and conceptual relationships (Solan 1987b; Rourke and Finlayson 1978).

Visual Attention

Visual processes such as vergence and accommodation, eye movements, spatial organization, central-peripheral integration, and adequacy of reach-grasp-release, are involved in the ability to selectively attend and to sustain visual attention. Deficits in any of these interrelated processes may contribute to attentional disorder and distractibility. Borsting (1991) reports that children with vergence or accommodative dysfunction perform poorer than normals on tasks that require coming to and sustaining attention.

The ability to control eye movements to selectively attend has a developmental component. Flax (1970a) notes that the infant's eye movements are generally directed to the areas of most intense physical stimulation. By first grade, the child must selectively control eye movements so as to respond to stimuli of cultural importance, rather than those which are brightest, loudest, or most novel. When development lags so that the first grade child is unable to override these primitive reflex mechanisms, his attention will be captured by noise, movement, and bright windows, rather than by the appropriate demands of the classroom. Consequently, the child will demonstrate attentional difficulty and distractibility.

Copying and Writing

The child must be able to neatly and accurately organize letters, words, and numbers on the page when copying from chalkboard or text to notebook, or when taking notes. Efficient performance requires adequate eye movement, vergence, accommodative, visual-spatial, and visual-motor skills. The Wold Sentence Copy Test (Treganza and Wold 1978–79) is a useful probe of speed and accuracy in copying. Visual-motor and eye-hand coordination skills also play an important role in handwriting and in drawing ability.

Spelling

Spelling involves a combination of visual and verbal processing. The good speller uses phonologic cues to break word sounds into their constituent letters, and at the same time visualizes the word being spelled. Mental imagery, or visualization, permits proper spelling despite the phonetic irregularities frequently encountered in the English language. The speller with inadequate visualization skill is excessively dependent on phonologic analysis and spells words exactly as they sound, misspelling irregular words with great frequency. Inadequate visualization skills should be suspected in the child who is a good reader, indicating that phonetic decoding skills are adequate, but who persistently spells poorly (Forrest 1981).

SUMMARY

Research indicates a high prevalence of hyperopia, accommodative dysfunction, high heterophoria (particularly exophoria at near), restricted fusional vergence ranges, convergence insufficiency, abnormal pursuit and saccadic eye movements, inadequate visual perceptual function, and deficits in transient visual system proccessing in reading-disabled individuals.

The visual requirements for reading vary with the nature and level of the reading demand. Visual perceptual deficits contribute to difficulty in learning to read; binocular and accommodative disorders are more likely to interfere with reading efficiency, comprehension, and ability to sustain in the later grades. The clinician must consider the nature of the individual child's reading difficulty to evaluate the degree to which diagnosed deficits in visual function may contribute.

Therapy to remediate visual dysfunction may lead to significant gains in reading in those cases in which reading disability is closely linked to visual deficit, and other contributing factors are minimal or absent. Deficits in visual function may also contribute to difficulties in mathematics, copying, writing, spelling, and sustaining visual attention.

SUGGESTED READING

Flax N (1970). The contribution of visual problems to learning disability. *J Am Optom Assoc* 41(10):841–845.

Flax N (1970). Problems in relating visual function to reading disorder. *Am J Optom Arch Am Acad Optom* 47(5):366–372.

Garzia RP, Nicholson SB (1990). Visual function and reading disability: An optometric viewpoint. *J Am Optom Assoc* 61:88–97.

Grisham JD, Simons HD (1986). Refractive error and the reading process: A literature analysis. *J Am Optom Assoc* 57(1):44–55.

Simons HD, Grisham JD (1987). Binocular anomalies and reading problems. *J Am Optom Assoc* 58(7):578–587.

Suchoff IB (1981). Research on the relationship between reading and vision—What does it mean? *J Learn Disab* 14(10):573–576.

Treganza A, Wold RM (1978–79). *Optometric Evaluation of Children with Academic Dysfunction.* Optometric Extension Program Continuing Education Courses, Santa Ana, CA: Optometric Extension Program Foundation, vol. 51, series 3, Oct. 1978–Sept. 1979.

REFERENCES

Adler-Grinberg D, Stark L (1978). Eye movements, scanpaths, and dyslexia. *Am J Optom Physiol Opt* 55:557–570.

Anapolle L (1967). Visual skills survey of dyslexic students. *J Am Optom Assoc* 38:853–859.

Andriola MR (1983). EEG and evoked potentials in learning disabilities. In: Hughes JR, Wilson WP (eds), *EEG and Evoked Potentials in Psychiatry and Behavioral Neurology*. Woburn, MA: Butterworth–Heinemann, pp. 211–229.

Apell RJ, Lowry RW (1959). *Preschool Vision*. St. Louis: American Optometric Association.

Ayers AJ (1969). Deficits in sensory integration in educationally handicapped children. *J Learn Disab* 2:160–168.

Bedwell CH, Grant R, McKeown JR (1980). Visual and ocular control anomalies in relation to reading difficulty. *Br J Educ Psychol* 50:61–70.

Bender WN, Golden LB (1990). Subtypes of students with learning disabilities as derived from cognitive, academic, behavioral, and self-concept measures. *Learning Disabilities Quarterly* 13:183–194.

Benton AL (1975). Developmental dyslexia: Neurological aspects. In: Friedlander WF (ed), *Advances in Neurology. Current Reviews of Higher Nervous System Dysfunction*. New York: Raven Press, 7(1):1–47.

Benton CD (1961). Ophthalmological approach to the problem of retarded readers among elementary school children. *J Florida Med Assoc* 47(10):1123–1125.

Benton C (1968). Management of dyslexias associated with binocular control abnormalities. In: Keeney A, Keeney V (eds), *Dyslexia: Diagnosis and Treatment of Reading Disorders*. St. Louis: C.V. Mosby, pp. 143–154.

Benton CD, McCann JW, Larsen M (1965). Dyslexia and dominance. *J Pediatr Ophthalmol* 2:53–57.

Betts E (1936). *The Prevention and Correction of Reading Difficulties*. Evanston, IL: Row, Peterson.

Birch HG (1962). Dyslexia and the maturation of visual function. In: J Money (ed), *Reading Disability*. Baltimore: Johns Hopkins Press, pp. 161–169.

Birch TF, Bateman GF, Griffin JR (1991). Dyslexia and vision perception: Is there a relationship? Presented at the Annual Meeting of the American Academy of Optometry, Section on Binocular Vision and Perception, Dec. 16, 1991, Anaheim, CA. Submitted for publication, *Optom Vis Sci*.

Birnbaum P, Birnbaum M (1968). Binocular coordination as a factor in reading achievement. *J Am Optom Assoc* 39:48–56.

Blika J (1982). Ophthalmological findings in pupils of a primary school with particular reference to reading difficulties. *Acta Ophthalmol* 60:927–934.

Bogacz J, Mendilaharsu C, de Mendilaharsu SA (1974). Electro-oculographic abnormalities during pursuit movements in developmental dyslexia. *EEG Clin Neurophysiol* 36:651–656.

Borsting E (1991). Measures of visual attention in children with and without visual efficiency problems. *J Behav Optom* 2(6):151–156.

Breitmeyer BG (1983). Sensory masking, persistence and enhancement in visual exploration and reading. In: Rayner K (ed), *Eye Movements in Reading: Perceptual and Language Processes*. New York: Academic Press, pp. 3–30.

Brown B, Haegerstrom-Portnoy G, Yingling CD, et al. (1983). Tracking eye movements are normal in dyslexic children. *Am J Optom Physiol Opt* 60:376–383.

Bryant ND (1964). Characteristics of dyslexia and their remedial implications. *Except Child* 31:195–199.

Buzzelli AR (1991). Stereopsis, accommodative and vergence facility: Do they relate to dyslexia. *Optom Vis Sci* 68(11):842–846.

Christenson GN, Griffin JR, Wesson MD (1990). Optometry's role in reading disabilities: Resolving the controversy. *J Am Optom Assoc* 61(5):363–372.

Clark B (1935). The effect of binocular imbalance on the behavior of the eyes during reading. *J Educ Res* 26:530–538.

Cohen J (1980). Cerebral evoked responses in dyslexic children. In: Kornhuber HH,

Deecke L (eds), *Motivation, Motor and Sensory Processes of the Brain.* (*Prog Brain Res,* vol. 54) Amsterdam: Elsevier, pp. 502–506.

Coleman HM (1968). Visual perception and reading dysfunction. *J Learn Disab* 2:498–503.

Cotter SA, Rouse MW, DeLand PN (1987). Comparative study of the Jordan Left-Right Reversal Test, the Reversals Frequency Test, and teachers' observations. *Am J Optom Physiol Opt* 64(3):195–203.

Dalton MM (1943). A visual survey of 5000 children. *J Educ Res* 36:81–94.

Dautrich B (1990). Evidence of aberrant patterns of visual peripheral sensitivity in the dyslexic reader in response to color and letter stimuli. Unpublished doctoral dissertation. Springfield, MA: American International College.

Dearborn W, Anderson I (1938). Aniseikonia related to disability in reading. *J Educ Psychol* 23:559–577.

Dunlop D (1976). The changing role of orthoptics in dyslexia. *Br Orthopt J* 33:22–28.

Dunlop D, Banks E (1973). New binocular factors in reading disability. *Aust Orthopt J* 13:7–11.

Eames TH (1932). A comparison of the ocular characteristics of unselected and reading disability groups. *J Educ Res* 25:211–215.

Eames TH (1934). Low fusional convergence as a factor in reading disability. *Am J Ophthalmol* 15:709–710.

Eames TH (1935). A frequency study of physical handicaps in reading disability and unselected groups. *J Educ Res* 29:1–5.

Eames TH (1948). Comparison of eye conditions among 1000 reading failures, 500 ophthalmic patients, and 150 unselected children. *Am J Ophthalmol* 31:713–717.

Eames TH (1949). The effect of glasses for the correction of hypermetropia and myopia on the speed of visual perception of objects and words. *J Educ Res* 42:534–540.

Eames TH (1955). The influence of hypermetropia and myopia on reading achievement. *Am J Ophthalmol* 39:375–377.

Eames TH (1964). The effect of anisometropia on reading achievement. *Am J Optom Arch Am Acad Optom* 41:700–702.

Elterman RD, Abel LA, Daroff RB, et al. (1980). Eye movement patterns in dyslexic children. *J Learn Disab* 13:11–16.

Evans JR, Efron M, Hodge C (1976). Incidence of lateral phoria among SLD children. *Academ Ther* 11:431–433.

Farris LP (1936). Visual defects as factors influencing achievement in reading. Ph.D. theses, Berkeley: University of California.

Fendrick P (1935). *Visual Characteristics of Poor Readers.* New York: Teachers College, Columbia University Contributions to Education no. 656.

Fisher DF, Frankfurter A (1977). Normal and disabled readers can locate and identify letters: Where's the perceptual deficit? *J Reading Behav* 9:31–43.

Flax N (1968). Visual function in dyslexia. *Am J Optom Arch Am Acad Optom* 45(9):574–587.

Flax N (1970a). The contribution of visual problems to learning disability. *J Am Optom Assoc* 41(10):841–845.

Flax N (1970b). Problems in relating visual function to reading disorder. *Am J Optom Arch Am Acad Optom* 47(5):366–372.

Forrest EB (1981). *Visual Imagery: An Optometric Approach.* Santa Ana, CA: Optometric Extension Program Foundation.

Frankling SR (1961). A study of reading difficulties in Toronto school children. *Can Med Assoc J* 85:237–239.

Gaarder KR (1975). *Eye Movements, Vision, and Behavior: A Hierarchial Visual Information Processing Model.* Washington Hemisphere Pub. Corp. Distributed by Halsted Press, New York.

Gardner RA (1978). *Reversals Frequency Test.* Cresskill, NJ: Creative Therapeutics.

Garzia RP, Nicholson SB (1990). Visual function and reading disability: An optometric viewpoint. *J Am Optom Assoc* 61:88–97.

Garzia RP, Nicholson SB, Gaines CS, et al. (1989). Effects of nearpoint visual stress on psycholinguistic processing in reading. *J Am Optom Assoc* 60(1):38–44.

Garzia RP, Richman JE, Nicholson SB, et al. (1990). A new visual-verbal saccade test: The Developmental Eye Movement (DEM) Test. *J Am Optom Assoc* 61(2): 124–135.

Geiger G, Lettvin JY (1987). Peripheral vision in persons with dyslexia. *N Engl J Med* 315:1238–1243.

Getman GN (1960). *Techniques and Diagnostic Criteria for the Optometric Care of Children's Vision.* Santa Ana, CA: Optometric Extension Program Foundation.

Getz DJ, McGraw L (1980). Phorias and reading. *J Optom Vis Dev* 11(3):21–25.

Gibson EJ, Gibson JJ, Pick AD, et al. (1962). A developmental study of the discrimination of letter-like form. *J Comp Physiol Psychol* 55:897–906.

Ginsberg GP, Hartwick A (1971). Directional confusion as a sign of dyslexia. *Percept Mot Skills* 32:535–543.

Glatt LD, Glatt MM (1956). Visual efficiency in the classroom. *Opt J Rev Optom* 93:37–39,52.

Goldrich SG, Sedgwick H (1982). An objective comparison of oculomotor functioning in reading disabled and normal children. *Am J Optom Physiol Opt* 59:82P.

Good GH (1939). Relationship of fusion weaknesses to reading disability. *J Exp Educ* 8:115–121.

Griffin DC, Walton HN, Ives V (1974). Saccades as related to reading disorders. *J Learn Disab* 7:310–316.

Grisham JD, Simons HD (1986). Refractive error and the reading process: A literature analysis. *J Am Optom Assoc* 57(1):44–55.

Gross K, Rothenberg S (1979). An examination of methods used to test the visual perceptual deficit hypotheses of dyslexia. *J Learn Disab* 12(10):670–677.

Grosser GS, Spafford CS (1989). Perceptual evidence for an anomalous distribution of rods and cones in the retinas of dyslexics: A new hypothesis. *Percept Mot Skills* 68:683–698.

Grosser GS, Spafford CS (1990). Light sensitivity in peripheral retinal fields of dyslexic and proficient readers. *Percept Mot Skills* 71:467–477.

Haddad H, Isaacs N, Onghena K, et al. (1984). The use of orthoptics in dyslexia. *J Learn Disab* 17:142–144.

Helveston EM, Weber JC, Miller K, et al. (1985). Visual function and academic performance. *Am J Ophthalmol* 99(3):346–355.

Hoffman LG (1974). The relationship of basic visual skills to school readiness at the kindergarten level. *J Am Optom Assoc* 45:608–614.

Hoffman LG (1980). Incidence of vision difficulties in children with learning disabilities. *J Am Optom Assoc* 51(5):447–451.

Hoffman LG, Rouse MW (1987). Vision therapy revisted: A restatement. *J Am Optom Assoc* 58(7):536–541.

Ilg FL, Ames LB (1972). *School Readiness. Behavior Tests Used at the Gesell Institute.* New York: Harper and Row.

Jones A, Stark L (1983). Abnormal patterns of eye movements in specific dyslexia. In: Rayner K (ed), *Eye Movements in Reading: Perceptual and Language Processes.* New York: Academic, pp. 481–498.

Kagan J (1965). Reflection-impulsivity and reading ability in primary grade children. *Child Dev* 36:609–628.

Kavale K (1982). Meta-analysis of the relationship between visual perceptual skills and reading achievement. *J Learn Disab* 15(1):42–51.

Kelly CR (1957). *Visual Screening and Child Development*. Raleigh, NC: Department of Psychology, North Carolina State College.

Kephart NC (1953). Visual skills and their relation to school achievement. *Amer J Ophthalmol* 36:794–799.

Kephart NC (1960). *The Slow Learner in the Classroom*. 2nd ed. Columbus, OH: Charles E. Merrill, pp. 86–96.

Kephart NC, Manas L, Simpson D (1960). Vision and achievement in kindergarten. *Am J Optom Arch Am Acad Optom* 37(1):36–39.

King JW, Michael LD (1969). Near binocular performance as it relates to reading. In: Wold RM (ed), *Visual and Perceptual Aspects for the Achieving and Underachieving Child*. Seattle: Special Child Publications Inc., pp. 129–139.

Larsen SC, Hammill DD (1975). Relationship of selected visual perceptual abilities to school learning. *J Spec Educ* 9:281–291.

Lesevre N (1968). L'organisation du regard chez des enfants d'age scolaire, lecteurs normaux et dyslexiques. *Rev Neuropsychiatr Infant Hyg Ment Enfance* 16:323–349.

Letourneau J, Lapierre N, Lamont A (1969). The relationship between convergence insufficiency and school achievement. *Am J Optom Physiol Opt* 56:18–22.

Livingstone MS, Hubel DH (1987). Psychophysical evidence for separate channels for the perception of form, color, movement and depth. *J Neurosci* 7:3416—3468.

Lowry RW (1970). *Handbook of Diagnostic Tests for the Developmental Optometrist*. Worthington, MN: author.

Lovegrove W, Brown C (1978). Development of information processing in normal and disabled readers. *Percept Mot Skills* 46:1047–1054.

Lovegrove WJ, Garzia RP, Nicholson SB (1990). Experimental evidence for a transient system deficit in specific reading disability. *J Am Optom Assoc* 61:137–146.

Lovegrove W, Martin F, Slaghuis W (1986). A theoretical and experimental case for a visual deficit in specific reading disability. *Cogn Neuropsychol* 3:225–267.

Lyon GR, Watson B (1981). Empirically derived subgroups of learning disabled readers: Diagnostic characteristics. *J Learning Disabilities* 14:256–261.

Mann GT (1969). Reversal reading errors in children trained in dual directionality. *Reading Teacher* 22:646–649.

Maples WC, Ficklin T (1989). A preliminary study of the oculomotor skills of learning-disabled, gifted and normal children. *J Optom Vis Dev* 20:9–14.

Maples WC, Ficklin T (1990). Comparison of eye movement skills between above average and below average readers. *J Behav Optom* 1(4):87–91.

Marcus SE (1974). A syndrome of visual constrictions in the learning disabled child. *J Am Optom Assoc* 45(6):746–749.

Mattis S, French JH, Rapin I (1975). Dyslexia in children and adults: Three independent neuropsychological syndromes. *Developmental Med Child Neurol* 17:150–163.

McKinney JD (1984). The search for subtypes of specific learning disability. *J Learn Disab* 17(1):43–50.

Mecacci L, Sechi E, Levi G (1983). Abnormalities of visual evoked potentials by checkerboards in children with specific reading disability. *Brain Cognition* 2:135–143.

Norn MS, Rindziunski E, Skydsgaard H (1969). Ophthalmologic and orthoptic examinations of dyslexics. *Acta Ophthalmol* 47:147–160.

O'Grady J (1984). The relationship between vision and educational performance: A study of year 2 children in Tasmania. *Aust J Optom* 67:126–140.

Olson RK, Kliegl R, Davidson BJ (1983). Eye movements in reading disability. In: Rayner K (ed), *Eye Movements in Reading: Perceptual and Language Processes.* New York: Academic, pp. 481–498.

Orton ST (1925). Word blindness in school children. *Arch Neurol Psychiatry* 14:581–615.

Park G (1948). Reading difficulty (dyslexia) from the ophthalmic point of view. *Am J Opthalmol* 31(1):28–34.

Park G (1969). Functional dyslexia (reading failures) vs. normal reading. *Eye Ear Nose Throat Monthly* 2:189–198.

Park GE, Burri C (1943a). Relationship of various eye conditions and reading achievement. *J Educ Psychol* 34:290–299.

Park GE, Burri C (1943b). Eye maturations and reading difficulties. *J Educ Psychol* 12:535–545.

Pavlidis GT (1985). Eye movement differences between dyslexics, normal, and retarded readers while sequentially fixating digits. *Am J Optom Physiol Opt* 62(12):820–823.

Pierce J (1977). Is there a relationship between vision therapy and academic achievement? *Rev Optom* 114(6):48–63.

Pirozzolo FJ (1979). *The Neuropsychology of Developmental Reading Disorders.* New York: Praeger.

Poynter HL, Schor C, Haynes HM, et al. (1982). Oculomotor functions in reading disability. *Am J Optom Physiol Opt* 59(2):116–127.

Preston MS (1979). The use of evoked response procedures in studies of reading disability. In: Begleiter H (ed), *Evoked Brain Potentials and Behavior.* New York: Plenum, pp. 247–268.

Robertson KL, Zaborske-Roy L (1988). The relationship of academic achievement to visual memory. *J Optom Vis Dev* 19:12–15.

Robinson H (1946). *Why Pupils Fail in Reading.* Chicago: University of Chicago Press.

Robinson HM (1968). Visual efficiency and reading status in the elementary school. In: Robinson H, Smith H (eds), *Clinical Studies in Reading.* Chicago: University of Chicago Press, pp. 49–65.

Robinson H, Huelsman C Jr. (1953). Visual efficiency and progress in learning to read. In: Robinson H (ed.), *Clinical Studies in Reading II.* Chicago: University of Chicago Press, pp. 31–63.

Rosenbloom A (1968). The relationship between aniseikonia and achievement in reading. In: Robinson H (ed), *Clinical Studies in Reading III.* Supplementary Educational Monographs no. 97, Chicago: University of Chicago Press, pp. 109–116.

Rosner J, Rosner J (1987). Comparison of visual characteristics in children with and without learning difficulties. *Am J Optom Physiol Opt* 64(7):531–533.

Rosner J, Rosner J (1990). *Pediatric Optometry.* 2nd ed. Boston: Butterworth–Heinemann.

Rounds BR, Manley CW, Norris RH (1991). The effect of oculomotor training on reading efficiency. *J Am Optom Assoc* 62(2):92–99.

Rourke BP, Finlayson MA (1978). Neuropsychological significance of variations in patterns of academic performance: verbal and visual-spatial abilities. *J Abnorm Child Psychol* 6(1):121–133.

Satz P, Morris R (1981). Learning disability subtypes: A review. In: Pirozzolo FJ, Wittrock MC (eds), *Neuropsychological and cognitive processes in reading.* New York: Academic Press, pp. 109–140.

Satz P, Sparrow S (1973). Developmental dyslexia: A theoretical formulation. In: Bakker DJ, Satz P (eds), *Specific Reading Disability: Advances in Theory and Method.* Rotterdam: Rotterdam University Press, pp. 17–40.

Selzer CA (1933). *Lateral Dominance and Visual Fusion: Their Application to Difficulties in Reading, Writing, Spelling and Speech.* Harvard Monographs in Education, no. 12, Cambridge, MA: Harvard University Press.

Shearer RV (1966). Eye findings in children with reading difficulties. *J Pediatr Ophthalmol* 3:47–52.

Sherman A (1973). Relating vision disorders to learning disability. *J Am Optom Assoc* 44(2):140–141.

Silbiger F, Woolf D (1968). Fixation disparity and reading achievement at the college level. *Am J Optom Physiol Opt* 45:734–742.

Silver AA (1961). Diagnostic considerations in children with reading disability. *Bull Orton Soc* 11:91.

Simons HD, Gassler PA (1988). Vision anomalies and reading skills: A meta-analysis of the literature. *Am J Optom Physiol Opt* 65(11):893–904.

Simons HD, Grisham JD (1987). Binocular anomalies and reading problems. *J Am Optom Assoc* 58(7):578–587.

Skeffington AM (1946–50). *Analytical Optometry.* Optometric Education Program Continuing Education Courses, Santa Ana, CA: Optometric Extension Program Foundation, vol. 18–22, Jan. 1946–Sept. 1950.

Solan HA (1969). Visual processing training with the tachistoscope: A rationale and grade one norms. *J Learn Disab* 2(1):30–36.

Solan HA (1985). Eye movement problems in achieving readers: An update. *Am J Optom Physiol Opt* 62(12):812–819.

Solan HA (1986). Learning disabilities: The importance of considering sub-types in optometric research. *J Am Optom Assoc* 57(1):15–16.

Solan HA (1987a). A comparison of the influences of verbal-successive and spatial-simultaneous factors on achieving readers in fourth and fifth grade: A multivariate correlational study. *J Learn Disab* 20(4):237–242.

Solan HA (1987b). The effects of visual-spatial and verbal skills on written and mental arithmetic. *J Am Optom Assoc* 58(2):88–94.

Solan HA, Ficarra AP (1990). A study of perceptual and verbal skills of disabled readers in grade 4, 5 and 6. *J Am Optom Assoc* 61:628–634.

Solan HA, Mozlin R (1986). Correlation of perceptual-motor maturation to readiness and reading in kindergarten and the primary grades. *J Am Optom Assoc* 57:28–35.

Solan HA, Mozlin R, Rumpf DA (1985). Selected perceptual norms and their relationship to reading in kindergarten and the primary grades. *J Am Optom Assoc* 56:458–467.

Solan HA, Sutija VG, Ficarra AP, et al. (1990). Binocular advantage and visual processing in dyslexic and control children as measured by visual evoked potentials. *Optom Vis Sci* 67(2):105–110.

Spache GD, Tillman CE (1962). A comparison of the visual profiles of retarded and nonretarded readers. *J Dev Reading* 5:101–109.

Spafford C, Grosser GS (1991). Retinal differences in light sensitivity between dyslexic and proficient reading children: New prospects for optometric input in diagnosing dyslexia. *J Am Optom Assoc* 62(8):610–615

Stanley G (1975). Visual memory processes in dyslexia. In: Deutsch D, Deutsch J (eds), *Short-Term Memory.* New York: Academic Press, pp. 181–194.

Stanley G, Hall R (1973a). A comparison of dyslexics and normals in recalling letter arrays after brief presentations. *Br J Educ Psychol* 43:301–304.

Stanley G, Hall R (1973b). Short-term visual information processing in dyslexia. *Child Dev* 44:841–844.

Stanley G, Smith GA, Howell EA (1983). Eye movements and sequential tracking in dyslexic and control children. *Br J Psychol* 74:181–187.

Stein J, Fowler S (1986). Occlusion treatment. *Optician* 11:16–22.

Stein JF, Riddell PM, Fowler S (1986). The Dunlop test and reading in primary school children. *Br J Opthalmol* 70:317–320.

Stein JF, Riddell PM, Fowler S (1988). Disordered vergence control in dyslexic children. *Br J Ophthalmol* 72:162–166.

Stolzberg ME, Ritty JM, Cohen A, et al. (1989). Effects of ocular functioning and time upon reading proficiency. *J Am Optom Assoc* 60 (2):122–126.

Stromberg EL (1937). The relationship of lateral muscle balance and the ductions to reading speed. *Am J Optom* 14:415–420.

Stromberg E (1938). Binocular movements of the eyes in reading. *J Gen Psychol* 18:349–355.

Suchoff IB (1975). *Visual-Spatial Development in the Child. An Optometric Theoretical and Clinical Approach*. New York: State University of New York College of Optometry.

Suchoff IB (1981). Research on the relationship between reading and vision—What does it mean? *J Learn Disab* 14(10):573–576.

Swanson DE, Tiffin J (1936). Betts' physiological approach to the analysis of reading disabilities as applied to the college level. *J Educ Res* 29:433–438.

Symann-Lovett N, Gascon G, Matsumiya Y, et al. (1977). Wave form difference in visual evoked responses between normal and reading disabled children. *Neurology* 27:156–159.

Taylor E (1937). *Controlled Reading: A Correlation of Diagnostic, Teaching and Corrective Techniques*. Chicago: University of Chicago Press.

Taylor EA (1966). *The Fundamental Reading Skill*. 2nd ed. Springfield, IL: Charles C. Thomas.

Thomson ME (1984). *Developmental Dyslexia: Its Nature, Assessment and Remediation*. London: Edward Arnold.

Treganza A, Wold RM (1978–79). *Optometric Evaluation of Children with Academic Dysfunction*. Optometric Extension Program Continuing Education Courses, Santa Ana, CA: Optometric Extention Program Foundation, Vol. 51, series 3, Oct. 1978–Sept. 1989.

Vellutino FR, Steger BM, Moyer SC, et al. (1977). Has the perceptual deficit hypothesis led us astray? *J Learn Disab* 10:54–64.

Walton HN, Schubert DG, Clark D, et al. (1978). Effects of induced hyperopia. *Am J Optom Physiol Opt* 55 (7): 451–455.

Watson BU, Goldgar DE (1983). Subtypes of reading disability. *J Clinical Neuropsychology* 5:377–399.

Weber G (1980). Visual disabilities: Their identification and relationship with academic achievement. *J Learn Disab* 13:13–19.

Williams MC, LeCluyse K (1990). The perceptual consequences of a temporal processing deficit in reading disabled children. *J Am Optom Assoc* 61:111–121.

Wilson K, Wold R (1972). A report of vision screening in the schools. *Academic Ther* 8:155–166.

Wirt S, Morgan C, Floyd W (1947). Visual reading achievement of grade school pupils in relation to visual performance. *Claremont Reading Conference* Vol. 11, pp. 59–66.

Witty P, Kopel D (1936a). Factors associated with the etiology of reading disability. *J Educ Res* 29:449–459.

Witty P, Kopel D (1936b). Heterophoria and reading disability. *J Educ Psychol* 27:222–230.

Wood C, Powell S, Knight RC (1984). Predicting school readiness: The validity of developmental age. *J Learn Disab* 17(1):8–11.

Zangwill OL, Blakemore C (1972). Dyslexia: Reversal of eye movements during reading. *Neuropsychologia* 10:371–373.

PART IV

Vision Therapy

Vision therapy is generally recommended when evaluation and case analysis indicate that lens application alone is insufficient to provide optimal visual function. In vision therapy, procedures are selected and organized in appropriate sequences to provide conditions optimal for the development of more adequate visual skills and abilities. The goal is to remediate existing vision disorder and/or enhance visual function.

Chapter 14 overviews the various models and approaches to vision therapy and summarizes principles that are fundamental to effective treatment. Specific vision therapy regimens are presented for treatment of oculomotor disfunction, accommodative disorder, convergence insufficiency, convergence excess, and binocular instability, as well as for management of the myopic patient. Chapter 15 describes a large variety of procedures for training pursuit, saccadic, accommodative, and fusional abilities, as well as the sequencing of these procedures. Chapter 16 reviews research documenting the effectiveness of vision therapy in remediating deficits in eye movement, accommodative, and binocular function.

14

Vision Therapy: Models, Approaches, and Principles

Vision therapy (vision training, visual training) involves the use of therapeutic procedures to modify visual function. Vision therapy is used to remediate eye movement, and accommodative and nonstrabismic binocular vision disorders (as well as strabismic and visual-perceptual-motor disorders not covered in this text), to relieve associated symptoms, and to permit efficient acquisition and processing of visual information (Flax 1986; 1986/87 Future of Visual Development/ Performance Task Force 1988; Peachey 1990).

Peachey (1990) notes that optometric visual training is an extension of the practice of traditional orthoptics, and identifies four major areas:

1. Developmental vision training, used for the guidance and development of visual abilities in young children.
2. Preventive visual training, used to prevent the development of vision disorders that might otherwise occur.
3. Rehabilitative vision training, used to remediate specific diagnosed vision disorders.
4. Enhancement visual training, used to enhance visual abilities required for specific sports, work, or academic demands.

DIVERSE APPROACHES TO VISION THERAPY

Nowhere in optometry is there greater diversity of approach than in vision therapy. This diversity emerges from differing concepts of the etiology of vision disorders, as well as conceptual differences regarding the nature of vision and how it relates to human performance.

Traditional Versus OEP Approaches

Practitioners schooled in traditional orthoptics view vision therapy primarily as a means to remediate strabismus and vergence dysfunction. Such practitioners may limit vision therapy to the treatment of sensory fusion anomalies

283

and expansion of restricted fusional vergence ranges. Other practitioners view vision therapy more broadly and treat disorders of ocular motility, accommodation, eye-hand coordination, visual-perceptual-motor function, visual attention, and visual cognitive function as well.

Practitioners who view oculomotor and vergence dysfunction primarily as products of genetic or random biologic factors typically offer treatment programs that are narrowly directed toward remediation of deficient findings. Treatment is frequently based on reserve-demand models so that if a patient demonstrates high exophoria with low PRC or receded convergence near point, exercises are prescribed solely to improve convergence. Similarly, if accommodative facility is poor, the patient is given accommodative exercises.

In contrast, adherents of the OEP model emphasize the role of environmental factors in the etiology of visual dysfunction. Most vision disorders are held to result from interference with normal development and from the impact of nearpoint stress. In treating nearpoint stress–induced vision disorders, therapy is not directed toward a specific deficient vergence as in reserve-demand systems, but rather to develop more adequate flexibility between vergence and accommodation and to remediate functional skews presumed to have developed in response to a drive for convergence to localize closer. In addition to the use of vision therapy, OEP-oriented practitioners frequently seek to modify adverse environmental influences through the use of nearpoint lenses; guidance regarding near-work posture and lighting; visual hygiene suggestions to reduce stress on the visual system; and guidance regarding environmental factors that promote optimal development in the early years of life.

Some practitioners view vision therapy as a last resort, to be prescribed only if lenses and prisms fail to remediate the patient's symptoms. Others view vision therapy as a means of improving visual function beyond levels achievable with lenses or prisms alone, and recommend vision therapy to remediate dysfunction, to prevent adverse adaptation, and to expand the ability to process visual information. In contrast with traditional practitioners who generally do not recommend therapy unless the patient complains of asthenopia, adherents of the OEP model offer vision therapy to remediate dysfunction even in the absence of asthenopia in patients whose visual function is inefficient or who cope with nearpoint stress by avoiding near work.

Skills-Oriented Versus Behavioral Approaches

Many practitioners apply their ministrations primarily within the oculomotor system, organizing treatment in relation to specific identifiable deficits of binocular, accommodative, and oculomotor function. Such an approach is sometimes referred to as *skills-oriented*.

Other practitioners are broader in their approach, emphasizing aspects related to visual information-processing, visualization, visual awareness, visual attention, visual-cognitive, visual-motor, and visual-spatial functions (Furth and Wachs 1974; Forrest 1976; Birnbaum 1978a; Getman 1984; Pepper 1986). Such treatment programs are often referred to as *behavioral*, since vision is considered in relation to organismic aspects of behavior.

Many practitioners combine skills-oriented and behavioral approaches, diagnosing and treating specific functional oculomotor disorders while at the same time emphasizing visual information-processing ability, awareness, central-peripheral organization, and visual-motor integration. While therapy is directed toward the remediation of specific oculomotor deficits, the organization of training is influenced by analysis of the patient's visual information-processing style (Forrest 1976; Birnbaum 1978a).

Sequential Versus Directional Training

Apell (1967) distinguishes between sequential and directional approaches to training. In *sequential training*, procedures with preset goals are used in a hierarchial order to develop more adequate visual skills and abilities. In *directional training*, in contrast, the sequence and nature of procedures is not predetermined, but rather evolves in various directions depending on the practitioner's observations and the patient's experiences and responses. The practitioner shapes the procedures to guide the patient toward desired goals. Training is more open-ended, with an emphasis on awareness and self-discovery as the patient seeks to resolve the problems presented by the various therapy procedures.

In practice, many clinicians combine sequential and directional approaches, programming procedures hierarchially yet emphasizing the patient's awareness of visual process and modifying the training sequence and instructions in directions indicated by the patient's performance and responses.

Author's Approach

The diversity of approaches to vision therapy makes it impossible to speak of a single "correct" treatment plan. Different practitioners bring their individual models, experiences, goals, and biases to vision therapy. This author's approach to the treatment of nearpoint stress–induced vision disorders incorporates both skills- and behavior-oriented training, sequentially using vision therapy procedures to remediate deficient vergence and accommodative functions, while simultaneously organizing therapy to optimize central-peripheral organization and visual information-processing.

A typical treatment sequence used by this author in the management of nearpoint stress–induced vision disorders is as follows:

1. Nearpoint lens prescription, if indicated by case analysis, to minimize nearpoint stress
2. Visual hygiene suggestions regarding posture, lighting, and work habits to further reduce stress on the visual system during near work
3. Vision therapy
   a. ocular motility skills (as needed)
   b. monocular accommodative facility

    c. expand fusional vergence ranges
    d. binocular, fused accommodative facility
    e. behavioral approaches
        a. relaxation and stress reduction for the very intense individual
        b. peripheral awareness for the central specific individual
        c. detail-oriented procedures for the global-peripheral individual

Diversity in Delivery of Vision Therapy Services

Considerable diversity also exists in the delivery of vision therapy services. Some practitioners emphasize office treatment, while others use primarily home-based therapy. Some practitioners see patients as often as three times a week; others schedule less frequent office visits. In some offices, training is performed by the doctor; in others, the doctor is assisted by one or a number of aides; and in still other offices, training is programmed by the doctor and performed by therapists.

In some offices, patients are scheduled one at a time for therapy; in others, a combination of doctors and aides treat a number of patients simultaneously. In some offices, treatment is solely optometric; in others, a variety of educational and interdisciplinary services may be available.

This author's approach to management may be summarized as follows:

1. Office-based therapy is the rule; home therapy offers less opportunity for doctor-patient interaction and for hierarchial sequencing, and hence is much less effective. Home therapy is used for practice and reinforcement between office sessions.
2. Most patients are seen twice a week. In this author's experience, twice-a-week therapy is considerably more effective than once-a-week, producing better results in a shorter time period. Since results are obtained more quickly, the benefits of therapy are more readily visible to both patients and parents, resulting in greater enthusiasm and compliance.
3. Most patients are scheduled for multiple therapy. The doctor and three or four assistants work with five or six patients in each 45-minute session. All programming is done by the doctor, who is present in the therapy room and actively involved in the therapy at all times. Patients who require individual therapy with the doctor, either because of the complexity of their vision problem or because of behavioral disorder, are so scheduled.

PRINCIPLES OF VISION THERAPY

In vision therapy, the practitioner arranges conditions so that the patient learns to modify visual performance in a manner deemed advantageous by the doctor. The practioner must identify those aspects of visual function that require remediation or enhancement, and determine appropriate goals for therapy. The clinician must not only select appropriate therapy procedures toward this end, but must also sequence those procedures in a manner consistent with the patient's abilities. Further, the procedures selected must provide appropriate feedback so that the patient can adequately monitor performance.

For any given procedure, the optometrist must first make certain that the patient is aware of the visual process being trained, and then must guide the patient toward developing control of the process, with skill and eventually with stamina. The goal of therapy is that visual function will be so automatic that the process is controlled subconsciously (Peachey 1990, 1991).

Instructional Set

Birnbaum (1977) emphasizes the importance of instructional set in assisting the patient to make changes in visual function. For any particular procedure the clinician should make the patient aware not only of the goal to be achieved, but also of the nature of the change in process desired. Further, the practitioner should make certain that the patient understands that the phenomena observed during vision therapy procedures (blur, diplopia, suppression), which seem to result from external changes in the environment, in fact result from the patient's visual function and are subject to the patient's control.

In an accommodative procedure, therefore, instead of asking the patient to "keep the letters clear," which implies that the letters themselves are blurring, the therapist might explain that the letters appear blurred only when the patient is focusing inappropriately for the particular lens power. To maintain clarity when switching from one lens to another, the patient must adjust focus nearer or farther. Such an instructional set creates greater awareness of the process involved, as well as awareness that the process is subject to the patient's control.

In fusional vergence procedures, the therapist should not ask the patient "to keep the picture single" as the targets are disparated, which implies an external event. Rather, the therapist should advise that as the targets are disparated base-out and base-in, the patient needs to look closer and farther. If the target appears to double, it is because the patient is not looking close enough or far enough away; to keep it single, the patient needs to adjust where he or she is looking in space.

Similarly, in an antisuppression procedure, the patient should not be told "not to let anything disappear," which implies an external change, but rather the therapist should advise that if parts of the picture seem to disappear, it is because the patient is tuning out one eye; to see the entire picture, the patient must keep both eyes "turned on." Such instructional sets communicate that the phenomena experienced by the patient are products of the visual process, rather than events occurring in the targets, and that they are subject to the patient's control.

Training procedures will be more meaningful to the patient, and more effective in achieving desired goals, if the therapist explains what the particular task requires, how it relates to other training procedures that the patient has experienced, and how it relates to the patient's visual problem and to the goals of therapy. At the same time, patients should be encouraged to discover relationships and generalizations for themselves. The discovery of similarities in the demands imposed and processes used in different procedures increases the likelihood that improved visual function will transfer readily to new situations and new tasks (Peachey 1990).

Selecting and Sequencing Procedures

The practitioner must select procedures at a level at which the patient is capable of performing. Demands that are too easy will not foster learning, and demands that are too difficult will generate frustration. As performance improves, procedures are sequenced so as to impose progressively greater demand levels in small, manageable increments. As training progresses, increased ability, facility, and stamina develop as a product of appropriate instruction, increased demand levels, and repetitive practice.

In general, training should

1. Begin at demand levels that the patient is capable of achieving, and proceed toward increasingly difficult levels of demand.
2. Begin with gross targets and proceed toward finer targets that require greater accuracy and attention to detail.
3. Initially provide maximum feedback and permit maximum use of kinesthetic support, and proceed to develop the ability to sustain accurate performance even in the absence of feedback and kinesthetic support.
4. Begin with demands to achieve desired performance for brief periods, and proceed to increase demands for sustained performance.
5. Initially permit the patient to concentrate fully on the visual demand, and then, as performance improves, add cognitive and motor distractors in order to develop better integrated, more automatic, visual function.

Vision training is most effective when a broad variety of procedures is applied, since variety facilitates transfer of learning and generalization of skills, as opposed to the development of splinter skills. The practitioner should have many training procedures available; know how to sequence them appropriately; and be capable of reducing demand levels when necessary to permit achievement, and increasing demand levels in small increments as the patient's visual abilities expand. This ability to sequence and shift demand level is learned only with experience, but is facilitated when the practitioner self-performs the procedures, as would a patient, to experience the nuances and obstacles imposed at each demand level.

Automaticity

Excess effort that is required to maintain visual function saps attentional and mental capacity which would otherwise be directed toward the task at hand, and hence interferes with information-processing. It is therefore desirable that visual skills reach effortless and automatic levels (Peachey 1990, 1991).

Automaticity is achieved by progressively increasing demand levels to maximize visual ability, through repetitive practice, and through the use of cognitive loading. Initially, it is desirable to train any visual skill while minimizing concurrent cognitive and motor demand, so that the patient can concentrate fully on visual performance. As the trained visual function improves, the clinician may increase concurrent demands for cognitive processing and motor involvement. Such loading imposes demands that themselves require attention and effort, so that less attentional capacity is available for visual functions, which must then be performed at increasingly subconscious levels (Peachey 1990, 1991). Pepper (1986) describes a variety of procedures in which demands for concurrent motor activity and cognitive processing are sequentially increased, in small increments, in order to develop automaticity, improve the ability to maintain visual skills while performing other tasks, and expand information-processing ability.

Patient Motivation

Typically, patients who elect vision therapy, and are willing to pay for it, are highly motivated and cooperative. Occasional patients are uncooperative and poorly motivated, usually because they are too young to understand the importance of treatment, or because of concurrent behavior problems.

Numerous methods have been proposed for improving motivation and cooperation when necessary, including the following:

1. The patient should understand the purpose of therapy and relate the treatment to specific goals. Goals may include improved performance in school or sports, relief from symptoms, or prevention. The challenge is to communicate with the young or uncooperative patient in such a manner as to create this understanding. The patient must perceive the treatment program as a means of achieving her goals, not merely as something that the doctor is concerned about.

2. The patient should understand that *she* has a problem. The problem is hers, not the doctor's and not the parents'. The uncooperative patient must come to see that vision therapy is not simply done to her, but that she is an active participant and bears responsibility for the outcome. If the treatment is successful, it is she who benefits; if unsuccessful, it is she who suffers the consequences (Birnbaum 1977).

3. Many practitioners attempt to select interesting therapy procedures to optimize patient cooperation. The use of games, toys, computers, and dynamic motor procedures tends to heighten involvement and cooper-

ation. Boredom is also reduced by using a broad variety of procedures and by changing them frequently. If patients work on four or five procedures in a 45-minute session, there is little opportunity for boredom even if individual procedures are unexciting.

4. Positive reinforcement is used to maintain motivation and to modify adverse and disruptive behavior. Social reinforcers such as verbal praise, a smile, or a pat on the back from the doctor, and more tangible rewards such as candy, toys, stars, and tokens that can later be traded for rewards have been used to reinforce high achievement, cooperation, and attention (Feldman 1981; Groffman 1969). The clinician should make every effort to compliment the patient each time she achieves a desirable performance. Even when desired achievement is not obtained, the patient should be complimented for her effort and for that which she has accomplished. Such positive feedback creates good feelings about vision therapy and sets the stage for continued improvement.

5. Family support may be helpful. Communication with parents regarding the child's attitude may help to foster increased cooperation.

Home Therapy

Practice at home between office visits reinforces the use of visual processes learned during office sessions and speeds progress considerably. Home therapy procedures should be varied frequently to permit generalization of performance. The patient is typically expected to spend anywhere from 15 minutes to 1 hour daily on home therapy.

Many practitioners use parents as home vision therapists, teaching them the home therapy procedures and training them to work with their children at home. Some parents are very effective in this role; however, time pressures, excessive emotional involvement, or a troubled relationship between parent and child may make such an arrangement unworkable. In today's busy society, a requirement that parents work with their children at home is often difficult or impossible; many practitioners therefore teach children to perform home therapy alone, and simply ask the parents to remind their children of the home therapy obligation. This is obviously not possible when working with very young, immature, irresponsible, or hyperactive children. Many practitioners issue vision therapy notebooks in which the patient or parent keeps a record of home therapy performed, results, and observations.

Some practitioners lend, rent, or sell home therapy equipment to patients. Others, including the author, assign home therapy procedures that require inexpensive materials, which are simply given away. Many procedures described in Chapter 15 require minimal equipment and are readily adapted for home training.

Home training is sometimes prescribed as a substitute for office therapy by practitioners who do not offer in-office therapy, or when patients' schedules make office-based therapy difficult. In this author's experience, therapy that is solely home-based is unlikely to be successful. Even patients who appear highly motivated are unlikely to follow through without the reinforcement that comes from frequent contact with the practitioner. Even for the occasional patient who faithfully performs the assigned home therapy, repetitive practice of a limited number of procedures is far less effective than an office-based regimen in which the patient is exposed to a broad variety of procedures, procedures are sequenced appropriately and modified as needed, and the patient benefits from interaction with an insightful clinician.

Home therapy is best used as a supplement rather than a substitute for office-based treatment. Home training provides opportunity for practice and for integration of learned visual skills. An effective home therapy program in which procedures are sequenced to match the changing needs of the patient can best be organized in conjunction with an office-based program, and contributes significantly to the results obtained.

Training Lenses

Many vision training procedures require the use of lenses and prisms. Accommodative rock procedures use plus and minus lenses to develop accommodative facility. Base-in and base-out prisms, prism bars, and prism flippers are used to extend vergence ranges and increase flexibility between vergence and accommodation.

In addition to these uses of lenses and prisms, many clinicians prescribe training lenses to be worn for home and office therapy, for near work, or even for general use, to facilitate reorganization of the visual system (Horner 1972–73). Low-plus lenses, generally $+0.50$ to $+1.00$ D, are often used to foster accommodative relaxation and increased plus acceptance. Low-plus and low-minus lenses are sometimes used as training lenses in exophoria and esophoria, respectively. Such lenses serve to increase rather than decrease the phoria, and thus create a stringer stimulus to train positive (through plus) and negative (through minus) fusional vergence. Prism base-in or base-out may similarly be prescribed therapeutically for office or home therapy, for near use or for limited periods of general use, to train increased fusional divergence and convergence in esophoric and exophoric cases, respectively.

Rationales for prescribing low-power yoked prisms are described in Chapter 9. Higher-power yoked prisms, 10^Δ to 20^Δ are used in active vision therapy to disrupt learned patterns of spatial organization and visual-motor matching, and to foster the ability to adjust and reorganize (Kaplan 1978–79). Such yoked prisms are used during procedures such as the walk rail, pegboard rotator, throwing a beanbag at a pitchback and catching it, and similar procedures that require active movement and spatial judgements. The patient seeks to adjust and maintain performance as the yoked prisms are interposed in the base left, right, up, and down positions.

Adult Vision Therapy

Although vision therapy is commonly associated with children, many adults require vision therapy as well. Indeed, adults constitute a significant percentage of the patients treated in many vision therapy practices.

Adults with functional vision disorder frequently experience asthenopic symptoms and inability to sustain at near work. Such symptoms are commonly experienced by college students, secretaries, VDT operators, accountants, computer programmers, and others who perform extensive close work. Asthenopic symptoms frequently ensue when vocational changes bring increased near-work demands.

Adult vision therapy is not limited to young adults. Numerous presbyopic and geriatric patients develop high exophoria and convergence insufficiency, apparently due to reduction in accommodative convergence as amplitude of accommodation decreases (Eames 1933; Morgan and Peters 1951; Hokoda et al. 1991). Wick (1977) and Cohen and Soden (1984) report greater than 90% success in treating such patients.

Cohen and Soden (1981) report the rehabilitative use of vision therapy in cases of ocular motor dysfunction and diplopia caused by stroke and other systemic diseases common to geriatric populations.

SEQUENCING VISUAL SKILLS THERAPY

Patients with visual skills disorders demonstrate various combinations of oculomotor, vergence, and accommodative dysfunction. Individuals commonly exhibit deficiency in several areas of visual function, rather than an isolated single deficit. Thus, it is uncommon to find a patient with convergence insufficiency who does not also demonstrate accommodative disorder (Duke-Elder and Wybar 1973; Cooper et al. 1983; Daum 1984), or an individual with accommodative problems who does not also exhibit vergence dysfunction (Daum 1983; Cooper et al. 1987). Eye movement disorder may be present in either or both conditions. Terms such as *accommodative insufficiency, convergence insufficiency, oculomotor dysfunction*, etcetera, are simplistic in that they suggest the existence of a unitary dysfunction, which in fact is seldom the case.

Traditional models resolve this issue by applying multiple labels to a given case as indicated. For example, a particular patient may be said to have convergence excess, accommodative infacility, and oculomotor dysfunction. Treatment sequences are organized for each disorder, and therapy is directed toward each deficient function.

Practitioners schooled in the OEP framework view vergence and accommodative anomalies as arising from nearpoint stress. Conditions such as myopia, accommodative insufficiency, convergence insufficiency, and suppression are not viewed as independent entities, but rather as varieties of adaptation. When several such conditions are present, it suggests that the patient has explored a variety of adaptive paths to permit function in the presence of nearpoint stress.

Since OEP practitioners view these disorders as etiologically related, a common treatment approach is used for nearpoint stress–induced vision disorders in general, with modifications for individual differences. Treatment includes

1. prescription of low-plus nearpoint addition, when indicated by case analysis, to relieve nearpoint stress–induced overconvergence;
2. monocular skills therapy to develop equal and adequate ocular pursuit, saccadic, accommodative, and eye-hand coordination abilities;
3. binocular vision therapy, including both base-in and base-out fusional vergence and binocular accommodative facility training, to remediate sensory and motor fusion disorder and develop adequate flexibility between vergence and accommodation;
4. visual hygiene recommendations to reduce nearpoint stress.

Although the emphasis may vary depending on the specific findings and the behavioral characteristics of the individual patient, many aspects of therapy will be similar regardless of whether the patient exhibits convergence insufficiency, accommodative insufficiency, or other nearpoint stress–induced disorder. Since most individuals with nearpoint disorder demonstrate anomalies of both vergence and accommodative function, it is important to incorporate both accommodative and vergence training (Saladin 1986; Cooper et al. 1987).

Sequencing Monocular and Binocular Phases

Practitioners who use therapy approaches derived from traditional orthoptics frequently ignore monocular skills therapy and emphasize fusional vergence range extension, usually to overcome high heterophoria, which is viewed as a source of vergence stress. In the earliest OEP literature on visual skills training, in contrast, Crow and Fuog (1937–39) emphasized the importance of monocular visual skills therapy. They trained monocular pursuit and saccadic eye movements, accommodative facility, and eye-hand coordination, largely to the exclusion of specific binocular fusion training. This approach is based on the assumption that adequate binocular fusion will emerge when monocular visual functions are adequate and equal. Shankman (1988) similarly attributes fusion difficulty to differences in monocular spatial perception between the two eyes, and emphasizes the use of procedures to equalize monocular spatial judgements.

This author advocates an approach somewhat between these two extremes. In treating nonstrabismic functional vision disorders, ocular pursuit and saccadic procedures are incorporated to the degree indicated for each individual case, and may be used extensively in some cases and minimally in others. Ocular motility procedures are usually performed monocularly until performance is equal and adequate for both eyes, at which time procedures are performed binocularly. It is generally desirable to incorporate monocular skills training early in therapy, since efficient binocular function is unlikely when monocular visual abilities (ocular pursuits, saccades, accommodation, eye-hand coordination, visual-spatial judgements) are inadequate or unequal.

Techniques that emphasize spatial judgements with each eye, and biocular procedures (which create simultaneous perception through dissociation with prisms or septum), are used to develop equal visual-motor matching and visual-spatial judgements between the two eyes.

Monocular accommodative training is important and should be incorporated in the early stages. Equal and adequate monocular accommodative ability is prerequisite for efficient binocular function. Binocular accommodative facility training requires flexibility between vergence and accommodation, and should not be undertaken until monocular accommodative abilities are equal and adequate.

Binocular Phase

Most patients with nonstrabismic, nonamblyopic visual skills disorder demonstrate neither deep suppression nor severe inequality in monocular visual abilities. Suppression if present is usually minimal in extent, and specific anti-suppression therapy is generally not required. In most cases, fusional vergence procedures can be incorporated from the beginning, along with monocular motility and accommodative procedures.

Fusional vergence is trained using strong stimuli for fusion initially (such as the Topper vectogram), and then weak stimuli. Finally, binocular accommodative facility and *BOP-BIM* (base-out range extension through plus lenses and base-in range extension through minus) procedures are used to increase flexibility and freedom of action between vergence and accommodation. Specific ocular motility, accommodative, and fusional vergence procedures and their sequencing are described in Chapter 15.

Discharging the Patient

By the time the patient completes the therapeutic sequence and develops adequate performance on the various procedures, symptoms usually have diminished or resolved. It is appropriate at this stage to schedule a progress evaluation to assess the effectiveness of treatment, to pinpoint areas in need of further therapy, and to determine the need for change in lens prescription. The progress evaluation generally includes the 21-point analytical examination plus selected supplementary performance tests, particularly those on which performance was initially inadequate.

Comparing the phorometric findings to those obtained prior to therapy provides an important index of improvement. Normalization of these findings suggests that binocular skills developed in the training room have habituated and transferred to the phorometric testing situation. Since the targets are weak stimuli for fusion, the normalization of phorometric findings suggests that binocular function is truly adequate, since good function is present even with weak stimuli.

It is important to determine the optimal nearpoint lens prescription as the patient nears the end of therapy. As binocular and accommodative function reorganize during training, the indicated nearpoint lens may differ from that initially prescribed. Appropriate nearpoint lens prescription serves to minimize nearpoint stress and reduce the likelihood of regression.

Once the presenting symptoms resolve, the patient may see little need to use nearpoint lenses. If the phorometric findings suggest that nearpoint lens use is still indicated, it is important that the patient be so advised. The patient is more likely to continue use of nearpoint lenses if he or she understands that their purpose is not solely to improve clarity or comfort, but to relieve visual stress and prevent recurrence.

Generally, vision therapy is concluded when performance is adequate on the various training procedures; when phorometric findings reach expected levels, indicating that improved visual function has habituated; and when initial presenting symptoms have been relieved and goals achieved. When it is not possible to achieve these criteria, treatment proceeds until a plateau is reached from which further progress is unlikely.

When full functional care has been achieved, the results of vision therapy are usually long-lasting. Patients who improve but do not achieve full functional cure status are more subject to long-term instability and regression (Pantano 1982; Bowman et al. 1983; Grisham 1988; Grisham et al. 1991). Grisham (1988; Grisham et al. 1991) emphasizes that patients must not simply achieve symptomatic relief to be discharged, but must achieve a complete cure with clinically desirable fusional vergence ranges to prevent regression of skills and recurrence of symptoms.

Continued home therapy is often helpful in maintaining newly developed visual abilities, and may be maintained for some time after the completion of active office therapy. Progress evaluation should normally be scheduled for about 6 months after dismissal, to monitor the patient's status.

Length of Treatment

The time required for successful therapy varies with the severity, complexity, and nature of the visual problem; the degree of embeddedness; and patient motivation, attendance, and compliance.

The model and philosophy of the practitioner also influence the length of treatment. Some studies report success with as little as 3 to 4 weeks of home training, with weekly office visits to monitor progress. Other studies report an average of about 25 office visits for completion. These marked differences in length of treatment reflect differing goals and perspectives on the part of the clinicians and researchers involved.

Those studies that report "cured" status with very brief treatment are generally performed by clinicians who set relatively limited goals, based on a traditional "reserve/demand" approach. Such intervention is usually designed to remediate specific deficient findings such as the convergence near point, positive fusional convergence, or accommodative amplitude or facility.

Many practitioners, including the author, believe that such brief treatment programs provide but minimal care. In most cases, multiple deficits are present and more extensive treatment is required to develop adequate ocular motility, accommodative, and vergence abilities; to develop adequate flexibility between vergence and accommodation; and to integrate and automate visual function so that visual information-processing is both comfortable and efficient. In the author's office, treatment of noncomplicated cases generally requires approximately 25 to 36 treatment visits, usually twice a week over a period of 3 to 4 months. Complicated cases may require significantly longer treatment periods. Behaviorally oriented vision training programs that seek to enhance visual information-processing, visual-motor, and visual-spatial organization may require longer periods. Minimal therapy to normalize specific deficient findings produces minimal results and leaves the patient subject to regression on continued exposure to nearpoint stress.

TREATMENT PLAN FOR SPECIFIC DISORDERS

Oculomotor Dysfunction

Oculomotor dysfunction is characterized by inadequate pursuit and saccadic eye movement skills. Treatment begins with pursuit and saccadic training procedures at a level at which the patient is barely able to succeed with conscious effort. It is important that each procedure provide feedback so that the patient is aware of inaccuracy. Use of arm and hand provides tactual/kinesthetic sensory support, and visual feedback is provided through the use of a flashlight or afterimage. As performance improves, the use of these sensory supports is reduced, and cognitive and motor distractors are added to bring function to a more automatic level. The goal is that eye movements be so automatic as to require little effort so that attention and mental effort can be fully directed toward cognitive aspects of the tasks performed in daily life (Richman and Cron 1988).

Procedures are usually performed monocularly initially so as to develop equal and adequate monocular skills before binocular training is introduced. Richman and Cron (1988) suggest that procedures be sequenced as follows:

1. Monocular pursuits and rotations with tactual/kinesthetic sensory support, using hand and arm with balance integrated.
2. Monocular saccadic fixations with tactual/kinesthetic support, emphasizing auditory integration with use of the metronome for rhythm.
3. Biocular pursuits and fixations with tactual/kinesthetic support, to equalize function of the two eyes and eliminate suppression.
4. Binocular pursuits, rotations, and saccades with tactual/kinesthetic support.
5. Binocular pursuits, rotations, and saccades with visual feedback only.
6. Binocular oculomotor skill integration with accommodative and fusional skills and tachistoscopic activities.

Ocular motility training is used not only to develop more adequate oculomotor control, but also to improve attentional ability, spatial judgements, and central-peripheral organization.

Although ocular motility disorders generally result from interference with development, rather than from nearpoint stress, inadequate motility may accompany or exacerbate nearpoint stress–induced vision disorder. In such cases, considerable emphasis is placed on ocular motility procedures early in therapy. Specific procedures and their sequencing are described in Chapter 15.

Accommodative Dysfunction

Disorders of accommodative function are among the most common functional vision disorders (Borish 1970; Duke-Elder and Scott 1971; Daum 1983). A high incidence of accommodative disorder has been reported in patients with reading and learning problems (Robinson 1973; Sherman 1973; Hoffman 1980).

Accommodative disorders are traditionally classified as accommodative insufficiency, characterized by low amplitude and low PRA findings; accommodative infacility (or inertia of accommodation), characterized by difficulty shifting focus from one distance to another, with consequent transient blur associated with change in fixation distance; ill-sustained accommodation, characterized by inability to maintain accommodation during prolonged near work; accommodative excess, in which a stimulus for accommodation generates excessive accommodative response; and spasm of accommodation, characterized by inability to relax accommodation and by excessive fluctuations in accommodation (Borish 1970; Griffin 1982; Richman and Cron 1988). In practice, accommodative insufficiency, accommodative infacility, and ill-sustained accommodation are usually found together, and are frequently accompanied by vergence dysfunction (Bugola 1977; Daum 1983).

Symptoms commonly associated with accommodative dysfunction include nearpoint blur; intermittent distance blur when looking up from near work; headache, eyestrain, burning, and/or tearing of the eyes when reading; diplopia; loss of concentration; inability to perform near work for prolonged periods; reduced reading comprehension; need to read the same material over and over; fatigue toward the end of the day; excessively close nearpoint working distance; and avoidance of near activities (Hoffman and Rouse 1980; Daum 1983; Hennessey et al. 1984; Levine et al. 1985). Hennessey et al. (1984) and Levine et al. (1985) document that symptomatic patients demonstrate accommodative facility rates significantly lower than do asymptomatic patients.

Treatment of accommodative dysfunction should not be limited to patients who report asthenopia. Many patients avoid reading due to vision disorder, and hence report little symptomatology. Treatment in such cases permits the patient to keep up as near-work demands increase through the school years, and may lead to heightened interest in reading.

When accommodative disorder is present, plus lens prescription for near is usually indicated by the analytical examination findings. Plus is usually well accepted, and is best prescribed early. In addition, vision therapy is frequently required to normalize accommodative and binocular function.

Accommodative rock training usually incorporates both accommodative stimulation with minus lenses and accommodative relaxation with plus. If one aspect is more difficult than the other for a particular patient, that aspect should generally be emphasized.

Monocular accommodative rock procedures are performed initially, to ensure that monocular amplitude and facility are adequate and equal before introducing binocular accommodative procedures, which require, in addition to accommodative ability, flexibility between vergence and accommodation.

Most patients with accommodative disorder demonstrate vergence dysfunction as well (Daum 1983; Cooper et al. 1987). Fusion range extension and binocular accommodative rock training are incorporated to enhance binocular function and to increase flexibility between accommodation and convergence.

Monocular amplitude and facility generally respond quickly to treatment. In those occasional cases that do not show rapid improvement, organic or psychogenic factors should be suspected. Although most cases of accommodative disorder are functional in origin, a variety of neurologic and systemic diseases adversely influence accommodative function and must be ruled out. These include traumatic brain injury, cerebral vascular disorder and tumor, cerebral palsy, myasthenia gravis, diabetes mellitis, and a variety of other diseases (see Ciuffreda 1990).

Treatment procedures for accommodative dysfunction may be organized in the following sequence, modified from Richman and Cron (1988):

1. Rule out possible systemic causes.
2. Initiate oculomotor procedures as necessary.
3. Monocular accommodative stimulation, plano to minus, emphasizing awareness of feedback of accommodative change.
4. Monocular accommodative relaxation, plano to plus, emphasizing awareness of feedback of accommodative change.
5. Monocular accommodative stimulation-relaxation, minus to plus, emphasizing awareness of feedback of accommodative change.
6. Biocular accommodative relaxation-stimulation using plus lenses before one eye and minus before the other with septum, anaglyph, or vertical prism dissociation, to alternate demands for accommodative relaxation and stimulation in an unfused state in which vergence imposes no constraints on accommodation.
7. Binocular accommodative flexibility, alternating plus and minus lenses under binocular, fused conditions with suppression controls, to develop binocular accommodative facility and flexibility between vergence and accommodation.
8. Binocular accommodative rock combined with fusional vergence procedures, in which binocular plus and minus lenses are alternated while

the targets are disparated base-in and base-out, to further expand flexibility between vergence and accommodation. BOP-BIM tasks in which plus lens power is added during base-out vergence and minus during base-in are the most difficult, since they exacerbate the demand for flexibility between vergence and accommodation.

Specific accommodative procedures and their sequencing are described in Chapter 15.

Accommodative Spasm

The term *spasm of accommodation* is commonly applied to a variety of conditions in which accommodation is hyperactive or fluctuates excessively, including (1) frequent variations in accommodation during static retinoscopy which make the test difficult or unreliable; (2) latent hyperopia, in which cycloplegic refraction shows substantially greater hyperopia than is manifest without cycloplegia; and (3) the early stages of functional myopia, sometimes referred to as *pseudomyopia*, in which patients show low degrees of reversible functional myopia, or complain of distance blur following sustained close work, prior to the onset of measurable myopia.

Rutstein et al. (1988) restrict use of the term *accommodative spasm* or *accommodative excess* to that condition in which the accommodative response to a stimulus is greater than normal so that dynamic retinoscopy performed through the distance refraction demonstrates against motion. Accommodative excess as defined by Rutstein et al. (1988) is a rare condition, often psychogenic in origin, and frequently accompanied by convergence spasm and pupillary miosis. It results from a true spasm of accommodation, in contrast with latent hyperopia in which the accommodative response occurs to compensate an underlying hyperopia. Differential diagnosis is on the basis of dynamic retinoscopy: latent hyperopes typically show a large lag, while patients with accommodative excess demonstrate against motion with distance refraction in place.

Management includes the use of plus lenses to relieve excess accommodation, and accommodative facility training emphasizing accommodative relaxation (see Chapter 15). Cycloplegic agents may be helpful in some cases.

In cases in which variability of accommodation interferes with static retinoscopy, it is helpful to provide a distance fixation target that will hold the patient's interest. This author has an office assistant stand 7 or 8 feet away and involve the child in finger-counting games.

Convergence Insufficiency

Convergence insufficiency is characterized by high exophoria at near, reduced PRC, and/or receded convergence nearpoint (Cooper and Duckman 1978). Since many patients exhibit some but not all of these findings, clinicians often apply the term *convergence insufficiency* to patients who show any of these characteristics. Many patients with convergence insufficiency show accommodative dysfunction as well (Prakash et al. 1972; Duke-Elder and Wybar 1973; Cooper and Duckman 1978; Cooper et al. 1983; Daum 1984).

Convergence insufficiency and related nonstrabismic binocular vision disorders are common. Clinical studies of the incidence of convergence insufficiency have produced estimates that vary widely, from as little as 1% to as much as 25% of the population studied. Most studies report an incidence of approximately 3%. Females exhibit convergence insufficiency more frequently than males, in a ratio of 3:2 (Cooper and Duckman 1978; Bennett et al. 1982; Daum 1984).

True and Pseudo Convergence Insufficiency

Traditional models view convergence insufficiency as a weakness of convergence. Treatment consists primarily of convergence push-up and base-out fusion exercises.

Richman and Cron (1988) distinguish "true" and "pseudo" types of convergence insufficiency. In true convergence insufficiency, the convergence problem is primary; in pseudo cases, inadequate convergence is secondary to accommodative disorder. In true convergence insufficiency, accommodative function is essentially normal; the convergence near point is receded even with accommodative targets; and plus lenses further reduce base-out vergence at near. In pseudo convergence insufficiency, poor accommodative facility, low PRA, and high lag indicate accommodative dysfunction; and both convergence near point and low base-out vergence at near may improve with plus lenses, if reduced accommodative demand permits heightened accommodative response and consequent increase in accommodative convergence.

In treating convergence insufficiency, Richman and Cron recommend the following sequences:

1. True convergence insufficiency
   a. Monocular and biocular rotations and saccades to improve monocular skills and reduce suppression. Emphasize base-out prism to develop monocular adductive fixation.
   b. Physiological diplopia techniques (such as Brock string), incorporating jump vergences with base-out binocularly and accommodative flexibility.
   c. Base-out fusion activities with antisuppression checks.
   d. Base-out fusion with accommodation in play.
2. Pseudo convergence insufficiency
   a. Monocular and biocular rotations and saccades, emphasizing monocular base-out prism jump movements with plus lenses.
   b. Accommodative flexibility (biocular and binocular).
   c. Plus acceptance at near with base-out jump vergence.
   d. Base-out fusion and accommodative activities through plus.

Treatment Based on Nearpoint Stress Model

Although the term *convergence insufficiency* is not part of the vocabulary of the Skeffington model, high nearpoint exophoria and low base-out vergence at near are viewed as common patterns of adaptation to nearpoint stress (Skeffington 1947–50).

Treatment based on the Skeffington model is designed to relieve underlying nearpoint stress, as well as to remediate deficient convergence. Plus lenses are prescribed for near use when indicated by case analysis. Vision therapy is initiated to improve convergence ability and to maximize flexibility between vergence and accommodation. The treatment sequence generally includes monocular accommodative rock; convergence training; fusion range extension both base-out and base-in; jump vergence; binocular, fused accommodative rock; and BOP-BIM procedures.

Some patients demonstrate a shift toward esophoria with poor base-in fusion as training proceeds. The OEP model holds that this occurs because the underlying overconvergence becomes manifest as inhibition of convergence breaks down. The development of adequate base-in vergence and the prescription of low-plus lenses for near use are important aspects of treatment in such cases.

Resistant Cases

Remediation of convergence insufficiency with vision therapy is successful in greater than 90% of cases (Cooper and Duckman 1978). Most cases demonstrate rapid improvement in convergence, normalization of phorometric findings, and amelioration of symptoms.

A small number of cases are highly resistant to therapy. This author suspects that these cases, in which convergence responds minimally and slowly, have an organic rather than a functional etiology and represent true weakness of convergence. These cases are frequently associated with organic conditions such as minimal brain damage, mild retardation, and cerebral palsy.

These resistant cases may correlate with the C-type case postulated by Skeffington (1947–50) to represent an atypical adaptation to nearpoint stress. Nearpoint plus lens application is typically contraindicated because plus increases the exophoria and further impairs convergence.

In contrast with the typical cases of convergence insufficiency that respond readily to treatment, these organically based cases are highly resistant. Treatment consists primarily of convergence exercises, and is usually prolonged. Gains are usually limited, and often not well retained. When maximum improvement is obtained and the patient is discharged, convergence exercises should be continued at home to prevent regression.

Nearpoint Plus Lenses in Convergence Insufficiency

In contrast with traditional models in which nearpoint plus lens prescription is expected to increase exophoria and is therefore contraindicated, OEP theory views such lenses as desirable, when indicated by the analytical examination findings, to relieve the drive toward overconvergence held to underlie nearpoint stress.

When high nearpoint exophoria reduces with low-plus, such lenses should be prescribed (see Chapter 9). Plus lenses for near use should also be prescribed for convergence insufficiency patients who shift into esophoria as training proceeds. When the NRA and PRA indicate no plus acceptance, or the near exophoria increases through plus, such prescription is contraindicated. Such cases should be monitored, since many will show indications for nearpoint plus lens prescription as vision therapy proceeds.

When nearpoint plus lenses are indicated because the patient shows signs of overconvergence, or because plus balances the NRA/PRA or reduces exophoria at near, it is important that they be prescribed. If nearpoint plus lenses are not prescribed when indicated, or if such lenses are prescribed but not used, patients frequently either regress or develop myopia following successful therapy. The Skeffington model suggests that such changes occur adaptively when plus lenses are needed to resolve the overconvergence held to underlie nearpoint stress, but are not prescribed and used.

Convergence Excess

The convergence excess patient shows high esophoria at near, and often at distance as well. Nearpoint plus is usually indicated by the phorometric findings, and should be prescribed to reduce overconvergence. Vision therapy is used to improve monocular accommodative function, improve sensory and motor fusion, and maximize flexibility between accommodation and convergence. Major emphasis is on base-in fusion.

Richman and Cron (1988) advise the following sequence for convergence excess:

1. monocular and biocular rotations and saccades with plus lenses, using monocular base-in prism to stimulate abductive fixation movements;
2. accommodative flexibility: monocular, biocular, and binocular;
3. negative fusional range development with accommodative convergence integration and antisuppression controls.

Patients with convergence excess are often intense individuals who apply themselves to near-vision tasks with strong concentration. Asthenopic symptoms may arise both from vergence dysfunction and from tension associated with intense concentration. Visual hygiene suggestions, peripheral awareness, relaxation exercises, and visual imagery are often helpful both in developing base-in fusional vergence and in fostering less intense, more relaxed use of vision during near-vision tasks (Birnbaum 1990).

Binocular Instability

Richman and Cron (1988) describe *binocular instability* as a condition characterized by small rather than large degrees of esophoria or exophoria at distance and/or near, with intermittent suppression, reduced stereoacuity, sluggish accommodative flexibility, unstable and/or restricted fusional vergence ranges (especially recoveries), and unstable and inconsistent oculomotor skills. Symptoms include asthenopia, intermittent blur and diplopia, inability to sustain nearpoint visual efficiency, loss of place, need to re-read, and reduced comprehension.

Such cases are often referred to as *general skills* cases, and are characterized by poor quality of function and instability, rather than by significant quantitative deficiencies in clinical findings. The OEP model views such deficits as products of a nearpoint stress—induced mismatch between vergence and accommodation.

When case analysis indicates that nearpoint plus is desirable to reduce accommodative demand or permit more adequate integration between vergence and accommodation, prescription of such lenses facilitates stable binocular function. Vision therapy is used to improve quality of performance; develop smoothness, efficiency, stability, and ability to sustain; and to habituate performance to levels of high automaticity, in each of the basic visual functions of ocular motility, accommodation, and binocular fusion. Richman and Cron (1988) recommend the following treatment sequence:

1. oculomotor skills: monocular, biocular, and binocular pursuits and fixations, with emphasis on sustained attention and automaticity;
2. accommodative flexibility: monocular, biocular, and binocular;
3. fusion skills: initial small jump vergence responses and antisuppression; then expand fusional vergence ranges and improve accommodative/convergence flexibility and stereopsis. The emphasis is on sustained attention at the automaticity level.

Management of Myopia

Considerable evidence, reviewed in Chapter 2, suggests that accommodation and use of the eyes for near work are important factors contributing to the development of myopia. Additional evidence, reviewed in Chapter 10, documents the efficacy of nearpoint lens addition in slowing myopia progression, particularly for myopes who demonstrate nearpoint plus acceptance and esophoria at near. As a consequence, many practitioners recommend therapeutic regimens designed to prevent myopia development and control progression. Such regimens generally include (1) plus lens addition to reduce accommodative demand and/or relieve nearpoint stress—induced drive for convergence to localize closer than accommodation; (2) visual hygiene suggestions to read in a more relaxed manner, in good posture with proper lighting, and to take short breaks and frequently look out to distance, to attempt to reduce adverse effects of sustained nearpoint application; and (3) vision therapy to remediate deficient vergence and accommodative function, and to increase plus acceptance.

Determination of the optimal nearpoint lens prescription is described in Chapters 8 and 9. Clinical issues specific to the use of bifocals in myopia are discussed in Chapter 10.

Vision therapy has been used to attempt to prevent myopia and to slow myopia progression, to reduce existing myopia, and to improve unaided visual acuity. The therapeutic approach used depends on the goals for a particular patient. Attempts to prevent myopia or control progression generally emphasize remediation of vergence and accommodative dysfunction, as well as prescription of nearpoint plus lens addition. Programs designed to reduce existing myopia emphasize accommodative relaxation procedures to eliminate functional myopia that is not yet embedded. Treatment procedures to improve unaided visual acuity include a variety of techniques that introduce blur which the myope seeks to resolve; acuity improvement is often obtained independent of refractive change. Accommodative relaxation and visual acuity improvement procedures are described in Chapter 15.

Incipient and Progressing Myopia

Myopia development is typically preceded by transient distance vision blur, especially when looking up from reading; low PRA; esophoria, or lowered exophoria at near; increased plus acceptance on the binocular cross-cylinder test (Goss 1991); and low against-the-rule astigmatism (Hirsch 1964; Birnbaum 1978b). Incipient myopes frequently hold reading material very close, and may demonstrate a tendency toward bookishness and family history of myopia. When such signs are present, it is desirable to initiate preventive care as early as possible, since myopia is extremely difficult to reverse once it has developed. Treatment generally includes

1. nearpoint plus lens addition;
2. visual hygiene suggestions regarding optimal near-work posture, lighting, and rest periods;
3. monocular accommodative facility to develop equal and adequate function;
4. specific accommodative relaxation and plus acceptance procedures;
5. fusional vergence range extension base-out and base-in, emphasizing base-in therapy to reduce any tendency toward overconvergence;
6. binocular, fused accommodative rock;
7. BOP-BIM training to maximize flexibility between vergence and accommodation.

Little research has been performed to document the ability to prevent myopia development. Streff (1978) reports a lower incidence of myopia, particularly among girls, following a school intervention program consisting of (1) homogeneous grouping according to developmental levels; (2) changes in classroom equipment, furniture, and lighting; and (3) one-half hour per day of motor-sensory developmental problem-solving activities.

Once myopia has developed small degrees, up to 0.50 or 0.75 D, can sometimes be reversed or eliminated in the early stages with nearpoint plus lens prescription and vision therapy. Treatment is similar to that described above for incipient myopia, with a strong emphasis on the use of accommodative relaxation and plus acceptance procedures.

Stoddard (1942) reports that orthoptic treatment often produces myopia reduction in patients who become less myopic with cycloplegia. He considers such cases as functional or pseudo myopia, which arises from extensive near work, and attributes them to accommodative rather than to anatomical change. He indicates that these cases, which generally do not exceed 0.75 D, usually respond well to orthoptic treatment, and advocates that such treatment be attempted in all cases of low myopia.

Other studies of the efficacy of training to reduce myopia have concluded that such training is ineffective (Woods 1946; Hildreth et al. 1947). However, some subjects in these studies showed small reduction in myopia of 0.50 to 0.75 D, consistent with the findings of Stoddard (1942).

Trachtman (1978; Trachtman et al. 1981) used the Accommotrac Vision Trainer (Biofeedtrac, Inc.) to provide auditory biofeedback to train relaxation of accommodation, and reported small but consistent reduction of myopia, of at least 0.50 D. However, using the same equipment, Gallaway et al. (1987) and Koslowe et al. (1991) found no reduction in myopia.

Higher degrees of myopia can rarely be eliminated. Once myopia is well established, it is generally best to prescribe minus lenses to provide adequate distance acuity. Bifocal lenses and vision therapy should be prescribed, when indicated, to attempt to control myopia progression.

Patients with progressing myopia frequently demonstrate vergence and accommodative disorder, often with signs of overconvergence. Common clinical findings include accommodative infacility, inadequate accommodative relaxation, low PRA, esophoria or lowered exophoria at near, esophoric shift during sustained attention, constricted fusional vergence ranges, and excessively close near working distance. Vision therapy is similar to that described for cases of incipient myopia, and is designed to remediate dysfunction and maximize nearpoint visual efficiency so that the system can more readily withstand stress (Birnbaum 1979).

In most cases in which myopia is developing or progressing, phorometric analysis indicates plus lens acceptance at near. However, in some cases, low NRA and MEM measures, inability to clear plus on the accommodative facility test, case analysis of the phorometric findings, and the patient's subjective reaction to plus contraindicate such prescription. In such cases, vision therapy is designed to develop plus acceptance so that plus lenses can ultimately be prescribed to relieve nearpoint stress.

Stone (1976) and Perrigin et al. (1990) report a reduced rate of progression among myopes wearing rigid contact lenses. This effect is only partially attributable to corneal flattening; both authors suggest that rigid lenses may in some way have an effect in controlling the axial length of the eye.

Stable Myopia

When myopia progression has run its course and the condition stabilizes, patients frequently demonstrate exophoria at near and equilibrium between the NRA/PRA findings, so that case analysis no longer indicates nearpoint plus lens addition. In this stage, single-vision lens prescription is generally optimal.

Vision therapy to reduce or eliminate myopia in this stage usually achieves very limited gains. However, substantial visual acuity improvement can frequently be obtained, usually in brief flashes rather than stable clear vision, even in the absence of refractive change, in myopic patients who are motivated to qualify for jobs that require specific levels of unaided acuity, as with the police or fire departments. This acuity improvement is achieved with plus acceptance, accommodative relaxation, and visual acuity training procedures described in Chapter 15.

Numerous studies document improvement in unaided visual acuity in myopic patients following visual training (Ewalt 1945; Woods 1946; Hildreth et al. 1947; Marg 1952; Epstein et al. 1978, 1981; Collins et al. 1981, 1982; Baillet et al. 1982; Gil and Collins 1983; Blount et al. 1984; Rosen et al. 1984; Berman et al. 1985). Ewalt (1945) and Baillet et al. (1982) report gains in unaided acuity in almost all subjects. These gains were frequently substantial in magnitude, occasionally as great as improvement from 20/800 to 20/25 or 20/30.

Visual acuity improvement in myopia tends to occur in clear flashes of brief duration, rather than as continuous clear vision. The mechanism for these "flashes" of clear vision is uncertain. They are not the result of squinting, and retinoscopy reveals no change in accommodation, refraction, or pupil size during the flashes (Marg 1952).

Since improvement usually occurs without significant reduction in myopia, it is often attributed to blur interpretation. However, interpretation of blur seems an unlikely mechanism, since improved acuity usually comes in flashes in which the entire chart suddenly clears, rather than as a result of effort to gradually distinguish each individual optotype. Psychologic factors and changes in tear film distribution have been proposed as mechanisms. However, these explanations are not wholly satisfactory and the issue remains unresolved (Marg 1952; Graham and Leibowitz 1972; Baillet et al. 1982; Press 1987).

Clinicians may question the usefulness of acuity improvement that occurs without actual myopia reduction, since flashes of clear vision are usually brief in duration, and clear vision may not be present during everyday seeing, and may regress after training. Clinical experience suggests that acuity improvement diminishes once training is discontinued, unless home therapy is maintained.

However, several of the studies cited indicate that many subjects report substantial improvement in their daily vision. Further, although partial regression is common, follow-up studies indicate that acuity gains are often partially retained without further training (Hildreth et al. 1947; Baillet et al. 1982; Collins et al. 1982). Thus, visual acuity training may be useful for those myopes who desire to be less dependent on their glasses, as well as for those with specific vocational requirements.

Visual Hygiene Suggestions

Adverse near-work posture (Harmon 1958) and intense concentration (Forrest 1988; Birnbaum 1990) each increase sympathetic activation and exacerbate the nearpoint stress response (see Chapters 3 and 5). In addition to prescribing the optimal nearpoint lens (which fosters proper near-work posture and reduces physiologic activation [Pierce 1966–68; Greenspan 1970]) and using vision therapy procedures to remediate deficient vergence and accommodative function, the optometrist should counsel patients regarding near-work habits to minimize tension and reduce stress activation (Birnbaum 1985, 1990; Francke and Kaplan 1978).

Patients are advised to read in a relaxed manner, in good posture with proper lighting, to take short breaks, and to frequently look out to distance to reduce adverse effects of sustained near work.

In the physiologically optimal near-work posture described by Harmon (1958), near work is inclined 20 degrees from the horizontal, in a plane parallel to the face, at a working distance equal to the distance from the elbow to the second knuckle. Patients should be advised to work in a comfortable chair at an appropriately sized desk to permit a proper working distance, and to arrange adequate and glare-free lighting (see Chapter 5).

When working with a VDT, it is important to design the workstation so that the operator works at appropriate viewing distances in a comfortable, relaxed posture without interfering glare and reflections (Miller 1984; Margach 1988). A well-designed workstation is depicted in Figure 14.1. The screen, keyboard, and copy should ideally be at approximately equal distances from the eyes. A working distance of 40 to 50 cm is usually considered optimal, with the screen slightly below eye level.

Prolonged concentration associated with sustained near work generates tension, physiological activation, and nearpoint stress. Whether reading text or working at the VDT, maintaining a relaxed attitude helps to relieve tension and to reduce the visual stress response. The patient should be advised to assume a comfortable posture, to relax muscular tension in the body, and to maintain general awareness of the surround. Birnbaum (1990) suggests the use of deep breathing, progressive relaxation, and peripheral awareness procedures to aid the patient to be more aware of bodily tension while reading, and to be better able to reduce it.

Intense individuals, who frequently hold reading material at excessively close working distances, are advised to read in a relaxed posture and to hold

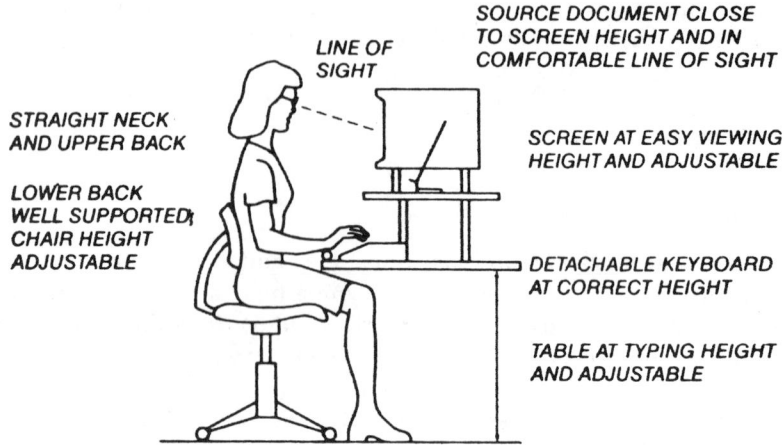

Figure 14.1 A well-designed video display terminal workstation. (Reprinted with permission of the publisher from VDTs and Vision, Santa Ana, CA: Optometric Extension Program Foundation, Inc.)

reading material at the Harmon distance. The recommendation to maintain a longer working distance is designed to promote general relaxation and reduce intensity of application, as well as to reduce accommodative demand.

Patients who work or read intensely are advised to look at a distant object momentarily at the end of each page. Such gaze-shifts reduce intensity of application, facilitate maintenance of accommodative flexibility, and may help to reduce incomplete relaxation of accommodation associated with fixation at near (Ebenholtz 1983). If possible, the work area should face into an open space rather than toward a wall, to facilitate looking out frequently.

Francke and Kaplan (1978) indicate that the capacity for concentration is no longer than 20 minutes for elementary students, 40 minutes for high school students, and 40 to 45 minutes for adults. Individuals should determine their own duration, and stop for a break before feeling tired. When the individual stops for a break prior to the onset of fatigue, both the quality and quantity of work performed improves.

Birnbaum (1990) advises that patients who read intensely for sustained periods get up and move about for a minute after each 10 or 15 minutes of near work. Sustained immobilization increases sympathetic activation; moving about serves to reduce physiological stress activation. The patient is advised to walk about, to do aerobic exercises, or to briefly perform stretches designed to relieve upper body tension.

Individuals who apply themselves very intensely to near work frequently experience severe asthenopia. Symptoms may be out of proportion to the optometric findings, and may persist even after appropriate lenses and vision therapy have been applied. Guidance as to reading in proper, relaxed posture with reduced muscular tension, and advice to look up frequently during near work and to take short breaks involving movement, are frequently effective in relieving symptoms. Birnbaum (1990) recommends the use of such guidance in patients suspected of extreme intensity in their near-work application, including those who demonstrate myopia or esophoria at near; patients who hold reading material excessively close; and patients whose asthenopic symptoms are out of proportion to the optometric findings, or persist after appropriate vision therapy and lens application.

VISUAL INFORMATION-PROCESSING STYLES

Several authors suggest that individuals differ in their preferred approach to gathering and processing visual information, and that these visual information-processing styles are related to ocular and oculomotor status, as well as to broader aspects of cognition and behavior. The management of vision disorders (as well as the efficiency of visual information-processing) may be enhanced by the selection of vision therapy procedures in relation to these information-processing styles, as well as to the patient's specific oculomotor disorder (MacDonald 1975; Forrest 1976, 1981; Birnbaum 1978a; Sutton 1985).

Central-Peripheral Organization

Central-peripheral organization is an important aspect of visual information-processing style. Central-peripheral organization refers to the way in which people derive, use, and integrate information obtained from figure (the area of primary attention at a given moment) with that obtained from ground (background). Individuals who are more central prefer to gather and process information in small bits, with greater emphasis on detail. This approach fosters the sequential processing of input from small areas of space, gathered on successive fixations. Individuals who are more peripheral, in contrast, prefer to gather information from broad areas of space, favoring a simultaneous, all-at-once, global approach (MacDonald 1975; Forrest 1976; Birnbaum 1978a; Sutton 1985).

These differences in central-peripheral organization may relate to ocular and oculomotor status, as well as to broader aspects of behavior. It has been suggested that individuals who prefer a peripheral approach are often hyperopic or exophoric; emphasize simultaneous processing, intuitive thinking, experiential learning, and visual imagery; tend to be global rather than specific in verbal communication and in listening; demonstrate a looser posture; tend to be more flexible in their opinions and thinking patterns; and tend to be less bookish, more physical, and demonstrate low stress reactivity. Individuals who prefer a more central, detail-oriented approach to gathering visual information, in contrast, are often myopic or esophoric; emphasize logical, analytical, and verbal thinking; tend to be precise, specific, and detail-oriented in their verbal communication and listening; demonstrate a tighter posture; are often more rigid in their attitudes and opinions; tend to be less physical and more bookish; and demonstrate high stress reactivity (Forrest 1976; Forkiotis 1977; Birnbaum 1978a; Sutton 1985).

Clinically, it is not difficult to identify individuals who are significantly skewed toward one or the other extreme. Central individuals tend toward myopia and esophoria, are sensitive to small differences, and typically observe blurs during vergence tests and discriminate fine differences in clarity between lenses during subjective refraction. When performing a task such as the Topper vectogram, the central individual may inquire as to precisely where to look. Verbal communication is usually precise, logical, and well structured.

Individuals who are global in their processing tend toward hyperopia and exophoria, emphasize background rather than detail, and may not notice blurs during vergence tests. They may be insensitive to small lens changes, since they are less attentive to detail. They are sensitive to the periphery, may be easily distracted, and may have difficulty sustaining visual attention. Verbalization tends to be more diffuse and random, less organized and to the point. The individual may be easily distracted and lose track, both in speaking and in listening. In listening, the global individual tends to get the general idea, but fails to get the details. When reading, global children make excessive small word errors and confuse similar looking words because they fail to note differences in fine detail.

Each of these extremes imposes limitations on visual information-processing and, indeed, on thinking ability. The individual who is highly central and detail-oriented may be excessively rigid and insensitive to broad relationships and divergent ideas. The individual who is excessively global may be insensitive to detail, fail to note and detect fine differences, and have greater difficulty organizing material in an orderly sequence. For most efficient function, it is desirable that an individual be well balanced and able to integrate both modes, with an ability to emphasize one mode or the other as required at any particular moment.

Vision Therapy and Central-Peripheral Organization

Vision therapy may be designed to enhance weak or underused processing strategies. The individual who prefers or emphasizes central, specific processing may benefit from procedures emphasizing peripheral awareness, visual imagery, and tachistoscopic training, to improve ability to use peripheral, global, and simultaneous processing. The goal is not to change the individual's processing style, but rather to expand abilities and permit greater flexibility. Similarly, the patient who emphasizes peripheral, global, simultaneous processing may benefit from procedures that emphasize attention to detail, sequential processing, and visual analysis (Forrest 1976, 1981; Birnbaum 1978a).

Significant behavioral changes frequently result from vision therapy, including changes in attitude and personality, intellectual capacity, verbal communication and comprehension, attentional skills, classroom behavior, sports performance, and posture. Such changes may result not only from remediation of specific visual deficits, but also because vision therapy procedures impact central-peripheral organization and other aspects of organismic behavior.

Garzia and Nicholson (1990) suggest a possible physiologic basis for such changes. They note that vision therapy procedures routinely require the patient to make figure-ground decisions and respond to changes in spatial-temporal stimulus properties. Procedures involving central-peripheral organization, tachistoscopic presentation, movement, and high and low spatial and temporal frequencies may differentially stimulate the sustained and transient visual mechanisms, improve their response characteristics and integration, and hence lead to improved performance on tasks far removed from the specific therapy procedures used.

The use of procedures selected in relation to central-peripheral organization may facilitate the remediation of specific oculomotor deficits, as well as the enhancement of visual information-processing ability. In patients with over-convergence, restricted base-in range, or myopia, peripheral awareness, visual imagery, and relaxation procedures frequently aid the development of accommodative relaxation and base-in fusional vergence. In patients with accommodative and convergence insufficiency, procedures that emphasize careful looking, attention to detail, and visual analysis may facilitate the development of positive vergence and accommodation (Forrest 1976, 1981; Birnbaum 1978a).

Training the Central Specific Processor

In treating the patient with myopia, esophoria, and restricted base-in vergence, therefore, as well as the patient who appears overly detail-oriented, intense, or verbal-analytical-sequential in processing style, the practitioner should incorporate procedures that emphasize peripheral awareness, simultaneous (all-at-once) processing, visual imagery, and visualization. Instructions to maintain peripheral awareness may be incorporated with any standard therapy procedure. Specific peripheral awareness procedures may also be prescribed (see Chapter 15), with the goal of expanding peripheral awareness in everyday seeing (Birnbaum 1978a, 1990; Marrone 1991). Tachistoscopic and visualization procedures are used to foster simultaneous visual processing; in using such procedures, the practitioner must instruct the patient to use visual imagery in solving the particular problems presented, since analytical individuals will generally attempt to use a verbal-sequential approach.

Training the Global Processor

Procedures typically used for gross motor, eye movement, eye-hand, accommodative, fusion, and visual perceptual training may be used to train not only these functions, but also the ability to look carefully, to notice and discriminate detail, to analyze similarities and differences, to sustain visual attention, and to organize sequentially. In training excessively global individuals, these aspects should be emphasized.

Gross motor procedures that foster internal awareness and feedback lead to improved ability to notice and analyze fine differences. Use of metronome or yoked prisms with such procedures adds demands for monitoring external stimuli and resolving mismatches, and contributes to the development of analytical processing. Pursuit eye movement procedures incorporate demands to sustain visual attention, while saccadic procedures foster selective attention and sequential fixation. The pegboard rotator and Ann Arbor Letter Tracking procedures foster careful looking and attention to detail. In working with accommodative procedures and with vectograms and other fusional vergence procedures, the clinician may emphasize awareness of changes in size and distance, and enhance the ability to discriminate barely noticeable differences. A variety of visual form perception and visual memory tasks require attention to detail and analysis of similarities and differences. In each of these procedures, a requirement to verbally describe the differences noted adds to the demand for awareness of detail and for visual analysis.

Visual Imagery

Forrest (1976, 1981) emphasizes the importance of visual imagery as a modality for thinking and processing information. As with central-peripheral organization (and frequently related to it), an individual's preferred approach may be categorized on a visual-verbal continuum with a preference for spatial imagistic processing at one extreme and verbal-linguistic processing at the other. One achieves the highest capacity for effective thinking and information-processing through the effective use and integration of these complementary modes. Central, specific individuals who are overly specialized for sequential processing frequently prefer the verbal analytical mode and may use visual imagery less effectively. Forrest (1981) describes procedures for developing and enhancing the use of visual imagery.

Conceptual Tempo

In responding to problems that have several possible solutions, some individuals, termed *reflective*, take the time to analyze alternate hypotheses before responding. They respond slowly, but make few errors. Impulsive individuals, in contrast, react quickly when presented with a problem, and respond without considering alternative solutions. They consequently make numerous errors, and often demonstrate reading and learning difficulty, attentional deficit, and distractability (Kagan 1965).

Vision therapy can be designed to modify impulsive behavior. Motor procedures such as the walk rail, balance board, and hand-foot tapping patterns are used to develop awareness and organization. As ability improves, the patient is asked to synchronize performance with the beat of a metronome which is set at progressively slower speeds to guide the patient to learn to delay response. The Ann Arbor Tracking series introduces a requirement for careful, accurate scanning to correctly locate the alphabet embedded in a paragraph of nonsense words.

Perceptual matching tasks such as parquetry blocks, which require the patient to look carefully and analyze alternative choices for correct performance, promote a more reflective style. Whatever procedures are performed, the impulsive child should be taught to delay his or her response, and to carefully consider all possible alternatives before responding.

At the other extreme, excessive reflectivity is characterized by extremely slow response, as the overly reflective child excruciatingly analyzes each of the possible choices before responding. Extremely reflective individuals may be excessively analytical and specific. Reading may be labored, one word at a time, despite the existence of adequate phonics and sight recognition skills. In training the overly reflective patient, the optometrist should use tachistoscopic procedures to facilitate rapidity of response, and visual imagery and peripheral awareness procedures to foster simultaneity and all-at-once seeing.

SUMMARY

Vision therapy is used to remediate vision disorder, to develop and enhance visual skills, and to prevent the development of vision disorders that might otherwise occur. Approaches to organizing and sequencing vision therapy are diverse; these variations result from differing concepts of the etiology of vision disorder and conceptual differences regarding the nature of vision and how it relates to human performance. Proper selection and sequencing of procedures, effective instructional set, patient motivation, and effective use of home therapy and training lenses each contribute to the success of therapy. Specific regimens are presented for remediation of oculomotor dysfunction, accommodative disorder, convergence insufficiency, convergence excess, and binocular instability, as well as for management of the myopic patient. Counseling regarding appropriate conditions for performing near work, and vision therapy procedures organized in relation to the individual's cognitive-perceptual style, may each contribute to more effective visual function.

SUGGESTED READING

Peachey GT (1990). Perspectives on optometric vision training. *J Behav Optom* 1(3):65–70.

Richman JE, Cron MT (1988). *Guide to Vision Therapy*. South Bend, IN: Bernell.

REFERENCES

1986/87 Future of Visual Development/Performance Task Force (1988). The efficacy of optometric vision therapy. *J Am Optom Assoc* 59(2):95–105.

Apell RJ (1967). *Sequence Versus Direction in Optometric Visual Training*. Eastern Seaboard Conference on Visual Training, Washington, DC, Jan., transcript by Caryl Croisant, Santa Ana, CA.

Baillet R, Clay A, Blood K (1982). The training of visual acuity in myopia. *J Am Optom Assoc* 53:719–724.

Bennett GR, Blondin M, Ruskiewicz J (1982). Incidence and prevalence of selected visual conditions. *J Am Optom Assoc* 53 (8):647–656.

Berman PE, Levinger SI, Massath NA, et al. (1985). The effectiveness of biofeedback visual training as a viable method of treatment and reduction of myopia. *J Optom Vis Dev* 16:17–21.

Birnbaum MH (1977). The role of the trainer in visual training. *J Am Optom Assoc* 48(8):1035–1039.

Birnbaum MH (1978a). Holistic aspects of visual style: A hemispheric model with implications for vision therapy. *J Am Optom Assoc* 49(10):1133–1141.

Birnbaum MH (1978b). Functional relationship between myopia, accommodative stress, and against-the-rule astigmia: A hypothesis. *J Am Optom Assoc* 49(8):911–914.

Birnbaum MH (1979) Management of the low myopia pediatric patient. *J Am Optom Assoc* 50(11): 1281–1289.

Birnbaum MH (1985). Nearpoint visual stress: Clinical implications. *J Am Optom Assoc* 56(6): 480–490.

Birnbaum MH (1990). The use of stress reduction concepts and techniques in vision therapy. *J Behav Optom* 1(9):3–7.

Blount RL, Baer RA, Collins FL (1984). Improving visual acuity in a myopic child: Assessing compliance and effectiveness. *Behav Res Ther* 22:53–57.

Borish IM (1970). *Clinical Refraction*. 3rd ed. Chicago: Professional Press.

Bowman, M, Owyang L, Grisham D (1983). Vergence orthoptics: Persistence of the training effect. O.D. thesis, Berkeley: University of California.

Bugola, J (1977). Hypoaccommodation and convergence insufficiency. *Am Orthopt J* 27:85–90.

Ciuffreda KJ (1990). Accommodation and its anomalies. In: Charman WN (ed), *Vision and Visual Dysfunction, vol. 1: Visual Optics and Instrumentation*. London: MacMillan, pp. 227–275.

Cohen AH, Soden R (1981). An optometric approach to the rehabilitation of the stroke patient. *J Am Optom Assoc* 52(9):795–800.

Cohen AH, Soden R (1984). Effectiveness of visual therapy for convergence insufficiencies for an adult population. *J Am Optom Assoc* 55(7): 491–494.

Collins FL, Epstein LH, Hannay HY (1981). A component analysis of an operant training program for improving visual acuity in myopic students. *Behav Ther* 12: 692–701.

Collins FL, Ricci JA, Burkett PA (1982). Behavioral training for myopia: Long-term maintenance of improved acuity. *Behav Res Ther* 19:265–268.

Cooper J, Duckman R (1978). Convergence insufficiency: Incidence, diagnosis and treatment. *J Am Optom Assoc* 49(6):673–680.

Cooper J, Feldman J, Selenow A, et al. (1987). Reduction of asthenopia after accommodative facility training. *Am J Optom Physiol Opt* 64(6):430–436.

Cooper J, Selenow A, Ciuffreda KJ, et al. (1983). Reduction in asthenopia in patients with convergence insufficiency after fusional vergence training. *Am J Optom Physiol Opt* 60(12):982–989.

Crow G, Fuog HL (1937–39). *Basic Orthoptics and Reconditioning*. Optometric Extension Program Continuing Education Courses, Santa Ana, Ca: Optometric Extension Program Foundation, Oct. 1937–Sept. 1939.

Daum KM (1983). Accommodative insufficiency. *Am J Optom Physiol Opt* 60(5):352–359.

Daum KM (1984). Convergence insufficiency. *Am J Optom Physiol Opt* 61:16–22.

Duke-Elder WS, Scott GI (1971). *System of Ophthalmology, vol. XII, Neuro-ophthalmology*. London: Henry Kimpton, pp. 698–709.

Duke-Elder WS, Wybar K (1973). Ocular motility and strabismus. In: Duke-Elder WS (ed), *System of Ophthalmology.* vol. 6. St. Louis: C.V. Mosby, pp. 564–572.

Eames TH (1933). Physiological exophoria in relation to age. *Arch Ophthalmol* 9:104–105.

Ebenholtz SM (1983). Accommodative hysteresis: A precursor for induced myopia. *Invest Ophthalmol Vis Sci* 24(4):513–515.

Epstein LH, Collins FL, Hannay HJ (1978). Fading and feedback in the modification of visual acuity. *J Behav Med* 1:273–287.

Epstein LH, Greenwald DJ, Hennon D, et al. (1981). Monocular fading and feedback: Effects on vision changes in the trained and untrained eye. *Behav Modif* 5:171–186.

Ewalt HW (1945). The Baltimore Myopia Control Project. *J Am Optom Assoc* 17(5):167–185.

Feldman J (1981). Behavior modification in vision training: Facilitating prerequisite behaviors and visual skills. *J Am Optom Assoc* 52:329–340.

Flax N (1986). *Vision Therapy and Insurance: A Position Statement.* New York: State University of New York, State College of Optometry.

Forkiotis CJ (1977). Behavioral characteristics of the exophore: Perceived observations. *J Optom Vis Dev* 8(3):35–46.

Forrest E (1976). Clinical manifestations of visual information processing. *J Am Optom Assoc* 47(1):73–80; 47(4):499–507.

Forrest E (1981). *Visual Imagery: An Optometric Approach.* Santa Ana, CA: Optometric Extension Program Foundation.

Forrest E (1988). *Stress and Vision.* Santa Ana, CA: Optometric Extension Program Foundation.

Francke AW, Kaplan WJ (1978). Easier and more productive study and desk work. *J Am Optom Assoc* 49 (8):931–939.

Furth HG, Wachs H (1974). *Thinking Goes to School: Piaget's Theory in Practice.* New York: Oxford University Press.

Gallaway M, Pearl SM, Winkelstein AM, et al. (1987). Biofeedback training of visual acuity and myopia: A pilot study. *Am J Optom Physiol Opt* 64(1):62–71.

Garzia RP, Nicholson SB (1990). Visual function and reading disability: An optometric viewpoint. *J Am Optom Assoc* 61:88–97.

Getman GN (1984). *How to Develop Your Child's Intelligence.* 8th ed. Santa Ana, CA: VisionExtension, Inc.

Gil KM, Collins FL (1983). Behavioral training for myopia: Generalization of effects. *Behav Res Ther* 21:269–273.

Goss DA (1991). Clinical accommodation and heterophoria findings preceding juvenile onset of myopia. *Optom Vis Sci* 68 (2):110–116.

Graham C, Leibowitz HW (1972). The effect of suggestion on visual acuity. *Int J Clin Exp Hypnosis* 20:169–186.

Greenspan SB (1970). Effects of children's nearpoint lenses upon body posture and performance. *Am J Optom Arch Acad Optom* 47(12):982–990.

Griffin JR (1982). *Binocular Anomalies: Procedures For Vision Therapy.* 2nd ed. Chicago: Professional Press.

Grisham JD (1988). Visual therapy results for convergence insufficiency: A literature review. *Am J Optom Physiol Opt* 65(6):448–454

Grisham JD, Bowman MC, Owyang LA, et al. (1991). Vergence orthoptics: Validity and persistence of the training effect. *Optom Vis Sci* 68(6):441–451.

Groffman S (1969). Operant conditioning and vision training. *Am J Optom Arch Am Acad Optom* 46(8):583–594.

Harmon DB (1958). *Notes on a Dynamic Theory of Vision.* Austin, TX: author.

Hennessey D, Iosue RA, Rouse MW (1984). Relation of symptoms to accommodative infacility of school-aged children. *Am J Optom Physiol Opt* 61:177–183.

Hildreth HR, Mainberg WH, Milder B, et al. (1947). The effects of visual training on existing myopia. *Am J Ophthalmol* 30:1563–1576.

Hirsch MJ (1964). Predictability of refraction at age 14 on the basis of testing at age 6— Interim report from the Ojai longitudinal study of refraction. *Am J Optom Arch Am Acad Optom* 41(10):567–573.

Hoffman LG (1980). Incidence of vision disabilities in children with learning disabilities. *J Am Optom Assoc* 51(5):447–451.

Hoffman LG, Rouse M (1980). Referral recommendations for binocular function and/or developmental perceptual deficiencies. *J Am Optom Assoc* 51(2):119–125.

Hokoda SC, Rosenfield M, Ciuffreda KJ (1991). Proximal vergence and age. *Optom Vis Sci* 68(3):168–172.

Horner SH (1972–73). *The Use of Lenses and Prisms to Enhance Vision Training*. Optometric Extension Program Continuing Education Courses, Santa Ana, CA: Optometric Extension Program Foundation, Oct. 1972–Sept. 1973.

Kagan J (1965). Reflection-impulsivity and reading ability in primary grade children. *Child Dev* 36:609–628.

Kaplan M (1978–79). *Vertical Yoked Prisms*. Optometric Extension Program Continuing Education Courses, Santa Ana, CA: Optometric Extension Program Foundation, vol. 51.

Koslowe KC, Spierer A, Rosner M, et al. (1991). Evaluation of Accommotrac biofeedback training for myopia control. *Optom Vis Sci* 68(5):338–343.

Levine S, Ciuffreda KJ, Selenow A, et al. (1985). Clinical assessment of accommodative facility in symptomatic and asymptomatic individuals. *J Am Optom Assoc* 56:286–290.

Macdonald L (1975). Presentation at Eastern States Optometric Congress, New York.

Marg E (1952). Flashes of clear vision and negative accommodation with reference to the Bates method of visual training. *Am J Optom Arch Am Acad Optom* 29(4):167–184.

Margach CB (1988). *Video Display Terminals—II*. Optometric Extension Program Continuing Education Courses, Santa Ana, CA: Optometric Extension Program Foundation, 60(7):37–41.

Marrone MA (1991). Peripheral awareness. *J Behav Optom* 2(1):7–11.

Miller SC (1984). Meeting the eye care needs of video display terminal operators. *J Am Optom Assoc* 55(8):611–618.

Morgan MW, Peters HB (1951). Accommodative-convergence in presbyopia. *Am J Optom Arch Am Acad Optom* 28:3–10.

Pantano F (1982). Orthoptic treatment of convergence insufficiency: A two year follow-up report. *Am Orthopt J* 32:73–80.

Peachey GT (1990). Perspectives on optometric vision training. *J Behav Optom* 1(3):65–70.

Peachey GT (1991). Minimum attention model for understanding the development of efficient visual function. *J Behav Optom* 2(8):199–206.

Pepper RC (1986). *Developmental Vision: A Multisensory Approach to Stress Therapy*. Santa Ana, CA: Optometric Extension Program Foundation.

Perrigin J, Perrigin D, Quintero S, et al. (1990). Silicone-acrylate contact lenses for myopia control: 3 year results. *Optom Vis Sci* 67(10):764–769.

Pierce JR (1966–68). Research on the relationship between nearpoint lenses, human performance and physiological activity of the body. In: *Research Reports and Special Articles Pertaining to Vision and Its Care*. Optometric Extension Program

Postgraduate Courses, Santa Ana, CA: Optometric Extension Program Foundation, series 1, no. 1–12, Oct. 1966–Sept. 1967; series 2, no. 1–5, Oct. 1967–Feb. 1968.

Prakash P, Agarwaz, LP, Nag SG (1972). Accommodational weakness and convergence insufficiency. *Orient Arch Ophthalmol* 10(5):261–264.

Press LJ (1987). Myopia. *J Optom Vis Dev* 18:1–17.

Richman JE, Cron MT (1988). *Guide to Vision Therapy*. South Bend, IN: Bernell.

Robinson BN (1973). A study of visual function in institutionalized juveniles who are demonstrated underachieving readers. *Am J Optom Arch Am Acad Optom* 50(2):113–116.

Rosen RC, Schiffman HR, Meyers H (1984). Behavioral treatment of myopia: Refractive error and acuity changes in relation to axial length and intraocular pressure. *Am J Optom Physiol Opt* 61:100–105.

Rutstein RP, Daum KM, Amos JF (1988). Accommodative spasm: A study of 17 cases. *J Am Optom Assoc* 59(7):527–538.

Saladin JJ (1986). Convergence insufficiency, fixation disparity, and control systems analysis. *Am J Optom Physiol Opt* 63(8):645–653.

Shankman AL (1988). *Vision Enhancement Training*. Santa Ana, CA: Optometric Extension Program Foundation.

Sherman A (1973). Predicting vision disorders with learning disability. *J Am Optom Assoc* 44(2):140–141.

Skeffington AM, Lesser SK, Barstow R (1947–50). *Near Point Optometry*. Santa Ana, CA: Optometric Extension Program Foundation.

Stoddard KB (1942). Physiological limitations on the functional production and elimination of ametropia. *Am J Optom Arch Am Acad Optom* 19(3):112–118.

Stone J (1976). The possible influence of contact lenses on myopia. *Br J Physiol Opt* 31(3):89–114.

Streff JW (1978). The Cheshire study: Change in incidence of myopia following program intervention. In: Cool SG, Smith EL (eds), *Frontiers of Visual Science*. vol. 8. New York: Springer-Verlag, pp. 733–749.

Sutton A (1985). *Building a Visual Space World*. Optometric Extension Program Postgraduate Education Courses, Santa Ana, CA: Optometric Extension Program Foundation, vol. 57, series 1, no. 8, pp. 47–54, May.

Trachtman JN (1978). Biofeedback of accommodation to reduce functional myopia: A case report. *Am J Optom Physiol Opt* 55(6):400–406.

Trachtman JN, Giambalvo V, Feldman J (1981). Biofeedback of accommodation to reduce functional myopia. *Biofeedback Self-Regul* 6(4):547–564.

Wick B (1977). Vision training for presbyopic nonstrabismic patients. *Am J Optom Physiol Opt* 54(4):244–247.

Woods A (1946). Report from the Wilmer Institute on the results obtained in the treatment of myopia by visual training. *Am J Optom Arch Am Acad Optom* 29(4):167–184.

15

Vision Therapy: Procedures and Sequencing

Procedures to develop more adequate pursuit, saccadic, accommodative, and fusional abilities lie at the heart of vision therapy. Although this chapter describes a variety of vision training procedures and their sequencing, no one text can present all the procedures and variations that have been successfully used. Numerous texts and manuals present a variety of additional procedures. A listing of such texts and procedure manuals is provided in Appendix I.

OCULAR PURSUIT TRAINING

Pursuit training is performed to develop ocular motor control and ability to sustain visual attention. Pursuit activities require sustained fixation of a moving target, in contrast with saccades, which require shifts of fixation from one target to another.

In training pursuit eye movements, as well as other visual abilities, it is important to vary the task demands so as to broaden the base from which skills can be generalized. This avoids the development of splinter skills that can be applied only to the task at hand. Manual pursuits, thumb rotations, Marsden ball activities, and rotator pursuits are typical initial pursuit activities.

Manual Pursuits

In performing manual pursuits, the patient tracks a target that is slowly moved through the horizontal, vertical, and diagonal meridians, as well as through a circle. Suitable targets include a pen or pencil, Optistick, tongue depressor with pictures affixed, penlight, Wolff wand, Disney erasers, or small toy. The target is moved either by the therapist or the patient. The procedure is performed both monocularly and binocularly, lends itself well to home therapy, and can be used to emphasize peripheral awareness or plus acceptance when desired.

Flashlight pursuits is another procedure that lends itself to both office and home therapy. The therapist or parent holds a flashlight and moves the beam over the walls and ceiling of the room. The patient also holds a flashlight, and attempts to track the therapist's beam as it is moved.

Thumb pursuits require that the patient move one arm in circular, horizontal, vertical, diagonal, and random squiggle patterns while fixating the thumb. The technique requires no special equipment and is easily performed for home and office training. Use of the patient's own thumb facilitates performance, since kinesthetic input makes it easier to localize the target visually and to track it accurately, with hand leading eye.

Marsden Ball

The Marsden ball, a soft ball with vinyl letters affixed, is hung from the ceiling at or slightly below eye level. The ball is rotated in a wide arc while the patient tracks it. Following the ball with a hand-held flashlight or Russell ring adds attentional involvement and provides the patient with feedback as to accuracy of performance. The patient may be asked to read the letters on the ball or to locate letters in sequence to spell words.

Rotating Devices

Rotators such as those manufactured by Mast/Keystone (Figure 15.1) and Bernell provide excellent targets for pursuit training. As the disk rotates, the patient tracks a target located near its edge, and points a flashlight at the rotating

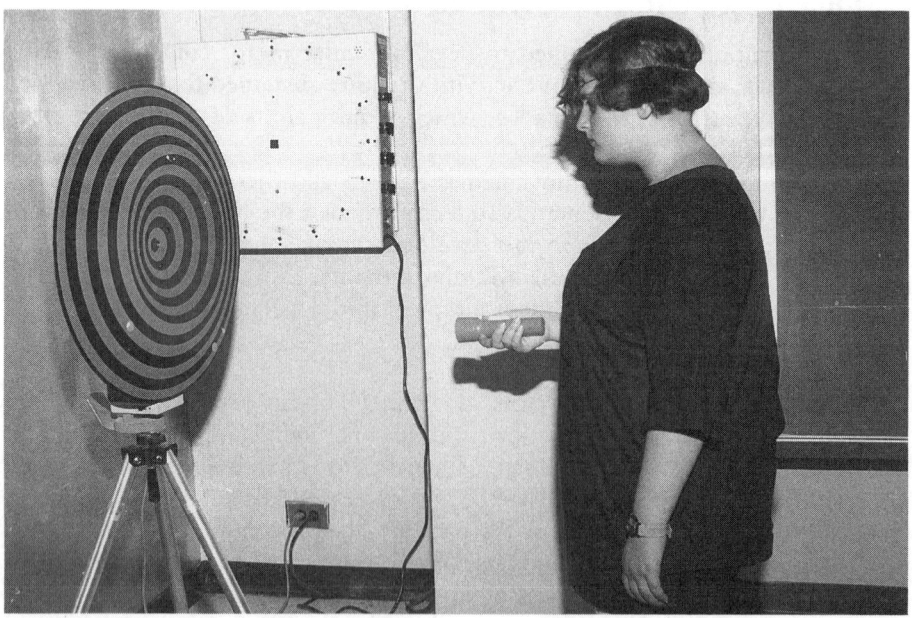

Figure 15.1 The patient tracks a target on the Keystone Rotator while using a flashlight to increase feedback as to accuracy.

target. The flashlight provides visual feedback so the patient can monitor and improve performance.

To evaluate the patient's performance, the examiner should observe both the eye movement and the accuracy with which the patient keeps the flashlight on target. Although eye movement accuracy and eye-hand coordination usually correlate, some patients demonstrate good eye-hand coordination despite the presence of jerky pursuits; others show good pursuit movements, but poor eye-hand coordination.

The Keystone rotator can be operated at varied speeds. Some patients perform better at slower and others at faster speeds. It is generally best to start the patient at the speed that permits best performance, and to work toward more difficult speeds.

A Branchaud light is affixed to the Keystone rotator. The light pulses at a rate just above the foveal critical flicker fusion frequency. Flicker is obliterated and the light is perceived as steady as long as the patient maintains foveal fixation as the target rotates. The light appears to flicker when foveal fixation is lost. The Branchaud light thus provides feedback regarding accuracy of fixation.

Demand is increased through use of a pegboard rotator, available from Bernell, JW Engineering, and Manico/Bloomington, a rotating disk with numerous holes. The patient attempts to accurately place pegs or golf tees in the holes as the disk rotates. The goal is to achieve such proficiency that the pegs are placed in the holes without hitting the wooden disk. This requires accurate tracking, good eye-hand coordination, and an ability to compute space-time relationships so as to accurately predict the location of the particular hole being fixated as the hand reaches it. It is easiest to begin with the more central holes, since they are moving more slowly than the peripheral holes.

Groffman Tracing

The Groffman Visual Tracing Program (Mast/Keystone) is more demanding and should not be introduced until the patient demonstrates adequate performance on manual pursuit and rotator procedures. The program consists of a series of plates that present increasingly complex, interweaving lines to be tracked (Figure 15.2). The program is useful in developing visual tracking, visual attention, visual grasp, ability to attend to detail, and the ability to maintain figural awareness in the presence of a complex background. The procedure may be performed in free space or as a cheiroscopic tracing procedure. A computerized procedure presenting similar demands is available from American Vision Training, Inc.

Chalkboard Racetrack

For patients who have difficulty with manual or rotator pursuit procedures, increasing kinesthetic involvement frequently aids performance. In the chalkboard racetrack procedure, the child drives a car (a piece of colored chalk) around a racetrack (outlined in white chalk) without crashing into the walls (Figure

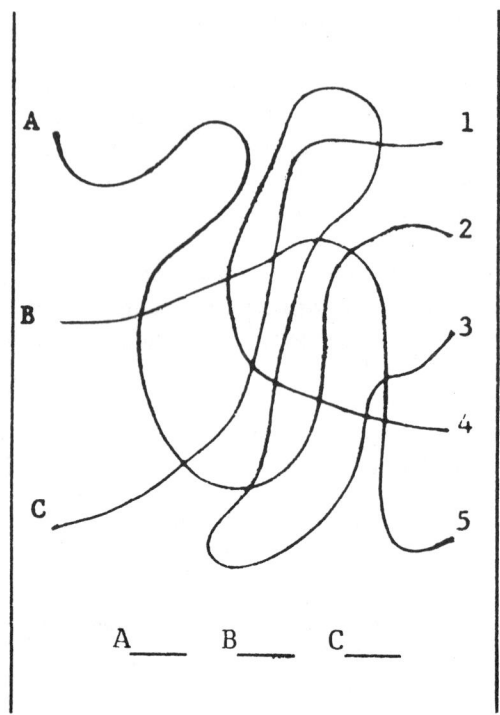

Figure 15.2 A plate from the Groffman Visual Tracing Program. (Reprinted with permission from Mast/Keystone.)

15.3). As performance improves, task difficulty is increased by changing the shape of the racetrack and by making it narrower.

The chalkboard racetrack is a lower-level training procedure in which the hand leads the eyes, and is useful for patients who require increased kinesthetic involvement to achieve good pursuits.

Sequencing Pursuit Procedures

In selecting pursuit training procedures, it is desirable to begin at a level appropriate for the patient. Each procedure may be considered in terms of the level of task difficulty; the feedback provided to the patient regarding accuracy of performance; the degree of kinesthetic involvement; concurrent demands for balance, awareness, and information-processing; and the degree to which the task stimulates interest and is motivating to the patient. Each of these factors may be manipulated so as to increase or decrease demand consistent with the needs of the particular patient. In general, when pursuit ability is poor, tasks are made less demanding by reducing task difficulty, increasing motivation and interest in the task, increasing the feedback the patient receives as to adequacy of

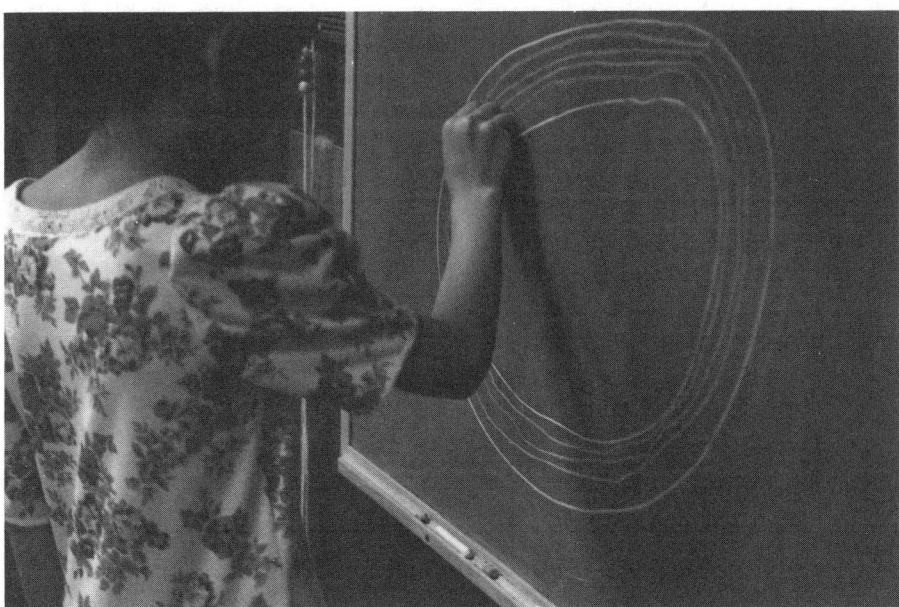

Figure 15.3 The chalkboard racetrack procedure.

performance, increasing kinesthetic involvement, and reducing concurrent demands for balance and information-processing. As ability improves, the patient is expected to be able to maintain accurate pursuit performance even when tasks are less interesting and less motivating; when task difficulty is greater; when feedback and kinesthetic involvement are decreased; and when demands for concurrent mental and physical activity are increased.

When performance is poor on a pursuit procedure, several approaches may be used to facilitate improvement:

1. Increase interest and involvement with the task

Bunting a Marsden ball with a dowel stick requires accurate tracking. The procedure stimulates a high degree of interest, which frequently leads to improved performance.

The Computer Orthoptor (American Vision Training Inc.) provides a pursuit task in which the patient tracks a target, and moves a stylus to keep the target within a moving square. Performance is scored as the percentage of time in which the target is maintained in the square. The task tends to be highly motivating.

2. Reduce task demand

The trainer should be able to make any vision therapy procedure more or less demanding as needed. With the Keystone rotator or pegboard rotator, task demand is reduced by slowing the rotator. In the case of the pegboard rotator, task demand may be reduced even further by stopping the rotator and asking the patient to accurately aim the pegs into the holes with the rotator stationary. The chalkboard racetrack procedure is made easier by increasing the width of the track.

3. Provide adequate feedback

Adequate feedback allows the patient to become aware of errors in performance, and hence to correct such errors. Training is more effective when adequate feedback and reinforcement are provided (Schroeder and Holland 1968, 1969; Punnett and Steinhauer 1984).

Feedback as to accuracy of performance is provided by observing the patient's performance and telling him when pursuits are inaccurate; by use of auditory feedback devices such as the Perceptuomotor Pen, available from Wayne Engineering, or the Groffman Visual Tracing program of the Computer Orthopter, each of which provides an auditory signal as to accuracy of performance; by use of afterimages to "tag" the fovea (the patient is asked to keep the afterimage on the target which is being tracked); and by use of a Russell ring (a piece of wire or a pipe cleaner bent into a ring) or a flashlight as one tracks the target.

The demand to keep the flashlight on the target, or to keep the target centered within the ring as one tracks, provides feedback as to accuracy of performance. The task may be made easier by using a larger ring or a wider beam flashlight so that there is greater tolerance for inaccuracy in the early stages of training.

Patients who demonstrate poor pursuits frequently also demonstrate poor awareness and ability to monitor feedback. In such cases, the trainer must increase the strength of the feedback to levels that can be appreciated by the patient, as by creating a larger, more intense afterimage; using a brighter, larger flashlight; and verbally exhorting the patient to stay on target. The chalkboard racetrack procedure is particularly effective in providing an appreciable feedback level even for children with poor ability to monitor; when the child's chalk goes outside the boundary lines of the racetrack, it leaves a visible chalk trace so that error can be pointed out to the patient (see Figure 15.3).

4. Increase kinesthetic involvement

Increased kinesthetic involvement often facilitates improved performance. In thumb rotations and the chalkboard racetrack procedure, the patient tracks his own hand and thus receives kinesthetic information regarding target location. Having the therapist or parent guide the movement initially, holding and moving the child's fist while the child fixates his outstretched thumb, relieves the child of the need to organize his arm movement and provides heightened tactual and kinesthetic support.

5. Reduce concurrent demands and distractions

The child with hyperkinesis, attentional, or motor organization difficulty commonly shows improved performance when distractors are removed, demands for balance are reduced, and potential for random, unrelated body movement is restricted. The patient may be asked to sit instead of stand, or to begin pursuit activity lying on the floor following a moving Marsden ball.

6. Develop steady position maintenance of a stationary target

Griffin (1982) indicates that the first step in pursuit training is to ensure that the patient has adequate position maintenance of a stationary target. The patient should be able to monocularly fixate a target for at least 5 seconds without noticeable drift or eye movement from the target.

This ability may be improved by using a stronger stimulus (for example, a strong light or a favorite toy); by increasing attentional demand (for example, have the patient read the letters on a stationary Marsden ball, or aim pegs at the holes of a stationary pegboard rotator); by increasing kinesthetic involvement (ask the patient to fixate his thumb to increase kinesthetic support); and by increasing feedback (urge the patient to fixate steadily and keep an afterimage, Russell ring or flashlight beam centered on the target).

Some patients demonstrate poor performance even when task demands are reduced, increased kinesthetic support and feedback are provided, and efforts are made to maximize interest and motivation. Although neurologic deficits may underlie some such cases, in other instances poor pursuit ability reflects poor general motor skills and inadequate spatial organization. In such cases, a developmental approach emphasizing gross motor skills, motor planning, and spatial organization may establish a foundation for the development of improved eye movement ability.

As performance improves, the practitioner should modify the task demands so as to shape further improvement in pursuit ability. The patient is asked to perform progressively more difficult tasks; to maintain pursuits as feedback and kinesthetic support are reduced; and to maintain good pursuit performance in the presence of increasing demands for balance and for concurrent mental activity:

1. Reduce use of tasks that stimulate high interest and patient motivation

As performance improves, the patient should be able to maintain good pursuits even when the task is less interesting and motivating.

2. Increase task difficulty

As performance improves, more complex tasks such as the pegboard rotator or Groffman tracing procedure (see Figure 15.2) may be attempted. A modified Groffman tracing procedure may be performed using the chalkboard.

3. Reduce kinesthetic support

The patient is expected to perform accurately with progressively less kinesthetic support. For the patient who initially requires considerable kinesthetic support, the emphasis will gradually change from procedures such as thumb rotations and chalkboard racetrack to tracking a Marsden ball or following a target on the rotator, procedures in which judgements are made on a more strictly visual basis.

4. Reduce feedback

It is desirable that the patient be able to sustain accurate pursuits with reduced need for feedback. In tracking a target on the rotator, for example, the patient who initially uses a flashlight to provide feedback may begin to track with the flashlight off, turning the beam on periodically to monitor accuracy. If performance is accurate, the beam will be on target each time the patient turns the light on. Eventually the patient should be able to sustain accurate pursuits without need for the flashlight at all.

5. Increase concurrent demands for balance, movement, awareness, fusional vergence, and information-processing

In typical eye movement tasks, all of the patient's attention can be directed toward maintaining accuracy. The addition of task demands to maintain peripheral awareness; to keep one's balance on a balance board, walk on a walk rail, or bounce on a trampoline; to carry on a conversation, read aloud letters on a Marsden ball, spell words, or solve continuous arithmetic problems; and to maintain fusion despite the addition of loose prisms that create base-in and base-out fusional vergence demand, requires that attention be allocated to these supplementary tasks, and detracts from that available for performing the pursuit. Consequently, pursuit performance is more difficult. Once pursuit performance is adequate, incorporation of such "distractors" helps to develop greater automaticity of eye movements and to facilitate their integration with general movement and problem-solving activities. Such automaticity is necessary so that in daily life, when one cannot concentrate on eye movements, eye movement performance can be sustained in the presence of other demands.

Monocular Versus Binocular Training

Equality of monocular function is important for normal binocular vision. When spatial localization and visual judgements are more accurate with one eye than the other, efficient binocular integration is difficult. Motility training is thus usually initiated under monocular conditions to ensure that monocular visual abilities are adequate and equal. The monocular phase of therapy will be relatively brief in duration if performance is equal for the two eyes, and more prolonged when monocular abilities are unequal.

Getman (1964) suggests that when pursuits are better binocularly than monocularly, the implication is that adequate performance has not been achieved within each ocular circuit; with both eyes open, one eye reinforces the other so that binocular performance is better. Getman indicates that training should begin monocularly in such cases, to develop more adequate performance in each ocular circuit.

Better performance under binocular than monocular viewing conditions may also occur because spatial localization is more accurate under binocular conditions, or may indicate that pursuit ability has not developed to an adequate level of automaticity. Testing with one eye covered presents a novel situation in which the patient has had little prior experience. A decrement in performance suggests that pursuit ability is fragile and easily broken down. In such cases, it may be best to begin ocular motility training binocularly, where performance is stronger, and to introduce monocular motility work later in therapy as oculomotor and spatial localization functions improve.

Poorer binocular than monocular performance suggests the presence of a binocular vision dysfunction that interferes with pursuit efficiency. Under monocular test conditions, binocular perturbating factors are eliminated and performance improves. Getman (1964) suggests that training in such cases emphasize binocular routines. Since each ocular mechanism has achieved its own adequate motility, the need is for practice in coordination and interweaving.

In the early stages of monocular motility training, procedures are organized so that the patient works with each eye, with greater emphasis on the poorer eye if inequality exists. The patient should work with the better eye first on each procedure, and then attempt to do as well with the poorer eye.

Biocular Training

As monocular motility improves, biocular (simultaneous perception) training is introduced to facilitate equalization. Biocular procedures present stimuli to the two eyes simultaneously without opportunity for fusion. For example, the patient may follow a rotating target (using a flashlight to provide feedback) while wearing vertical dissociating prisms, switching fixation periodically from one target to the other. Biocular procedures with the Marsden ball require that the patient follow the moving ball while wearing dissociating vertical prisms, shifting fixation from one diplopically perceived ball to the other; use a dowel stick to alternately bunt the diplopic balls; or follow the ball while holding a vertical septum so that the eyes alternately fixate as the ball moves back and forth between the left and right fields.

Biocular procedures permit the patient to directly compare eye movement accuracy, eye-hand coordination, and spatial localization ability with each visual circuit, and to more effectively equalize performance. The trainer should encourage the patient to notice and describe differences in visual perception and performance obtained with the two eyes. This helps to increase awareness and facilitate equalization of monocular visual skills.

Once monocular motility skills are equal and adequate, ocular motility procedures are performed binocularly to ensure smooth and efficient performance. Little binocular motility training is usually needed once monocular abilities normalize.

Pursuits and Head Movement

The patient should be able to move eyes independent of head. The patient who moves the head excessively, using head movements to replace or to lead eye movements, should be asked to reduce head movement and to try to move the eyes primarily.

When head movements are excessive, this author prefers not to hold the child's head immobile, or to place a book on the child's head with instructions not to let it fall. Although these procedures are commonly used, such restraint produces an undesirable rigidity. It is preferable for the trainer to gently and briefly place one hand on the child's head, providing a gentle reminder to reduce head movement.

When the child is unable to move the eyes independent of the head, head rotations often help to develop greater freedom between the eye and head transport systems. The child maintains fixation on a stationary target such as a Marsden ball, and moves the head from side to side, up and down, and then in a circle. He then tracks a rotating target or a moving Marsden ball, moving the head rather than the eyes. The experience of moving the head with the eyes fixed often leads to better ability to move the eyes independent of head movement. When the child cannot perform at this level, developmental training is indicated to teach more adequate gross and fine motor skills, so that the child can ultimately differentiate fine motor systems.

Pursuits, Visual Attention, and Central-Peripheral Organization

Patients with inadequate visual attention ability often demonstrate poor grasp and difficulty sustaining ocular pursuit movements. Since pursuit training requires that the patient maintain ocular fixation while tracking a visual target, improved ability to sustain visual attention is a frequent concomitant of pursuit training.

Central-peripheral organization involves the ability to appropriately select figure for attention, monitor background information, and shift attention when appropriate. When patients lack adequate ability to integrate the processing of detail with peripheral awareness, vision therapy should be directed toward the development of more adequate visual information-processing (MacDonald 1965; Forrest 1976; Birnbaum 1978; Sutton 1985).

For individuals who are relatively peripheral, processing visual information globally with little attention to detail, pursuit training should emphasize attention to detail. Individuals who are less peripherally aware and tend to concentrate on detail are encouraged to broaden peripheral awareness while performing pursuits.

Effort, stress, and tension are characterized by narrowing of the perceptual field (Easterbrook 1959; Kahneman 1973); expansion of the perceptual field is associated with a more relaxed, passive form of concentration. The ability to expand peripheral awareness while performing ocular pursuits signals that the task is being performed with ease, in a more relaxed state, without undue effort or strain (Birnbaum 1978, 1990).

SACCADIC EYE MOVEMENT TRAINING

In training saccades, as in training pursuits and other visual abilities, a variety of procedures should be used so as to generalize performance. Among the many procedures commonly used to train accurate saccadic eye movements are manual saccades, use of a sequential fixator or the Wayne Saccadic Fixator, Hart chart, chalkboard and AN star saccades, Ann Arbor tracking, prism saccades, and large oculomotor calisthenics.

There are many ways to perform manual saccadic eye movements. Since kinesthetic feedback facilitates awareness of position, the patient may use his thumbs as targets, holding them apart to create horizontal targets initially, and then training vertical and diagonal saccades as well. When such feedback is no longer necessary the parent or therapist holds two targets (for example, pen and pencil, pencils with animal erasers, small toys, or tongue depressors with pictures affixed) and positions them so that the patient practices horizontal, vertical, and diagonal saccades (see Figure 11.3).

The Wayne Saccadic Fixator (Figure 15.4), available from Wayne Engineering, is an automated device that presents a lighted target for fixation each time the patient successfully locates and touches the previously lighted target. The instrument is programmed to present targets in clockwise, counterclockwise, or random sequence, and keeps score of the number of successful saccades per unit of time. Rapid performance requires good peripheral awareness, short reaction time, accurate saccades, and good eye-hand coordination. The procedure provides auditory and visual feedback, as well as manual involvement. The competitive aspect of attempting to achieve the highest possible score, and the automaticity and "hi-tech" character of the instrument make it particularly interesting and motivating.

An AN star printed on 8-by-11-inch paper serves as a convenient target for saccadic fixation training, and lends itself to both office and home therapy. The patient shifts fixation from one number to the next. With each saccadic fixation, the patient touches the tip of the star at the appropriate number with a pointer, incorporating kinesthetic support, visual feedback, and eye-hand coordination. Demands for organization and control may be increased by using a metronome and instructing the patient to touch the tip of the star at each number in a four-beat, "ready, aim, touch, back" sequence, in time with the metronome.

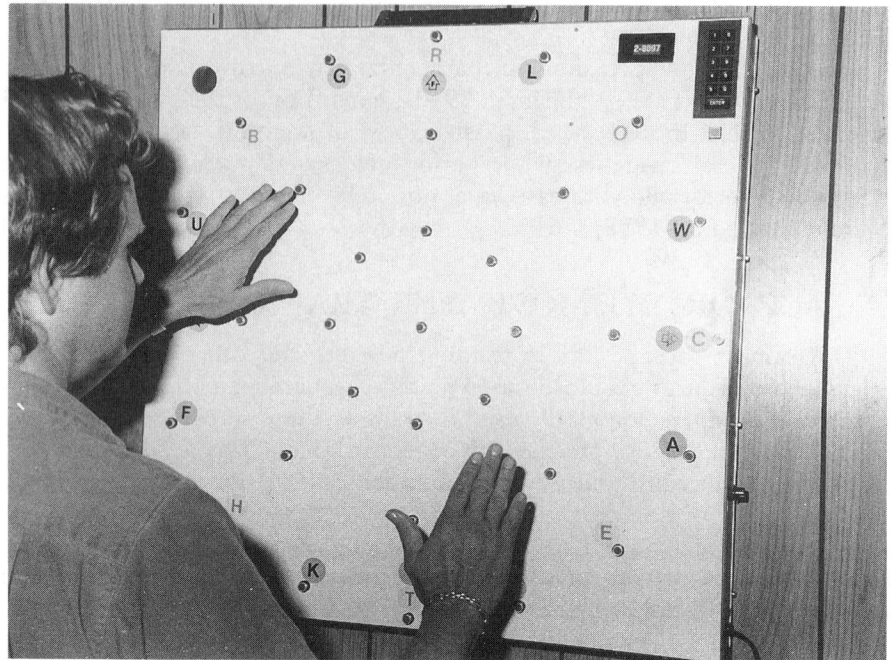

Figure 15.4 Wayne Saccadic Fixator. (Photo courtesy of Wayne Engineering Co.)

The sequential fixator is a clear acetate or plexiglass sheet upon which fixation targets are printed. A design commonly used for saccadic training presents five lines, each of which contains five targets. A transparent sequential fixator permits the doctor to view the patient's eyes to evaluate accuracy of eye movements (see Figure 11.4).

Letters or numbers on a chalkboard or on index cards affixed to the wall may be used as saccadic fixation targets for office and home training. Targets are placed in a variety of horizontal, vertical, diagonal, or random patterns. Kinesthetic support and visual feedback are provided by having the patient aim a flashlight at each target, or touch each target with dowel sticks held one in each hand.

The following chalkboard saccadic sequence is organized to develop adequate visual attention and central-peripheral organization:

1. Chalkboard saccadics

    The numerals 1, 2, 3, and 4 are placed near the corners of a chalkboard. The patient, holding a dowel stick in each hand, sequentially fixates the numbers and touches each number with the two dowel sticks simultaneously (Figure 15.5).

    When performance is adequate, a metronome is added. The patient touches a number on each beat. The demand level is varied by

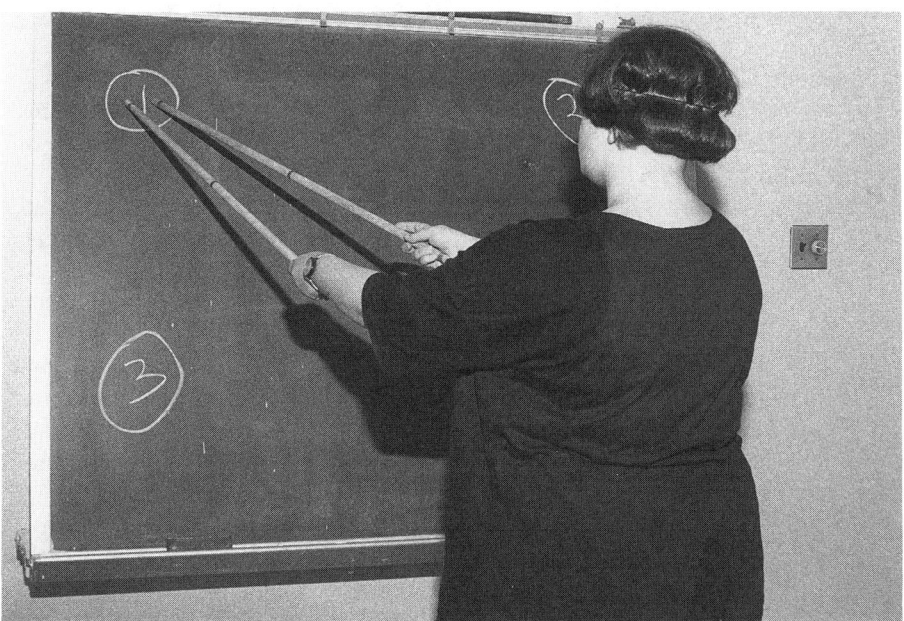

Figure 15.5 Chalkboard saccades.

changing the speed at which the metronome beats, or by changing the instruction from "touch a number on each beat" to "touch a number every other beat," "every fourth beat," etcetera. The metronome provides an external stimulus to which the patient must match his performance, and increases demands for attention and control.

The metronome should initially be set at that speed at which performance is best. When working with lethargic, passive, slow-acting children, the metronome is introduced at a slow rate and the speed is increased as performance warrants. With hyperactive or impulsive children who have difficulty slowing down, the metronome is initially set at a rapid rate and the patient is trained to perform at progressively slower speeds.

2. Peripheral awareness

An X is placed in the center of the chalkboard. The patient fixates the X and attempts to maintain peripheral awareness of the surrounding numbers, and to touch the numbers sequentially with the dowel sticks.

Distractable or impulsive children typically find it difficult to maintain fixation on the X while pointing to the peripheral numbers. Such children typically shift attention to each new stimulus that enters their perceptual field, and frequently demonstrate attentional difficulty in the classroom. This procedure helps to develop the ability to sustain central visual attention and monitor with the periphery.

3. Central-peripheral saccadics

The central X is erased. The patient is instructed to fixate number "1" and to touch it with both dowel sticks. He is to be aware of "2" out of the corner of his eyes, and then to accurately move the dowel sticks to touch "2" while maintaining visual fixation at "1." He then shifts visual fixation to "2." The patient then maintains visual fixation at "2" while shifting the dowels to "3," and then fixates "3" to verify accuracy of performance. The procedure continues in this "touch-look" sequence as the patient touches "4"; then looks at "4"; then moves the dowels back to "1," using peripheral vision; and then shifts fixation to centrally fixate "1" and begin the cycle again.

Performance requires peripheral monitoring with continual restraint of the tendency to centrally fixate the target upon which one is acting. This is particularly difficult for the impulsive, distractable child, who must inhibit the urge to look at the stimulus of most intense demand. This procedure is used to develop control over fixation and visual attention. When adequate performance is achieved, a metronome is introduced and the child attempts to organize the look-touch sequence to the beat of the metronome.

Prism saccadic training (Flax 1963a) is performed to develop accurate spatial judgements, as well as saccadic eye movements. The patient fixates a small muscle light in a dimly lit room monocularly while a 15^Δ loose prism is interposed before the fixing eye base-up, base-down, base-left, or base-right. The patient refixates the visually displaced target, points or directs a flashlight toward it, and reports the direction in which the target is perceived to have moved.

The ability to interpret directional shifts is poor in many developmentally immature youngsters. Training should begin in the direction in which movement is easiest to perceive, usually the vertical. When the patient can readily perceive vertical shifts, training is performed in the horizontal meridian, where perception is more commonly confused, and even in oblique directions. Awareness of target movement is heightened, if necessary, by increasing the prism power; by performing the procedure in a dark room using a light as the target, so that the moving target clearly stands out from the background; and by having the patient point at the target as the prism is interposed. As performance improves, prism power is reduced so that the patient becomes sensitive to smaller increments of movement.

The Hart chart (see Figure 11.5) lends itself well to saccadic eye movement training. The patient is asked to read the first and last letters in each row. If this is too difficult, a chart is provided in which alternate rows have been erased to reduce confusion. When the patient can read the first and last letter of each row of the standard Hart chart without loss of place, task demand is increased to reading the second and next-to-last letter in each row; the third and third-from-last; second and third-from-last; and so on. Task difficulty increases with the increased potential for spatial confusion and loss of place as the patient is asked to shift fixation within the interior letters.

Hart chart saccadic training need not be limited to the horizontal meridian. The patient may be asked to perform vertical saccades, and ultimately to read letters in diagonal patterns (for example, alternately reading down the first vertical row of letters and up the last row, "O, L, Y, B, E, G, etc."). A pair of Hart charts placed on a wall 2 or 3 feet apart provides a variety of potential saccadic demands.

As ability improves, the patient is asked to maintain accurate saccades even when concurrent motor and cognitive demands are added. The patient may be directed to read the letters of the Hart chart in time with a metronome; to clap, or to say boy's or girl's names when a letter is reached that is in the child's name; to walk on a rail, maintain balance on a balance board, or bounce on a trampoline; and at the same time maintain accurate performance on the Hart chart saccadic task. The ability to maintain performance in the presence of such distractors signals that saccadic eye movement ability is well organized, automatic, and can be readily integrated with performance of other tasks.

The Ann Arbor Letter Tracking program (Figure 15.6), published by Academic Therapy Publications, consists of workbooks that present paragraphs of nonsense words in which the letters *a* through *z* are embedded in order. The patient finds and circles the first *a*; then locates the first *b* after the *a*; then the next *c*, and so on, until each letter of the alphabet has been located in sequence. The paragraphs are constructed so that there is only one correct solution. Any error will cause a failure to reach *z* at the end of the paragraph. This procedure requires accurate saccadic eye movements, careful looking, and the ability to notice fine detail while scanning and processing information.

The workbooks are printed in various type sizes. Children often perform better on the large print paragraphs initially. As performance improves, smaller

a b c d e f g h i j k l m n o p q r s t u v w x y z

Himz kolle dunth nocke horb kily Cith pyl mofod
kuh ther nurvik dit lazop juf Gulo phots taj panil rok
doj brux. Kalb neb metar tobe. Pord api wens suh
terbod gaiw reaz bis duig. Tympes galue quez lers kugi
zalc wod snote. Dowil geb kunch nim morb. Lavih dran
wilk romop. Nefag gurf nexap morc mayed lozorf geeb

Min____ Sec____

Figure 15.6   A paragraph from the Ann Arbor Letter Tracking program. (Reprinted with permission of the publisher, Academic Therapy Publications, Novato, CA.)

print is used. Motivation is increased by timing each paragraph so that the patient continually strives to improve performance.

Workbooks printed in red ink are used to reduce suppression, training monocular function in a binocular field with red-green anaglyph glasses. To see the paragraphs, the patient must maintain central visual perception in the suppressing eye despite the inhibitory influence of the open dominant eye.

The saccadic movements required for reading may be trained with the Guided Reader (Instructional Communications Technology), a projection device that presents lines of print at regulated speeds. Material is initially projected at a slow speed, and the speed of presentation is increased as performance improves.

The OPTI-MUM Vision Training System (Learning Frontiers) and the Computer Orthoptor (American Vision Training) each provide computer programs for training saccadic fixations. Fujimoto et al. (1985) report the successful use of videocassette techniques for the enhancement of saccadic eye movements.

Large-angle oculomotor calisthenics are performed to optimize oculomotor flexibility (Peckham 1931). The four corners of a wall are used as fixation targets. The patient fixates each corner in order, pointing at each corner to add kinesthetic support. A typical daily home training sequence would require 25 clockwise and 25 counterclockwise cycles with each eye and then binocularly. The patient moves closer to the wall as performance improves, increasing the angular subtense of the saccadic movements.

Sequencing Saccadic Procedures

It is important to train at a demand level appropriate for the patient. Griffin (1982) indicates that development of the ability to maintain steady fixation on a stationary target (position maintenance) should be the first step. Training then proceeds to gross (large) saccades (for example, targets on a wall or chalkboard) and then to fine saccades (for example, Ann Arbor Letter Tracking). Training emphasizes the development of increased speed and efficiency of saccadic performance, and of equal saccadic ability for each eye. Training should be organized so that the patient develops good eye-hand coordination during saccadic demands, and is ultimately able to perform without hand support. Training generally proceeds from monocular to binocular saccades, and toward elimination of head movement. As performance improves, Griffin adds demands to integrate performance with external stimuli, introducing auditory stimuli such as that provided by the metronome, and seeks to develop the ability to sequence motorically from left to right, as in reading the English language. Cognitive and motor demands are added to develop automaticity and the ability to sustain accurate eye movements even in the presence of potential distractors.

When saccadics are poor, the therapist should

1. Decrease task difficulty
   A task such as chalkboard saccadics uses relatively large targets and gross saccades, and is therefore easier than Ann Arbor Letter

Tracking, which requires fine saccades and careful attention to detail. If performance is very poor, the chalkboard saccadic targets are made large enough to permit achievement, and then generally reduced in size.

2. Increase kinesthetic involvement

Kinesthetic involvement is introduced through the use of dowel sticks or pointers with chalkboard saccades; pushing the buttons of the Wayne Saccadic Fixator; or having the patient hold the targets used for manual saccades. Kinesthetic involvement provides additional input as to the spatial location of the target and feedback as to accuracy of performance, and also generates heightened involvement with the task. Each of these factors serves to facilitate performance.

3. Increase feedback

Feedback as to accuracy of performance permits the patient to become aware of error. Feedback is provided through the use of after-images, dowel sticks, pointers, or a flashlight during chalkboard saccades; auditory feedback on the Wayne Saccadic Fixator; and the therapist's verbalization as to accuracy of performance with manual saccades. When performance is inadequate, the therapist should make every effort to increase feedback; as performance improves, the patient is expected to maintain accurate saccades with progressively less feedback.

4. Increase interest, involvement, and motivation

Performance tends to improve when interest in the task and patient motivation are high. Use of sophisticated instruments such as the Wayne Saccadic Fixator; timing performance on the Ann Arbor Letter Tracking paragraphs so that the patient is competing against himself; and increasing kinesthetic involvement and feedback tend, in general, to stimulate greater patient interest and motivation.

5. Minimize distractions and concurrent demands

When working with a child who is overactive, easily distracted, or whose motor organization is poor, the therapist should eliminate stimuli that are unrelated to the task, and work in a quiet room without other vision therapy patients, with as little extraneous equipment, noise, or other distraction as possible. Performing saccadic procedures while seated reduces the need for balance and may help to reduce random activity and improve performance in the early stages.

ACCOMMODATIVE FACILITY TRAINING

Monocular accommodative facility (accommodative rock) training is initiated early in treatment, to develop adequate function within each ocular circuit prior to the development of binocular skills. Monocular accommodative training always precedes binocular training. Binocular accommodative rock training requires flexibility between vergence and accommodation, and should not be initiated until adequate flexibility exists within each accommodative circuit. Even when monocular accommodation is adequate, some monocular training is generally included early in treatment to ensure flexibility and equality.

Accommodative rock is performed to develop both amplitude and facility. Many patients have difficulty relaxing accommodation after it is stimulated; for this reason, most procedures are organized in cycles of alternate stimulation and relaxation.

The goals of monocular accommodative training, as given by Pierce and Greenspan (1971) and Griffin (1982), include

- normalize amplitude of accommodation for each eye;
- achieve a monocular accommodative facility range of ± 2.50 D for each eye;
- achieve an accommodative facility rate of 20 cpm monocularly;
- achieve the ability to rapidly clear both the stimulatory and inhibitory phases;
- achieve equal facility for the left and right eye;
- increase the ability to sustain clear vision.

Sequencing Monocular Accommodative Procedures

Monocular accommodative procedures begin at low levels of demand and proceed to progressively greater demand levels as performance improves. Procedures are generally sequenced as follows:

1. The demand to shift focus from one distance to another in real space provides better cues to the direction and magnitude of the accommodative response required than is provided by the interposition of a lens. Therefore, this author prefers to initially stimulate accommodative change in real space, by requiring shifts in focus back and forth between distance and near targets. When performance is adequate, plus and minus lenses are used to vary accommodative demand; this is more difficult because lenses provide blur, but no proximal cues for accommodation. Procedures in which lenses are used to vary accommodative demand in enclosed instruments are even more difficult, since such instruments provide an artificial environment with few cues for accommodation.
2. Use large letters as targets initially, and introduce progressively finer targets as therapy proceeds.
3. Begin with low-power lenses that impose minimal accommodative demand, and increase lens power as training proceeds.
4. Begin with procedures that require a change in accommodation but impose little or no concurrent information-processing demand. As training proceeds, increase demands for eye movement, peripheral awareness, balance, and cognitive processing in conjunction with accommodative training.

Near-Far Monocular Accommodative Procedures

The Hart chart contains 100 letters, arranged in rows of 10 letters each. The Hart chart focus-change procedure requires that the patient shift focus between a distance chart and a hand-held chart with identical letters, reduced in size for near viewing (Figure 15.7). The patient reads three letters on one chart and the next three letters on the other. In addition to accommodative demand, the procedure requires accurate saccadic fixation and spatial localization to accurately shift fixation from one chart to the other.

If the patient has more difficulty clearing one chart than the other, a greater emphasis may be placed on accommodative stimulation or relaxation. The patient who has difficulty clearing the distance chart should start close to the chart and attempt to maintain clarity while gradually moving away. The patient who has difficulty clearing the near chart should attempt to trombone the target toward and away from the eyes, seeking to clear the chart at progressively closer distances. When this can be achieved a demand for flexibility is added, to maintain clarity while shifting focus from one chart to the other.

The Wayne Saccadic Fixator contains a remote unit that allows distance-to-near accommodative training. A letter lights on the wall unit; the patient, seated 6 to 8 feet away, locates the same letter on the hand-held unit and presses the corresponding button, scoring a point and activating another letter on the distance unit.

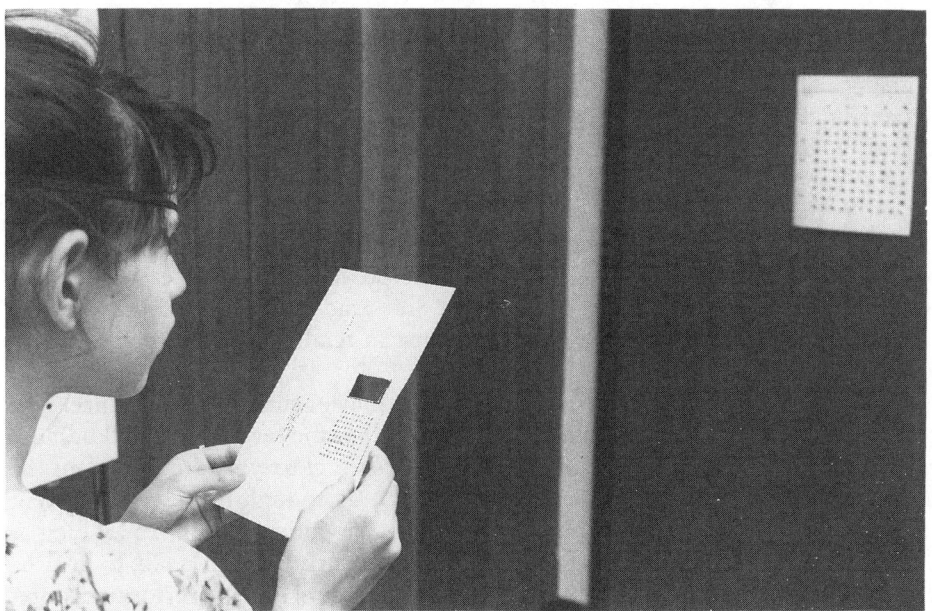

Figure 15.7 Hart chart near-far focus change procedure.

For preschoolers who do not know letters, playing cards are used for monocular accommodative facility training. Playing cards are arranged in random order on a shelf 6 to 8 feet away. The child's task is to arrange the cards in his hand in the same order, requiring numerous fixation shifts from the distance to the near cards to accomplish the task. The Sherman V.T. Playing Cards, available from Mast/Keystone, are anaglyphic cards that can be used for fusion and anti-suppression, as well as for accommodative rock training.

Monocular Accommodative Procedures with Lenses

Monocular accommodative facility training is performed with uncut ophthalmic lenses, loose trial case lenses, or lens flippers. Accommodative lens flippers, available from Bernell, GTVT, OEP, and Pacific Prisms, are convenient and widely used. Flippers with pairs of lenses in the following powers provide an effective set for accommodative rock training:

$+0.50/-0.50$	$+2.00/-4.00$
$+1.00/-1.00$	$+2.50/-4.00$
$+1.50/-1.50$	$+2.00/-6.00$
$+2.00/-2.00$	$+2.50/-6.00$
$+2.00/-2.50$	$+2.00/-8.00$
$+2.00/-3.00$	$+2.50/-8.00$

An additional flipper with two pairs of plus lenses ($+1.25/+2.50$) may be used to emphasize accommodative relaxation and plus acceptance.

Initial procedures should use large targets and low-power lenses to facilitate performance. Training is begun using either a Hart chart with large letters or a Marsden ball with large vinyl letters affixed. The Marsden ball, a three-dimensional object in real space, provides a strong stimulus for accommodation. It also facilitates training accommodative relaxation; because the ball is not affixed to the wall but hangs from the ceiling in the center of the room, it is easier for the patient to learn to focus beyond the target.

A variety of techniques may be used to facilitate accommodative relaxation in patients who are unable to clear plus lens power. It is often easier to clear plus if the patient starts close to the target and gradually moves away. The use of transparent acetate targets that the patient can readily look through also aids accommodative relaxation.

The instructional set used by the trainer may facilitate performance. The patient who cannot clear plus should be advised that the target is blurred because he is not focusing far enough away; in order to see clearly through the lens, he needs to look farther away, through the target, as though it were transparent (Birnbaum 1977). Imagery techniques in which the patient visualizes looking at distant objects may also aid performance, as may instructions to relax, to breathe deeply, and to expand peripheral awareness (Birnbaum 1990). Performance frequently improves when the patient is instructed to look at a distant object for a moment, and then to maintain the same feeling while looking at the near target through the plus lens.

The patient who has difficulty clearing minus lens power will often benefit from repetition and practice with lower-power lenses and with targets at longer working distances. As performance improves, lens power is increased and target distance decreased. The ability to clear minus lens power is facilitated, when necessary, by viewing the target through a minus lens held at arm's length, where the effective power of the lens is reduced, and gradually moving the lens in toward the eyes.

The patient who has difficulty with minus should be advised that the blur he perceives is the result of focusing too far away; to clear the target he needs to focus closer. Asking the patient to concentrate intensely, to touch the target, to visualize something very close, and to pay careful attention to the detail of the target often aid performance, as does holding a real object 3 or 4 inches from the patient's eyes so that he can experience what it feels like to focus at such a close distance.

As performance improves, plus and minus lens powers are increased, and the patient attempts to maintain clarity and facility. Accuracy of accommodative response can be monitored with the retinoscope if the patient's subjective report of clarity is unreliable (Eskridge 1989). Facility is indicated by the speed with which clarity is obtained as lenses are flipped.

When the patient demonstrates good accommodative facility with large letters as targets, small letters that require more precise accommodation are introduced. The nearpoint Hart chart, newspaper, book, magazine, nearpoint reading card, or the Ann Arbor Letter Tracking paragraphs may be used as targets.

Alternate monocular rock may be performed with lenses in a trial frame or refractor. The patient views nearpoint material at the habitual reading distance. A low-power plus lens is placed before one eye and a low-power minus lens before the other. The patient moves an occluder from one eye to the other and clears the target material. The patient attempts to maintain clarity and facility as the plus and minus lenses are reversed and the lens powers are increased.

The Ann Arbor Letter Tracking paragraphs (See Figure 15.6) may be used with flippers to combine accommodative rock training with demands for accurate saccades, scanning, and information-processing. The patient alternately flips so as to locate *a* and *b* while looking through the plus lens, *c* and *d* through the minus lens, etcetera. Training begins with low-power flippers and progresses to higher powers as performance permits.

When the patient is able to clear plus and minus lenses in free space, training may be performed in instruments such as the refractor, Tel-Eye-Trainer, Titmus Biopter, Telebinocular, Prism Reader, and Computer Orthoptor. Instrument procedures are frequently more difficult than those performed in free space, because it is more difficult to relax accommodation beyond the plane of regard and because the enclosed environment provides fewer cues to accommodation.

Allen (1988) gives a computer program for training accommodative facility using the Commodore 64, 64C, or 128 computer.

Biocular Accommodative Procedures

Biocular (unfused binocular) procedures are used to eliminate suppression and foster binocular awareness. Biocular accommodative rock is introduced once monocular facility is adequate and equal for the two eyes. Biocular procedures provide a bridge between monocular and binocular fused training. They require simultaneous perception, yet vergence exerts no constraint on accommodation since they are performed under dissociated conditions. Biocular procedures are therefore less demanding than binocular fused accommodative rock.

Robbins' rock is a biocular procedure in which the patient views a near-point card through the refractor. Plus lens power is placed before one eye and minus before the other. Dissociating vertical prisms are placed before each eye. The patient sees two charts, one through plus and one through minus, and attempts to alternately clear the two charts as he shifts fixation from one to the other. When this is achieved, lens power is increased and plus and minus lenses are alternated before the two eyes. A similar procedure may be performed in real space with a trial frame, vertical dissociating prisms, and loose trial lenses.

Biocular accommodative training can be performed in free space using a −6.00 D lens and a Marsden ball or other target. The patient views the ball with both eyes open while holding the lens at arm's length along the visual axis of the right eye. The patient sees two balls: one ball is seen through the lens with the right eye, and one ball is seen outside the lens through the left. The patient alternately fixates the two balls and attempts to change focus to maintain clarity. When the patient can clear each ball, he slowly moves the lens toward the right eye, gradually increasing the effective lens power. The procedure is then repeated with the lens in front of the left eye.

In patients with low amplitude of accommodation, the gradual increase in effective lens power induced as the lens moves closer to the eye in this procedure may be easier to clear than the step increases in stimulus to accommodation produced when flippers or loose lenses are changed. This procedure is also advantageous in that the patient's accommodative response is readily monitored. As the −6.00 D lens approaches the eye, increasing accommodative convergence is generated and the fellow eye, without a lens, is readily observed to deviate inward.

Binocular Accommodative Rock Training

Binocular, fused accommodative rock training creates a demand for increased flexibility between vergence and accommodation. Binocular rock training is therefore not introduced until monocular accommodative function is adequate and the patient demonstrates adequate fusional vergence ranges.

In response to binocular minus lenses, the patient must shift accommodation closer than convergence. The demand created is similar to that induced by base-in prism. Plus lens demand, like base-out prism, requires an ability to shift convergence closer than accommodation. It is therefore incorrect to think of vergence range procedures as training vergence and binocular rock procedures as training accommodation; rather, each is concerned with developing flexibility between accommodation and convergence.

Binocular rock procedures are generally more difficult than vergence range procedures, since they use targets that are finer, present less stereopsis and less peripheral fusion lock, and are consequently weaker stimuli for fusion. Binocular accommodative rock procedures are therefore not generally introduced until performance is adequate on vergence range extension procedures.

Binocular accommodative rock procedures should begin at low demand levels. It is well to begin with low-power lenses and to increase lens power in small increments. Targets presenting large letters are used initially. Fine letters that require more precise accommodation are introduced when performance warrants.

As plus or minus lenses are introduced binocularly, a demand is created to shift accommodation beyond or closer than convergence. The individual who has inadequate flexibility to meet this demand may allow the target to blur or double, or may suppress to maintain clear, single vision. In binocular accommodative rock procedures, it is therefore important to incorporate suppression controls so that the practitioner can be certain that the patient's report that the target is clear and single truly signifies clear, single, *binocular* vision, rather than suppression.

A binocular accommodative rock training sequence commonly used by this author, proceeding from gross to fine target material and from strong fusion lock with stereoscopic targets to weak stimuli with little stereopsis, is as follows:

1. Polaroid vectograms

    As vergence ranges reach adequate levels, lens flippers are introduced to create binocular accommodative rock demand. Training should begin with Topper, the vectogram presenting the strongest stimulus for fusion, and proceed to the Mother Goose and ultimately the Spirangle vectograms. Lens powers of $\pm$ 0.50 D or $\pm$ 1.00D are used initially and increased as performance warrants. Training begins at the ortho setting; when performance is adequate, targets are disparated to incorporate BOP-BIM training, combining *base-out* with *plus* (BOP) or *base-in* with *minus* (BIM), so as to increase the demand for flexibility between accommodation and convergence. Readily visible suppression controls are built into the Mother Goose and Spirangle vectograms; awareness of stereopsis is the best suppression control with Topper.

2. Marsden ball with red-green glasses

    A Marsden ball covered with red and green vinyl letters serves as a useful target. The patient wears red-green anaglyph glasses and attempts to keep the letters clear and single while viewing the ball bi-nocularly at a 16-inch distance through flippers of increasing plus and minus lens power. The letters provide useful suppression controls, as does the perception of lustre, a blend of red and green in the white ball.

3. Polaroid vectogram #9 acuity-suppression target

The polaroid vectogram #9 acuity-suppression target (Bernell Corp.) (Figure 15.8) is an excellent target for binocular accommoda-tive training. The vectogram, designed for near use, presents seven rows of letters; the fourth and sixth are each perceived by one eye only and provide suppression control. The patient seeks to keep the rows of letters clear and single, with no rows disappearing, while viewing the target through lens flippers of increasing power.

4. Polaroid and red-green bar trainers

Bar trainers are composed of strips of red-green or Polaroid fil-ter material arranged so that target material viewed through the trainer (while the patient wears appropriate anaglyph or Polaroid glasses) is perceived in alternate bands by the right eye, both eyes, left eye, both eyes, etcetera. Bar readers, as well as Polaroid and red-green anaglyph glasses, are available from Bernell Corp., GTVT, and Mast/Keystone.

Bar trainers are commonly used with accommodative flippers for binocular rock. However, such trainers often induce retinal rivalry and exacerbate suppression. Bar trainers are thus more difficult than the #9 acuity-suppression vectogram, and are best used only after the patient has achieved adequate performance on less-demanding proce-dures.

5. Binocular lens and prism rock (BOP-BIM)

Flippers with base-in prisms on one side and base-out prisms on the other, designed for step vergence training, may be combined with

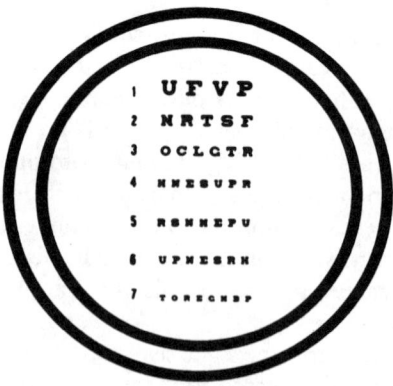

Figure 15.8 Acuity-suppression vectogram. (Photo courtesy Bernell Corp.)

accommodative lens flippers to increase demands for flexibility be-tween vergence and accommodation. The patient holds the flippers so that the plus lenses and base-out prisms are presented together (BOP), followed by the minus lenses and base-in prisms (BIM). The patient begins with gross targets such as the Marsden ball with red-green glasses, with low-power lens and prism flippers, and works toward maintaining clear, single vision without suppression as lens and prism powers are increased. When performance is adequate, finer targets such as the #9 acuity-suppression vectogram are introduced.

Accommodative Training and Spatial Effects

When viewed through a minus lens, objects and object distances appear smaller than they really are. Not only the size of the object, but also the distance between it and the observer is perceived as smaller. Thus, an object viewed through a minus lens is perceived as smaller and closer. A plus lens alters the input to the visual system so that an object viewed through it is perceived as larger and farther away. These effects are examples of the SILO (smaller-in, larger-out) phenomenon. SILO occurs when, as a result of artificially induced accommodative or vergence demands, an object appears to be located at a distance other than its actual location. This phenomenon stands in marked contrast to daily experience, since objects in real life appear smaller as they move away.

When accommodation or convergence is stimulated with minus lenses, base-out prisms, or vectograms, a conflict is thus created. The visual input suggests that the object of regard is smaller and closer (SILO), yet the logic of daily experience tells us that when objects appear smaller, they are farther away (SOLI; small-out, large-in). The logic of daily experience is thus in direct conflict with the visual input. The SILO response indicates that the individual's spatial judgement is based primarily on current visual input; a SOLI response suggests that greater emphasis is placed on logic and past experience.

When patients give persistent SOLI responses, it is desirable to create an opportunity to experience SILO. The value of the SILO response is twofold. First, the image viewed through the minus lens is perceived by the SILO re-sponder as both closer and smaller, and thus serves as a more appropriate stim-ulus for accommodation than the target that is perceived by the SOLI responder to be smaller and hence farther away. Second, the SILO response signals the ability to perceive events in the here and now, rather than through the filters of one's expectations, logic, and past experience.

Some procedures are more likely than others to yield a SILO response. In general, procedures that allow simultaneous comparison of the two targets fa-cilitate the perception of SILO. The previously described biocular Robbins's rock is one such procedure. Another is the monocular bifocal rock procedure, in which the patient holds a minus lens before the unoccluded eye so that the rim of the lens bisects the pupil. The target, a Marsden ball, is seen in monocular diplopia. The image viewed through the minus lens is usually seen as smaller and closer (SILO) than the image seen outside the lens. The simultaneous perception of the two images makes it difficult to override the visual cues. Hence, the visual cues predominate over the logic of daily experience, and the procedure is likely to elicit a SILO response.

Procedures that present no opportunity for simultaneous comparison of the images are more likely to elicit a SOLI response. In performing accommodative rock with flippers while viewing a Marsden ball or nearpoint card, for example, simultaneous comparison of the images is not possible. The input to the visual system regarding spatial localization is therefore less reliable, and the patient is more likely to rely on logic and past experience, reporting that the object appears farther away (SOLI) because it is smaller.

Accommodative procedures may also be structured to develop awareness of just noticeable differences. In procedures such as Robbins' rock and bifocal rock, the lenses create differences in size and spatial location of the diplopic images. To emphasize awareness, one begins with high-power lenses (provided that accommodative amplitude is adequate) and gradually reduces the lens powers. As lens power is reduced, it becomes more difficult to discriminate differences in size and location of the two images.

In a variation of this procedure, the patient is given an assortment of loose plus and minus lenses, and views a target through each. The patient attempts to arrange the lenses in proper dioptric sequence, based on observation of the size and localization changes induced by each lens.

Accommodative Relaxation/Plus Acceptance Training

Procedures to train accommodative relaxation or foster acceptance of plus lens power for near are used when patients show low NRA or inability to clear plus on the accommodative facility test; in cases of accommodative spasm; in cases in which the practitioner is attempting to reduce or reverse functional myopia; and in cases in which nearpoint plus lens prescription is desirable to reduce nearpoint esophoria, but case analysis or the patient's subjective response suggests that such lenses will not be well accepted.

Base-in prism may be used to facilitate acceptance of increased plus lens power for near use. The patient views small print on a nearpoint card through the phoroptor, and plus lens power is added binocularly until the print begins the blur. Base-in prism of 8 to 12^Δ is then added using Risley prisms. The patient must diverge to maintain fusion, and accommodation is simultaneously relaxed via convergence accommodation. Additional plus is added until the patient can just maintain clarity. The therapist then slowly reduces the base-in prism and the patient attempts to maintain clarity through the increased plus. The goal is for the patient to maintain clarity as the prism power is reduced to zero, at which point the patient is seeing clearly through greater plus power than was originally possible. The sequence is then repeated until maximum plus acceptance is achieved.

Accommodative relaxation procedures include the Hart chart walkaway, in which the patient views a distance Hart chart through low-plus fog and attempts to gradually increase the viewing distance over which the letters can be discriminated; and modified Updegrave or plus build-up procedures using the Telebinocular or refractor, in which the patient views a nearpoint target through high-plus lens power and attempts to maintain clarity as the target is gradually moved away.

Birnbaum (1990) suggests the use of relaxation, peripheral awareness, Plateau spiral, and visual imagery procedures to facilitate accommodative relaxation. Visualization of far scenes fosters the feeling of looking beyond the plane of regard, and helps to develop the ability to relax accommodation and maintain clarity through increased plus lens power.

Auditory biofeedback may also be useful in aiding accommodative relaxation. The Accommotrac Vision Trainer (Biofeedtrac, Inc.) has been used to attempt to reduce functional myopia. Trachtman (1978; Trachtman et al. 1981) obtained small but consistent reduction in myopia, of at least 0.50 D; however, Gallaway et al. (1987) and Koslowe et al. (1991) did not.

Friedman (1981) describes a procedure to teach accommodative control. Patients typically accommodate automatically to clear a target when a minus lens is interposed. Friedman asks the patient to interpose a minus lens, but not to clear the target; the patient is asked to inhibit accommodation so that the target remains blurred through the lens. Since accommodation tends to occur automatically, it is difficult to inhibit, especially when lens powers are small. It is best to start with a high-power lens, approximately -6 D, and reduce lens power as performance improves. Eventually the patient should be able to maintain blur with lens powers as low as 1.0 D, demonstrating a high degree of control over accommodation.

Many practitioners, when seeking to build plus acceptance, have the patient wear low-plus lenses for all office activities, for home vision training, and even for general wear. Cycloplegic therapy has been used to relieve accommodative spasm and latent hyperopia, and could be used to foster plus acceptance as well. Silbert and Alexander (1987) propose a protocol in which the manifest subjective refraction for maximum distance plus acceptance is first determined, and cycloplegic refraction is then performed 30 minutes after instillation of two drops of 1% cyclopentolate, administered 5 minutes apart. The authors report effective results in prescribing 80% to 85% of the full cycloplegic finding in single-vision form. To facilitate acceptance of the glasses, dispensing is scheduled early in the day; the patient is recyclopleged 30 minutes before dispensing, and instructed to wear the glasses constantly until bedtime. This eliminates the blur that may result from overfogging. The patient is instructed to return for further cycloplegia if distance blur is experienced through the new glasses on subsequent days.

FUSION AND FUSIONAL VERGENCE TRAINING

Authorities advocate differing approaches to training fusion and fusional vergence. The original OEP approach to visual skills training (Crow and Fuog 1937–39) views the development of adequate, equal monocular visual skills as prerequisite for adequate binocular function. This model holds that once adequate, equal monocular visual skills have developed, normal binocular function follows with little need for specific fusion training. Emphasis is therefore placed on the development of monocular pursuit and saccadic eye movement abilities, eye-hand coordination, monocular accommodative skills, and ability to localize and make visual judgements with each eye.

This premise underlies some modern optometric approaches to therapy, notably those of Wolff (1970) and Shankman (1988). Shankman suggests that fusion difficulty is caused by differences in monocular perception of size, distance, and color, and describes several procedures designed to allow the patient to become aware of and resolve these differences. These include procedures in which the patient compares judgements of size and distance with left and right eyes while viewing himself in a full-length mirror, and while making near-far saccadic eye movements between one Hart chart affixed to the mirror and another affixed to his chest and viewed in the mirror.

Although most clinicians agree that equal monocular abilities are important for efficient binocular function and therefore incorporate monocular activities in treating patients with binocular vision disorder, most clinicians also use binocular training procedures to develop adequate sensory and motor fusion. Approaches to therapy vary depending on the particular model to which the clinician adheres.

Classical Orthoptics

Classical orthoptics developed from strabismus therapy approaches pioneered by Javal (1896) and Worth (1903). The typical treatment sequence consists of

1. refractive correction
2. occlusion to eliminate amblyopia
3. antisuppression training
4. normalization of sensory fusion
5. normalization of fusional vergence ranges

This approach emphasizes the elimination of suppression and the sequential development of first-degree (simultaneous perception without fusion), second-degree (flat fusion of non-stereoscopic targets), and third-degree fusion (stereopsis), followed by the development of motor fusion ranges. Training usually takes place in instruments, particularly the major amblyoscope (Hugonnier and Clayette-Hugonnier 1969).

Although this model developed in relation to strabismus and amblyopia, it is commonly used in nonstrabismic binocular vision disorders as well. In treating patients with nonamblyopic visual skills disorders, proponents of this model commonly ignore monocular training and emphasize procedures to eliminate suppression and develop adequate sensory and motor fusion.

Simultaneous Perception Training

In patients with deep suppression arising from strabismus or anisometropia, simultaneous perception training is initiated to eliminate suppression before beginning fusional vergence range extension. However, deep suppression is unusual in visual skills or nearpoint stress–induced problems. As flexibility between accommodation and convergence improves with vision therapy, suppression generally disappears without need for specific antisuppression training. Only in unusual cases when suppression is deeply ingrained, as in binocular dysfunction caused by high anisometropia, is elimination of suppression a necessary prerequisite for the development of sensory and motor fusion.

Simultaneous perception procedures used to eliminate deep suppression include the following:

1. The Translid Binocular Interaction (TBI) trainer (Figure 15.9)
   Manufactured by Manico/Bloomington, the TBI consists of a pair of small light bulbs that provide intermittent photic stimulation

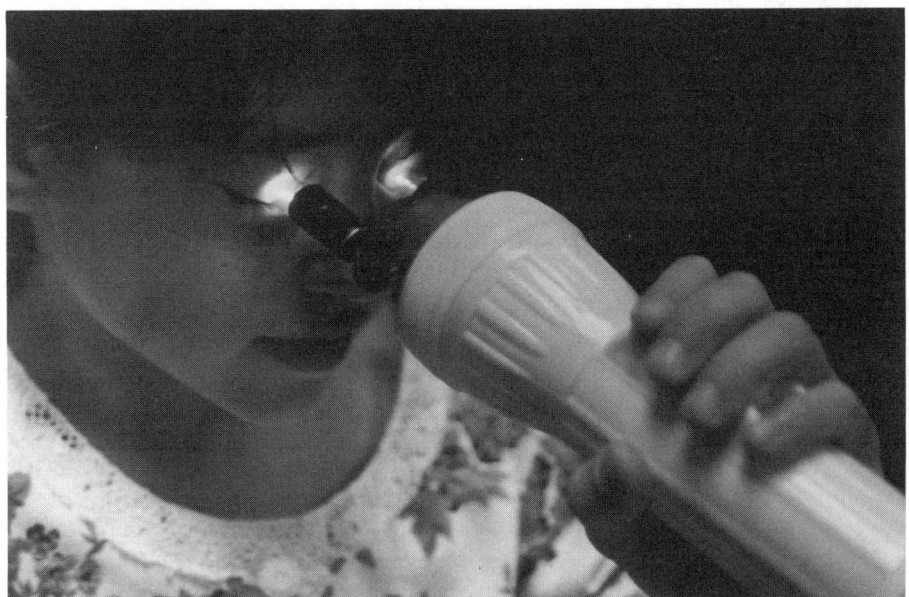

Figure 15.9 The TBI trainer.

at a rate of 7 to 10 cycles per second. The bulbs are placed over the patient's closed lids, and provide an intense flashing effect that is virtually impossible to suppress. Use of the TBI stimulates the two eyes so that suppression is often reduced on subsequent procedures (Allen 1966).

2. Monocular fixation in a binocular field

Both eyes are open in monocular fixation training in a binocular field, but filters are used to block the target from the dominant eye. For example, the patient may watch television, read letters on a Hart chart, or point at the numbers on an AN star covered with red plastic filter material. Red-green glasses are worn so that only the nondominant eye sees the television, Hart chart, or AN star, even though both eyes are open.

For patients with deep suppression, such procedures provide a useful transition between monocular and binocular training. In monocular training the dominant eye is occluded and therefore exerts no inhibitory influence on the nondominant eye. With both eyes open, the dominant eye inhibits the nondominant eye, resulting in suppression. Procedures that train monocular perception by the nondominant eye in a binocular field require that the nondominant eye maintain perception with both eyes open, despite the inhibitory influence exerted by the open dominant eye.

Both eyes are open in these procedures, but the central target is seen only by the nondominant eye. If it were to be suppressed, it would therefore seem to disappear. Such an experience would be inconsistent with reality; the patient knows that the target is really there. These procedures therefore serve as effective antisuppression agents. Numerous such procedures are described by Cohen (1981) and Colorado Vision Consultants (1985).

3. Red-green simultaneous perception

One half of a television screen, Hart chart, or AN star is covered with red and the other half with green filter material. The patient wears red-green glasses so that one half of the target is seen by each eye, and attempts to watch the television, read letters on the Hart chart, or touch the numbers on the AN star, while maintaining simultaneous perception of the two halves of the target. If one eye is suppressed, one half of the target is not seen.

4. Mirror transfer training

The patient views a target with the nonsuppressing eye at a distance of 5 or 6 feet while holding a small pocket mirror in front of the suppressing eye, inclined at an angle of 45 degrees to the nose. The mirror blocks the suppressing eye from seeing the fixation target. A penlight is held to the side of the mirror, pointing toward it at a distance of 2 feet, so that the penlight is seen in the mirror only by the suppressing eye (Figure 15.10). The patient adjusts the angle of

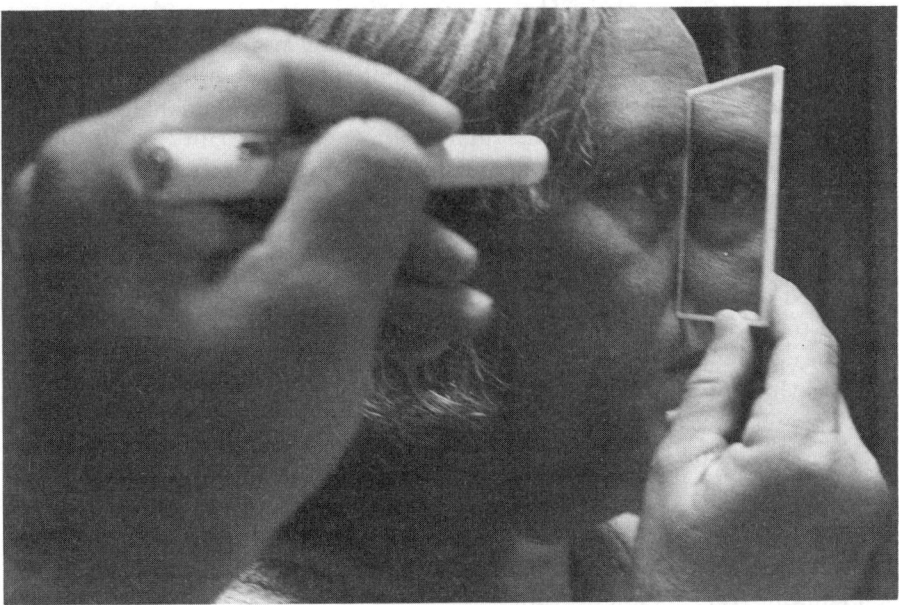

Figure 15.10   The mirror-light procedure is used for simultaneous perception training.

the mirror so as to superimpose the light onto the target without suppression.

5. Pola/Mirror training

The patient, wearing Polaroid glasses, views his face in a mirror and attempts to maintain perception of both eyes. Suppression of either eye causes the image of that eye to disappear.

Antisuppression training is facilitated by viewing dissimilar targets in orthoptic instruments far removed from the natural viewing conditions under which suppression is habituated; by increasing brightness and contrast of the target before the suppressing eye; by using large targets that cover the retinal periphery, as well as the fovea, providing stronger, harder-to-suppress stimuli; by flashing the targets, particularly before the suppressing eye; by asking the patient to blink rapidly, since intermittent stimulation is more difficult to suppress; and by shaking, oscillating, or moving the target before the suppressing eye to increase its attentional value. As simultaneous perception improves, training proceeds toward more natural viewing conditions; toward smaller targets that require bifoveal perception; and toward reduced flashing, blinking, target movement, and brightness differential, until the patient is able to maintain simultaneous perception under normal viewing conditions.

The effectiveness of any procedure is increased by an instructional set that informs the patient not only of the desired goals with the specific targets and instruments, but also of the changes in visual process that the patient must implement to achieve these goals. The patient who understands that the phenomena observed reflect that which is happening in the visual system can better learn to modify visual function. If, for example, the patient suppresses while viewing a red-green Hart chart through red-green glasses, he will be unable to simultaneously perceive both halves of the chart. It is well to explain that this occurs because the patient is ignoring the input from one eye. An instructional set that emphasizes the changes in the appearance of the target, such as telling the patient "Try not to let either color disappear," implies that the phenomenon is occurring externally, in the target. A more effective instructional set is: "When you see only the red or the green, it is because you are seeing with only one eye. What you need to do to see the red and green at the same time is to keep both eyes turned on. When you see one color disappear, increase your awareness of the eye that is shutting off. Try to feel both eyes, and to see with both at the same time." This instructional set informs the patient that the observed phenomena result from his visual function, and are subject to his control. Further, the instructional set informs the patient as to how to accomplish the desired goal (Birnbaum 1977).

Fusional Vergence Training

In traditional models based on Sheard's criterion and graphical analysis, heterophoria is viewed as a fusional demand (Hofstetter 1983). The primary goal of therapy is to increase the opposing fusional vergence to a level adequate to compensate high heterophoria. In treating patients with high exophoria, the emphasis is on base-out fusional vergence; in patients with high esophoria, base-in vergence is emphasized.

In the Skeffington model, fusional vergence training is performed not to compensate high heterophoria, but to develop flexibility between vergence and accommodation. High heterophoria and constricted vergence measures are each held to result from nearpoint stress and subsequent adaptation; fusional vergence training is performed to redress the adaptive skews that have occurred. In the Skeffington model, therefore, and in this author's approach, both base-in and base-out vergence ranges are usually trained, regardless of the direction of heterophoria (Birnbaum 1985a).

Disagreement exists as to whether fusional vergence training is more effective when base-in and base-out vergence are trained alternately, working in one direction until the limit is reached and then working in the other; or if sustained activity in one direction is more efficacious. Vaegan (1979) found that sustained effort in the direction being trained produced greater improvement than alternating movement in both directions. He concluded that sustained isometric activity in the desired direction is the optimal way to improve fusional vergence, particularly fusional divergence.

Nevertheless, many clinicians work both base-in and base-out to develop maximum vergence flexibility. Clinicians are concerned that training in one direction creates a tendency toward constriction of the opposite fusion range, particularly when training fusional convergence. However, Vaegan did not find a loss of the opposite function following sustained effort in one direction, and cites studies in which rapid alternation between extreme positions have led to decrements.

Since the goal is to develop adequate flexibility, it seems desirable to alternate base-in and base-out vergence training. However, Vaegan's research suggests that those patients who have particular difficulty in one direction may benefit from sustained activity in that direction in the early stages of training, until adequate function has developed.

Daum (1983) found a greater increase in fusional vergence with phasic training tasks such as prism flippers and the Aperture Rule Trainer (Bernell Corp.), which present rapid stepwise fusional vergence demands, than with tonic vergence tasks such as variable vectograms (Bernell Corp.) and convergence push-ups, which present smooth, slow changes in vergence demand. However, using computerized vergence therapy, Daum et al. (1987) found that slow training rates are more effective. In both studies, rapid and slow methods of increasing vergence demand each produced a substantial increase in fusional vergence. Sethi and North (1987) report that vergence adaptation develops most quickly when fusional vergence is trained by increasing vergence demand gradually in small increments that can be readily fused.

Grisham (1983) suggests the following sequence for fusional vergence training:

1. Smooth vergence, in which a disparity vergence stimulus is introduced slowly and smoothly, as with Risley prisms or variable vectograms.
2. Near-far tracking, in which the stimulus is moved smoothly toward and away from the patient, requiring accurate accommodative and vergence tracking. This may be performed with eccentric circles or variable vectograms, and may be combined with smooth vergence.
3. Step vergence, in which the patient views a target at a fixed distance while loose prisms or vectograms are used to introduce vergence stimuli in discrete steps of progressively increasing demand. The patient attempts to fuse and re-fuse as the prism is introduced and removed, to increase step vergence rate and improve velocity of the reflex fusion response.
4. Near-far jumps, in which the patient alternates between targets that present different fusional vergence demands at different distances. The patient may be asked to shift fixation from distance to a nearpoint variable vectogram as vergence demand is progressively increased, or to shift gaze back and forth between two pairs of variable vectograms that present differing base-in and base-out demands. Binocular lens flippers are used to increase demand for flexibility between vergence and accommodation.

Schor (1983) recommends different treatment strategies for vergence disorders depending on whether vergence adaptation is adequate. When vergence adaptation is adequate, as indicated clinically by flat forced vergence fixation disparity curves and the presence of little or no fixation disparity, therapy should emphasize training the fast-fusional vergence system, and therefore stress rapid, large fusional vergence responses to brief step presentations of lenses and prisms. Patients with reduced vergence adaptation ability, as indicated by a steep fixation disparity curve and the presence of significant fixation disparity, are best treated by training both the rapid fusional and adaptive vergence processes. Adaptive vergence is trained through procedures that emphasize slow, sustained responses to gradual increase in fusional vergence demand.

Wick (1985) reports that proximal vergence is an important contributor to the near-vergence response, and suggests that therapy procedures be organized so as to make optimal use of proximal vergence. For exophoric patients, he emphasizes (1) awareness of target distance; (2) use of large or medium-size targets that are moved closer to induce proximal vergence response; (3) use of maximum hand contact; and (4) accommodative accuracy and stereopsis. For esophoric patients he (1) avoids hand involvement; (2) deemphasizes accuracy of distance judgement, preferring to work in stereoscopes in which distance cannot be accurately judged; and (3) uses targets that are moved farther away as therapy is performed.

Norms and Goals

In training fusional vergence, the greatest possible blur, break, and recovery measures are sought in order to develop adequate flexibility between vergence and accommodation. On each procedure, the patient is encouraged to maintain fusion without blur or diplopia and to recover fusion as quickly as possible.

It is desirable to develop both fusional vergence amplitude and facility (Griffin 1982). With respect to fusional vergence amplitude, Morgan's norms (Morgan 1944a) and the OEP expecteds (Lesser 1969) are common goals (see Table 8.2).

For vergence facility, Griffin (1982) advocates as a goal that the patient be able to fuse over a range of 5^Δ base-in to 15^Δ base-out, at both distance and near, with a speed of 20 cpm. Rosner and Rosner (1990) indicate that the patient should be able to execute fusional vergence jumps from 6^Δ base-in to 12^Δ base-out at distance, and from 12^Δ base-in to 14^Δ base-out at near, and to achieve 60 cycles within 5 minutes.

Griffin (1982) points out that fusional vergence training should emphasize not only vergence facility and the amplitudes of blur, break, and recovery, but also the ability to sustain fusional vergence, to perform vergence tasks without discomfort, and to maintain fusional vergence without inducing fixation disparity. Fixation disparity tends to increase with increasing fusional vergence demand. Fusional vergence training is often effective in eliminating fixation disparity over a wide range of vergence demand. Griffin suggests as a goal that the fixation disparity–free range should be at least 75% of the blur-point range for a particular patient.

Instrument Versus Free-Space Training

Classical orthoptic and contemporary optometric approaches to vision therapy each use procedures performed in orthoptic instruments and procedures performed in free space. Classical orthoptics generally places greater emphasis on instrument training, while modern optometric approaches frequently place greater emphasis on training in free space.

The chief value of orthoptic instruments is that they provide an artificial environment in which flashers and oscillatory devices are used to create conditions far removed from everyday seeing; hence, such instruments facilitate the breakdown of perceptual adaptations such as deep suppression. However, visual skills learned in this artificial environment do not necessarily transfer readily to everyday seeing. In this author's view, free-space training is preferable in most cases of nonstrabismic vergence disorder, since deep suppression is the exception rather than the rule in such cases, and skills learned while standing and moving in free space are more likely to transfer to daily seeing.

Sequencing Procedures: Brock-Flax Model

Large stereoscopic targets that stimulate the retinal periphery constitute powerful fusional stimuli (Burian 1941, 1947; Kertesz 1981, 1982). Brock pioneered in the clinical use of such targets in strabismus therapy (Birnbaum 1981). Flax (1963b, 1968) notes that intermittent exotropes align their eyes in response to stereo cues, and advocates a treatment strategy using large stereoscopic targets to generate alignment. The patient is then trained to maintain alignment as stereoscopic cues are progressively reduced, until he or she can align with flat fusion targets with no stereo cues, and even maintain alignment in the absence of fusion (Cooper 1977).

As applied to nonstrabismic binocular vision disorders, the Brock-Flax model emphasizes the use of large stereoscopic targets that are strong stimuli for fusion. Treatment generally begins in free space, rather than enclosed instruments. As fusion improves, progressively smaller targets are used that present less stereopsis. Eventually the patient is expected to demonstrate adequate sensory and motor fusion even in instruments that present artificial demands and mismatches between perceived and actual target location. The ultimate goal is for the patient to sustain good binocular function even when the stimulus for fusion is relatively weak, as in reading small print on a two-dimensional page.

The binocular treatment sequence of the Flax-Brock model is virtually opposite that of traditional orthoptics. In classical orthoptics, treatment begins with first-degree fusion (simultaneous perception) and proceeds to second-degree (flat fusion) and third-degree fusion (stereopsis), primarily in orthoptic instruments. The Brock-Flax sequence, in contrast, begins with the use of large stereoscopic targets that serve as strong stimuli for fusion (usually in real space), and proceeds from third-degree to second-degree to first-degree fusion, developing the ability to maintain adequate binocular function as the strength of the stimulus for fusion decreases.

In this author's experience, the classical orthoptic approach is most effective in constant strabismus and in nonstrabismic patients with deep suppression secondary to high anisometropia or other sensory obstacle to fusion. The Brock-Flax approach has proved highly effective in the management of the great majority of functional, nonstrabismic binocular vision disorders in which there is no serious sensory impediment to fusion.

Training with Polaroid Vectograms

Polaroid vectograms, manufactured by Stereo Optical Co. and distributed by Bernell Corp., are a series of targets that differ considerably as to the strength of stimulus for fusion that they provide. These targets may thus be used in accord with the dictates of the Flax-Brock sequence. The Topper vectogram (which is no longer manufactured) and the Clown vectogram are large stereoscopic targets that stimulate peripheral as well as central retina, and which present considerable contour and textural variation. These vectograms thus provide strong stimuli for fusion. This author uses such targets in the early phase of fusional vergence training, and then seeks to train the patient to maintain fusional vergence ranges even when weaker stimuli for fusion such as the Mother Goose, Spirangle, and Quoits vectograms are used. The goal is to develop such efficient binocular function that the patient can maintain fusional vergence even when stimuli for fusion are weak.

Therapy generally begins with smooth vergence training. Step vergence and BOP-BIM demands are added as performance improves. Ultimately information-processing tasks and distractors are incorporated to integrate and automate vergence function.

Topper Polaroid Vectogram

Topper (see Figure 12.3) serves as a useful initial target. It is large, covers a wide retinal area, provides considerable detail and contour, and incorporates variations in disparity that create a stereoscopic texture. Each of these attributes enhances its effectiveness in creating a strong fusion lock. Consequently, most patients who demonstrate constricted prism vergence measures in phorometric tests (where target material consists of two-dimensional small print, which provides a weaker stimulus for fusion) will perform considerably better when tested and trained with the Topper vectogram.

In training fusion ranges with Topper, the first stage is to develop smooth vergence. The patient seeks to maintain clear, single vision as the targets are disparated base-out and base-in. The goal is to maximize motor fusion range for each patient, rather than to reach some arbitrary or normative value. In general, it is desirable (if possible) that patients reach at least 21 on the base-out scale and G on the base-in scale. Since each number and each letter represent 2^Δ at a 16-inch working distance, these values correspond to 42^Δ base-out and 14^Δ base-in, respectively. Performance with vectograms is often improved if the patient is permitted to disparate the targets himself, since he can control the speed and slow down when the task becomes difficult.

When performance is adequate, the task is changed from a smooth vergence to a jump vergence demand. Jump vergence training is not incorporated until smooth vergence ranges are adequate, since recovery of fusion during jump vergence training is more difficult.

In jump vergence training, the patient is instructed to disparate the vectograms in small increments, to look across the room, and then to look back at Topper and attempt to re-fuse. The patient should note where Topper is localized in space (how close or how far away), so that he knows where to look when he refixates.

An alternative method for jump vergence training is to place pairs of vectograms in the upper and lower units of the Polachrome Orthoptor. The patient disparates the upper-set base-in and the lower-set base-out, shifting gaze from one to the other until maximum base-in and base-out fusional vergence is achieved. This method is more demanding, since it requires a jump from high base-out to high base-in.

Some patients note a blur before the targets double, especially when working base-out. The presence of blur indicates that the limit of fusional convergence (convergence free of accommodation) has been reached. The patient should be instructed not to continue past the blur, but to stop when the target blurs or doubles, whichever comes first, and to attempt to expand the range of clear, single binocular vision.

Topper and SILO

The SILO phenomenon may be elicited whenever lenses, prisms, or target disparation cause an object to seem closer or farther than its actual physical location in space. When Topper is disparated base-out, the patient must converge to maintain fusion. The retinal input is the same as if there were a single Topper, closer and smaller than the actual vectograms (see Figure 12.4). As the targets are disparated base-in, the visual input is as if stimulation were coming from a single Topper, larger and farther away than the actual targets (see Figure 12.5). This perceptual phenomenon of small-in, large-out or SILO is expected when individuals respond on the basis of current visual input. The experience of SILO is contrary to that of everyday experience, in which objects appear smaller as they recede into the distance and larger as they move closer to the observer. Consequently, when Topper appears to become smaller as it is disparated base-out, some individuals perceive it as simultaneously moving away (small-out, large-in or SOLI). Some patients give a different SOLI response, perceiving spatial localization accurately, but distorting size to report that the target is larger and closer.

Topper presents a conflict between retinal input and daily experience. The

SOLI responder is typically a logical, analytical individual who interprets on the basis of that which he expects or thinks should be happening, rather than on the basis of current visual input.

Correct spatial localization with Topper facilitates the development of improved fusional vergence. As Topper is disparated base-out, the SILO responder perceives the target as moving closer. An effective instructional set is to inform the patient to "pull your eyes in to look closer." The patient should be told that Topper will appear single as long as he keeps looking closer; when Topper appears to double, it is because he is no longer looking close enough. The localization of Topper as closer and the awareness of the need to look closer facilitate the development of base-out fusional vergence range. When disparating base-in, the patient is asked to look farther away as the target is perceived to move away, and again the match between perceived distance and induced vergence facilitates fusional vergence development.

The typical SOLI responder, in contrast, perceives Topper as moving away as it is disparated base-out. As a result, the preceding instructional set cannot be used. Base-out stimulation requires that the SOLI responder make a convergence movement in response to a target that he perceives as moving away. Under such conditions, one may mechanically build vergence ranges, but is unlikely to create the desired internal feelings of convergence and divergence. Skills developed are less likely to be well integrated into daily performance. Consequently, it is desirable to elicit a SILO response when possible.

The most effective method to elicit SILO in a SOLI responder is to demonstrate the inconsistency between the patient's SOLI response and his actual spatial localization. The patient with visual skills disorder usually has adequate stereopsis, and will localize the target accurately with a pointer. As the target is disparated base-out, the patient generally moves the pointer to localize closer in space than the actual vectograms; as the target is disparated back toward the zero position, the patient moves the pointer farther away. This is inconsistent with the verbalized SOLI response that, as the target is disparated base-in, it moves closer. Demonstration of this inconsistency is usually sufficient to elicit a SILO response.

Mother Goose and Spirangle Vectograms

The Mother Goose (Figure 15.11) and Spirangle (Figure 15.12) vectograms present targets that are smaller than Topper and constitute weaker fusional stimuli. The Mother Goose vectogram targets are larger, stronger stimuli than those of the Spirangle, so the usual sequence is to work first with Topper, to introduce the Mother Goose vectogram when ranges are adequate with Topper, and to work with the Spirangle when adequate ranges are achieved with the Mother Goose vectogram.

The Mother Goose and Spirangle vectograms each present internal jump vergence demands. In working with the Mother Goose vectogram, the patient is asked to look from one target to another; with the Spirangle, the patient locates

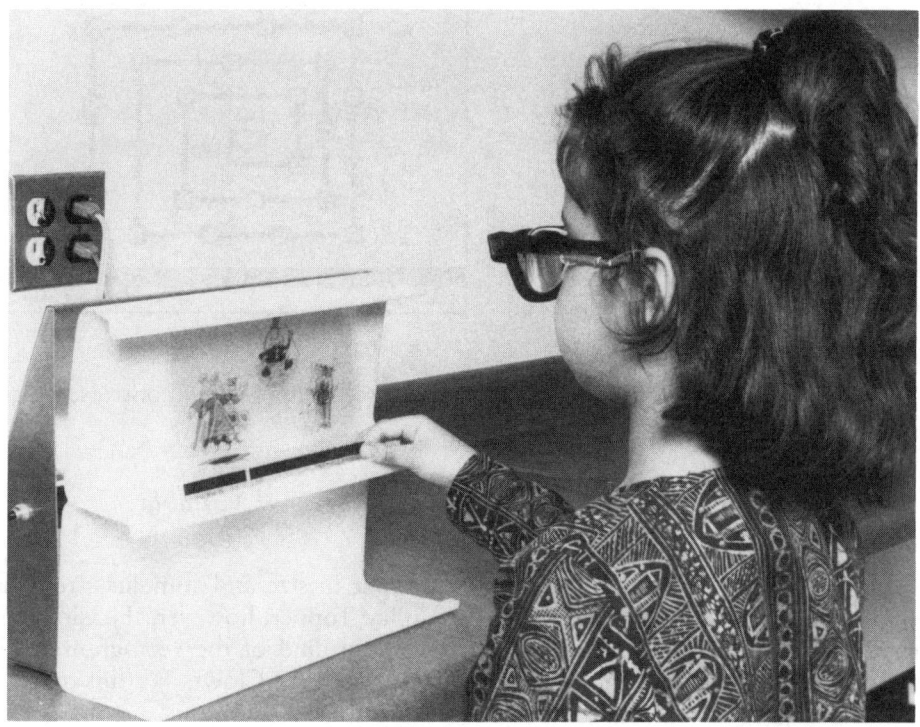

A

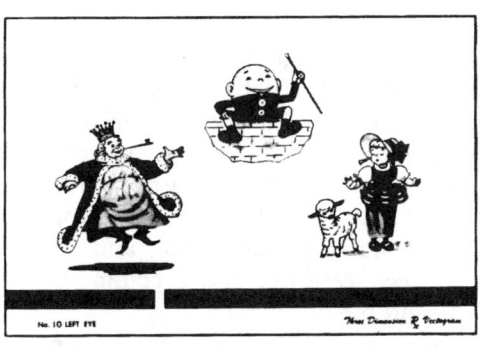

B

Figure 15.11 Mother Goose vectogram. *A*, Patient viewing Mother Goose vectogram in the polachrome orthopter. *B*, Left eye view. (Photo courtesy of Bernell Corp.)

the letters of the alphabet around the Spirangle, or looks from one to the other of the squares, which each contain three rows of letters. When performance is adequate with each vectogram, more difficult jump vergence demands are incorporated, looking away at the wall and then recovering fusion when gaze is shifted back to the vectogram; or shifting back and forth between two pairs of vectograms, one of which is disparated base-in and the other base-out. The Mother

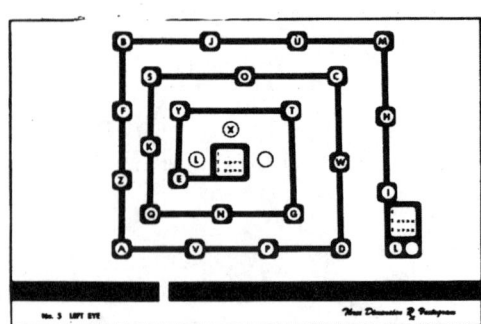

Figure 15.12 Spirangle vectogram, left eye view. (Photo courtesy Bernell Corp.)

Goose and Spirangle vectograms each provide useful suppression controls, which should be monitored.

Clown, Figure 8, Quoits, Chicago Skyline, and Variable Random Dot Vectograms

The Clown vectogram is similar to Topper in size and stimulus strength, and is often used interchangeably with it. Unlike Topper, however, the Clown is printed in the background rather than the foreground of the vectogram. This tends to make spatial localization more difficult with the Clown. For this reason, this author prefers to use the Topper vectogram.

The Figure 8 is a nonvariable vectogram that presents a large "8" in considerable stereoscopic depth. The patient scans the "8," localizing with a pointer and converging and diverging as the closest and farthest parts of the target are fixated. The letters of the alphabet are scattered throughout the vectogram and present considerable variation in vergence demand and perceived depth. Unlike variable vectograms such as Topper in which changes in localization are perceived through time as the targets are disparated, the Figure 8 presents substantial variation in localization all at once. It is often easier for patients to appreciate depth and learn to localize closer or farther than the plane of the vectogram when the Figure 8 is used. Although the vectogram is nonvariable and cannot be disparated, demands for flexibility between vergence and accommodation may be heightened through the use of lens and prism flippers.

The Quoits vectogram presents relatively little fusion lock and is hence a weak stimulus for fusion. It may be used after the other vectograms, to develop the ability to sustain fusional vergence even in the presence of weak stimuli.

The Quoits vectogram is often useful for patients who give persistent SOLI responses. Since there is little background to obscure the movement, correct spatial localization is more readily observed as the Quoits target floats toward and away from the observer.

The Chicago Skyline and Airplane vectogram incorporates jump vergence training at a very high level of demand. As the targets are disparated, base-in and base-out fusional vergence demands are induced in opposite directions for the Skyline and for the Airplane. This jump vergence demand makes performance quite difficult, and is best introduced in the later stages of therapy.

Variable random dot vectograms (Synthetic Optics, Bernell Corp.) are useful in developing the ability to sustain fusion, since perception of the figure is lost whenever fusion is not maintained.

Increasing Vergence Demands

In working with Polaroid vectograms, step vergence demands may be introduced through the use of flippers (Bernell Corp., GTVT) made up with varying amounts of base-in and base-out prism, or through the use of Polaroid viewers in which the direction of polarization is reversed in the top and bottom halves so that the demand changes from base-out to base-in as the patient alternately views through the top and bottom halves.

BOP/BIM training, in which *base-out* prism is combined with *plus* (BOP), and *base-in* prism is combined with *minus* (BIM), is performed to increase the demand for flexibility between vergence and accommodation. Plus lenses inhibit accommodation and accommodative convergence and make base-out prism–induced convergence more difficult; minus lenses stimulate accommodation and associated accommodative convergence, and hence make base-in prism–induced fusional divergence more difficult. BOP-BIM demands may be incorporated by combining lens and prism flippers, or by using lens flippers as the patient disparates base-out and base-in. Since BOP-BIM training creates increased demands for flexibility between vergence and accommodation, it should not be introduced until both smooth vergence and jump vergence performance are adequate.

Vectogram Training at Distance

Performance with vectograms is usually better at near than at distance, because of the greater angular size of the target and the heightened involvement that results from tactual manipulation at near. Polaroid vectogram training is therefore usually begun at near and extended to far as performance improves, even in cases in which the oculomotor imbalance is greater at near than at far.

The Brock Stereo-Motivator (used with the Keystone Overhead Projector) and the Stereo Project-Orthopter are instruments that use red-green anaglyph and Polaroid vectogram material, respectively, for distance vergence training. However, neither of these instruments is currently manufactured.

The most convenient currently available method of distance stereoprojection is to use Polaroid vectograms with a conventional overhead projector, projecting onto an aluminized screen, which will not alter the polarization of the incident light. A wall painted with aluminum reflectant paint may be used for this purpose. The vectograms, placed in a transparent plastic vectogram holder, can be readily disparated when placed on the table of the overhead projector. Dowel sticks are used to monitor spatial localization when training at distance.

Developing Automaticity

While working on fusional vergence procedures, the patient's attention is fully directed to the visual task. However, in everyday vision, the patient cannot concentrate solely on maintaining clear, single binocular vision; to do so would interfere with efficient performance of the task at hand. It is therefore desirable to automate fusion ability so that performance can be maintained during everyday tasks that impose their own demands for attention and information-processing.

To achieve such automaticity it is appropriate, once performance is adequate, to introduce other information-processing demands, movement activities, distractions, and confounding conditions. The patient may be asked to carry on a conversation while working with Polaroid vectograms; to maintain vergence while the vectograms are moved into different fields of gaze; to maintain fusional vergence while moving the shoulders and upper body, while moving the head up and down or left and right, while walking back and forth, while maintaining or shifting balance on a balance board, or while bouncing on a trampoline; and to look back and forth from a hand-held vectogram that is disparated base-in to a base-out disparated vectogram projected to distance, creating a paradoxical localization effect. The goal is to so habituate fusion that performance is automatic.

Polaroid Versus Anaglyph Materials

Polaroid vectograms are expensive to manufacture and curl, fade, and scratch easily. As a result, use of red-green anaglyphs instead of Polaroid vectograms has increased. However, red-green anaglyphs may be less effective in fusion training for several reasons:

1. Anaglyphs frequently do not filter out perfectly and are more prone to ghost images, especially when printed in high contrast shades. They are therefore usually printed in light, subdued colors that provide lower contrast, and serve as weak stimuli for fusion.
2. Unequal light transmission by the red-green filters creates inequality in brightness of the stimuli to the two eyes, which may exacerbate suppression (Bogdanovich et al. 1986).
3. While Polaroid vectograms such as Topper are printed so that the entire figure serves as a fusion target, red-green anaglyphs are printed in outline only. Anaglyphs therefore stimulate less retinal area and present weaker stimuli for fusion.
4. The variety of vectograms available makes the use of a gross-to-fine training sequence possible. Anaglyph materials do not lend themselves to such sequencing.

Since red-green anaglyph materials are weak stimuli for fusion and present brightness differences that may interfere with fusion, this author uses them as high demand targets toward the end of a fusional vergence training sequence, not as substitutes for Polaroid vectograms. Anaglyphs are also useful as inexpensive home-training materials.

Computer Vergence Training

Computers are useful for fusional vergence training because they generate high interest and motivation, and because they permit a broad variety of procedures (Somers et al. 1984; Press 1987–88; Cooper 1988). Commercially available computer packages include the Computer Orthopter (RC Instruments, Inc.) developed by Jeffrey Cooper, O.D.; the OPTI-MUM System (Learning Frontiers, Inc.) developed by William Ludlam, O.D.; Vergence 64, designed by and available from Michael Tyner, O.D.; and EyeTrix (VTC Enterprises), designed by William Somers, O.D.

Computer programs permit the presentation of large and small flat fusion, contoured and random dot stereopsis targets in both smooth and jump vergence formats. A large variety of targets and procedures are available, permitting sequencing from gross to fine targets and from smooth to jump vergence demands.

Brock String

The Brock string consists of a 10-foot length of string with movable beads at different fixation distances along the string. The patient holds one end to his nose; the other end is affixed to the wall or doorknob (Figure 15.13). As the

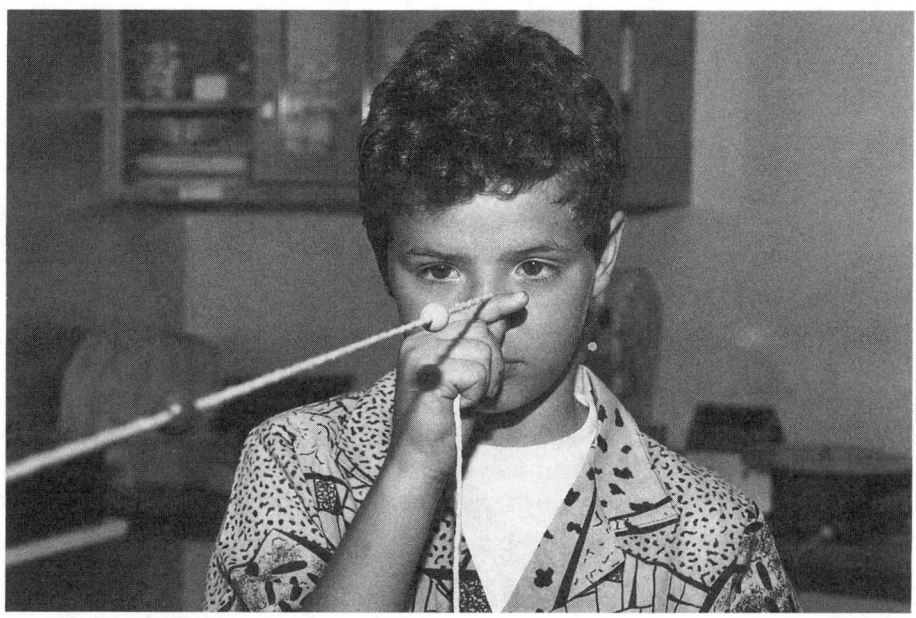

Figure 15.13 Brock string.

patient shifts fixation from one bead to another, the strings, seen in physiological diplopia, appear to cross at the fixation point, making an X when a near bead is fixated or a V when the bead at the end of the string is fixated.

The Brock string is extremely useful because it provides feedback as to accuracy of binocular fixation. The point at which the patient sees the strings cross is that at which the eyes are actually pointing. When the strings cross beyond the point of regard, the eyes are underconverged; when the strings cross closer than the bead being fixated, the eyes are overconverged.

When a patient demonstrates underconvergence, or exophoric posture, performance is aided by urging him to look closer, to pull the eyes in, to look hard, or to touch the near bead. When the patient shows overconvergence, or esophoric posture, performance is aided by asking him to relax, look easy, look farther away, and to imagine that the target is transparent and to look through it. Asking the patient to be more aware of peripheral vision also helps to reduce overconvergence, as does the use of visual imagery techniques in which the patient is asked to visualize a faraway scene (Birnbaum 1978, 1990). Standing in a relaxed, well-balanced posture with feet apart may facilitate relaxation and reduce esophoric posture.

When suppression is present so that the patient sees only one string, it is eliminated by creating viewing conditions that are far removed from habitual daily seeing. Suppression usually disappears if the patient wears red-green glasses. Cover first one eye and then the other, demonstrating the presence of a red string and a green string, and the patient will usually perceive both strings when the cover is removed. Most patients then retain the perception of two strings even after the red-green glasses are removed. Twanging the string to create movement, or placing flashing lights such as the bulbs of the TBI Trainer to the side of each eye, are also effective antisuppression procedures.

The Brock string is generally initiated as a jump vergence procedure in which the patient shifts fixation from one bead to another. The patient who has difficulty with jump fixation shifts may hold the near bead and slowly move it nearer and farther to first develop smooth vergence ability. As performance improves, demands are increased. Prism and lens flippers are added to develop flexibility between vergence and accommodation.

The "bug on the string" variation is used to develop greater control over vergence function. The patient is asked to imagine a ladybug at the end of the string, creeping toward him; to follow it slowly and smoothly, watching the crossing of the strings move closer as fixation shifts closer; to follow the bug up to a point 1 inch from the nose, and maintain fixation for 5 seconds; and finally, to follow the imaginary bug as it moves away along the string. The emphasis is on the quality of movement, which should be slow and smooth. Voluntary vergence in the absence of a real fixation target requires a high level of control.

The Brock string procedure is easily adapted for training fusion in various directions of gaze by having the patient turn the face to the left, right, up, or down while fixating the beads. Training in different directions of gaze is more demanding, because it imposes a requirement for asymmetric convergence. Such training is especially useful in the presence of noncomitancy.

The patient working with the Brock string should be encouraged to use peripheral vision to maintain awareness of the strings while fixating the bead. Patients with inadequate central-peripheral organization frequently look closer or farther to see the strings when asked where they cross; this causes a change in location of the perceived X. Brock string training thus facilitates improvement in visual attention and central-peripheral organization as well as fusion.

The Brock string may be used to aid performance on other procedures. For example, the patient who has difficulty disparating Topper base-out may work on the Brock string to develop awareness of the feeling tones associated with convergence. Afterwards the patient again works with Topper, and is asked to maintain the same feeling of looking closer; often, performance improves.

Other Fusional Vergence Procedures

When the patient can perform at adequate levels with Polaroid vectograms and with Brock string, training continues using other procedures to generalize performance and to develop the ability to maintain fusional vergence even when the stimulus for fusion is weak. A broad variety of procedures are commonly used, including red-green lustre training with anaglyph glasses and a flashlight; the Worth four-dot flashlight; Bagolini striated glasses; Pigeon-Cantonnet stereoscope; anaglyph training; eccentric circles and red-green "life saver" cards; the Aperture Rule Trainer; cheiroscopic tracing; and instruments such as the rotoscope, prism reader, and Keystone Telebinocular, among others.

In red-green lustre training, the patient views a flashlight while wearing anaglyph glasses. The size of the flashlight may be varied (or modified with masking tape) to increase or decrease the strength of stimulus. The desired response is for the patient to perceive a single light, with red and green blended together, a lustre response. The patient begins at the easiest distance for fusion, and moves toward and away from the light until he can maintain fusion at all distances. As performance improves, a Worth four-dot flashlight is substituted, presenting smaller targets that constitute weaker stimuli for fusion. Fusion training in real space may be similarly performed using Bagolini striated glasses. With each of these procedures, as well as while watching television or performing pursuit or saccadic training, fusional vergence demand may be increased through use of a prism bar, loose prisms, and prism or lens flippers, available from Bernell, GTVT, OEP, and Pacific Prisms. When performance is adequate, demand for step vergence is increased by having the patient cover one eye, uncover, and re-fuse the target.

The Variable Prismatic Stereoscope/Cheiroscope (Bernell Corp.) (Figure 15.14) is an inexpensive Pigeon-Cantonnet stereoscope that is used to expand base-out and base-in fusional vergence ranges. Transparent and opaque eccentric circles and red-green "life savers" cards, available from Bernell Corp., OEP, and

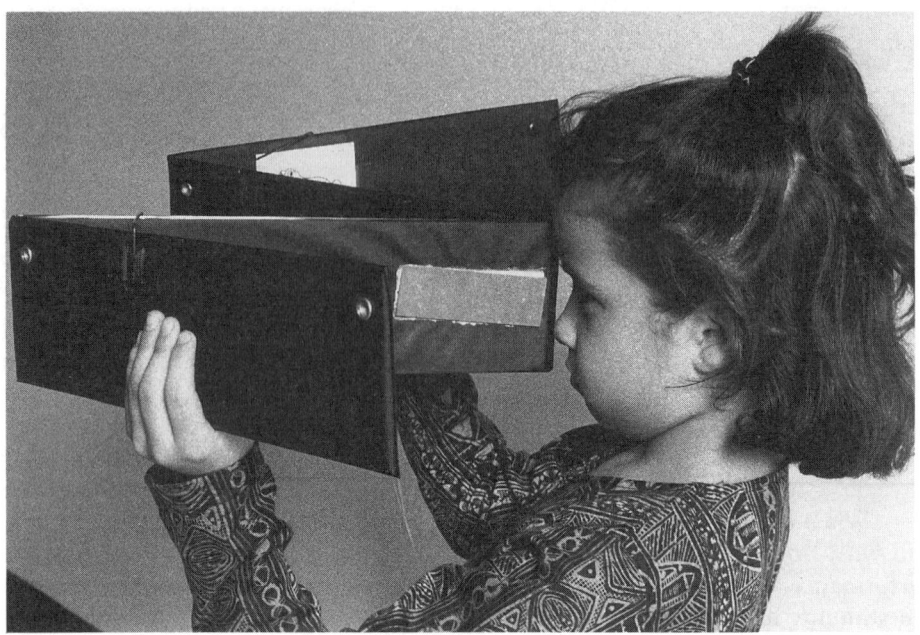

Figure 15.14 Variable prismatic stereoscope/cheiroscope.

Mast/Keystone, are used to train fusional vergence in free space. Opaque cards are used for base-out training (Figure 15.15). Transparent cards are used for base-in training, as they permit the feeling of looking beyond the plane of the target (Figure 15.16).

The Aperture Rule Trainer (Figure 15.17), available from Bernell Corp., is less artificial than many other instruments, since it is not fully enclosed and does not use lenses to simulate optical infinity. The Aperture Rule presents a range of demand from 30^Δ base-out to 30^Δ base-in, which may be increased with prism and lens flippers. As the patient views each target, the demand is to fuse, to sustain fusion, and then to look away and recover fusion.

The A.O. Wottring Rotoscope combines vergence range extension training with oculomotor rotations while following a moving target. The Prism Reader, a Controlled Reader with Risley prism head, allows for the introduction of prism vergence demand while the patient reads rows of print projected via a moving filmstrip. Both instruments are widely used, although neither has been manufactured for many years.

Brewster Stereoscope Training

Brewster stereoscope instruments such as the Keystone Telebinocular (Mast/Keystone) and the Bernell-O-Scope (Bernell Corp.) create a mismatch between visual and motor inputs. The targets are localized at optical infinity through

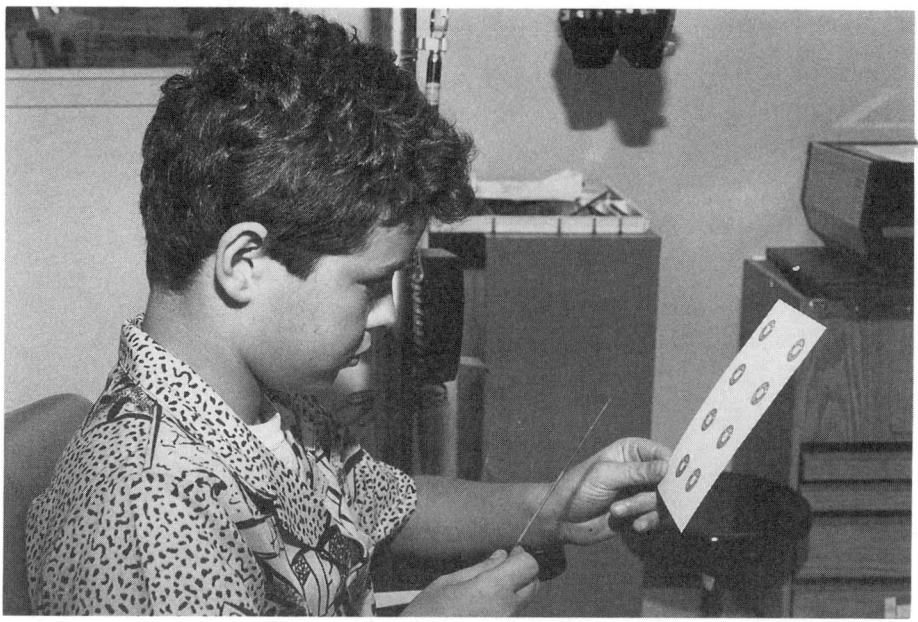

Figure 15.15 Base-out fusion training with the opaque red-green life savers card.

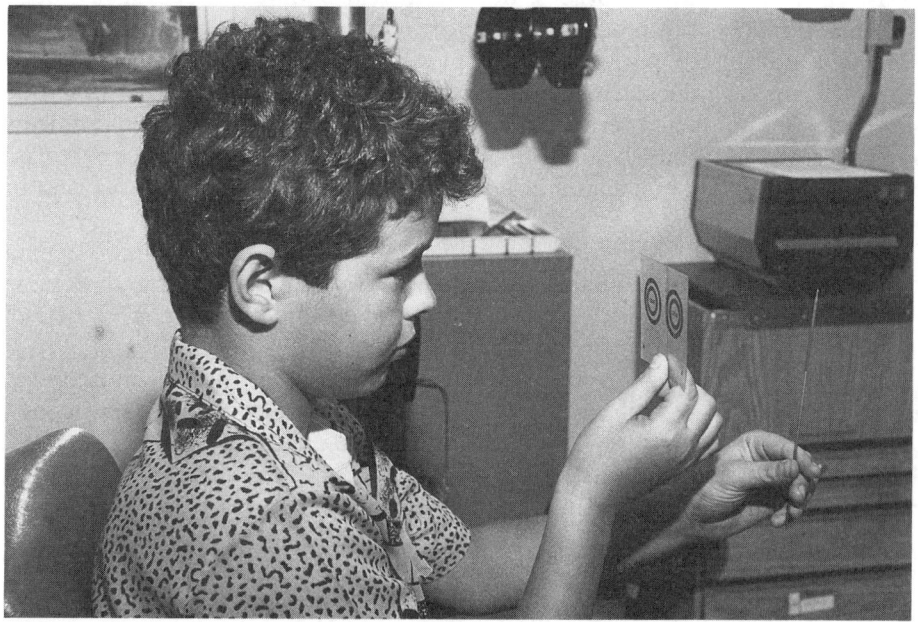

Figure 15.16 Base-in fusion training with transparent eccentric circles cards.

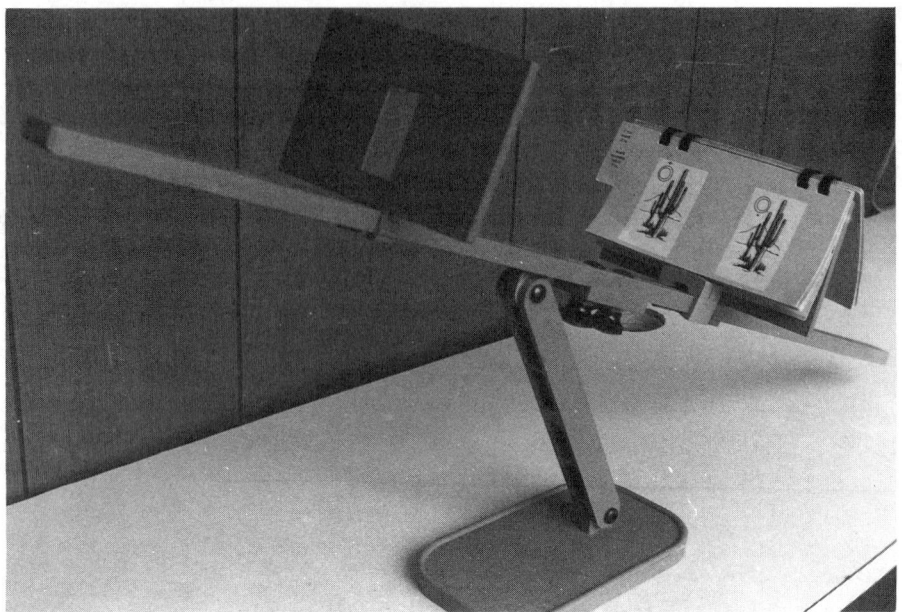

Figure 15.17 Aperture Rule Trainer.

the use of +5.00 D spheroprisms, but are in reality only 8 inches away. Such instruments induce proximal convergence and are therefore particularly demanding for esophoric patients. Overconvergence is exacerbated by the use of pointer techniques that increase kinesthetic awareness of proximity, and by the use of stereograms that present fine detail. This author uses such instruments toward the end of visual skills therapy, to develop such a high level of performance that the patient can maintain base-in vergence despite these visual-motor mismatch conditions.

Among the most popular stereograms are the AN, BU, EC, and Stepping Stones to Fusion series, available through Mast/Keystone and designed for use with the Keystone Telebinocular. Comparable slides are available from Bernell Corp. for use with the Bernell-O-Scope.

The AN series consists of 86 stereograms, including cards with scattered numbers or letters throughout the background, for use with pointers; stereoscopic scenic backgrounds with suppression controls; and jump vergence targets. The AN 1 through AN 4 stereograms present 12-pointed stars with numbers, and are commonly used for fusion and antisuppression training. The patient holds a pointer in each hand and touches corresponding points on the targets simultaneously, while maintaining awareness of both pointers.

The BU series, designed by Brock to foster sequential development of binocularity, consists of 38 cards that present stimuli for binocular luster and peripheral fusion, followed by gradually increasing demand for macular fusion and stereopsis. The EC Base-Out and EC Base-In series each contain 52 stereograms that present stereoscopic and jump vergence targets with increasing base-out and base-in fusion demand.

The Stepping Stones to Fusion are a series of split cards that can be disparated both base-in and base-out (Figure 15.18). With these cards, as with any of the other stereograms, demand for base-in vergence is increased by tromboning the slide holder toward the patient. This simultaneously increases both the stimulus to accommodation (which tends to cause increased accommodative convergence) and the demand for fusional divergence.

A great variety of stereograms exists, providing varied demand in terms of base-in and base-out fusion, step vergence increments, stereopsis, peripheral and central fusion, and lustre (Laxer et al. 1991). It is not necessary that the clinician use or own large numbers of stereograms, or entire series. A small, well-selected collection incorporating a variety of fusion demands is adequate.

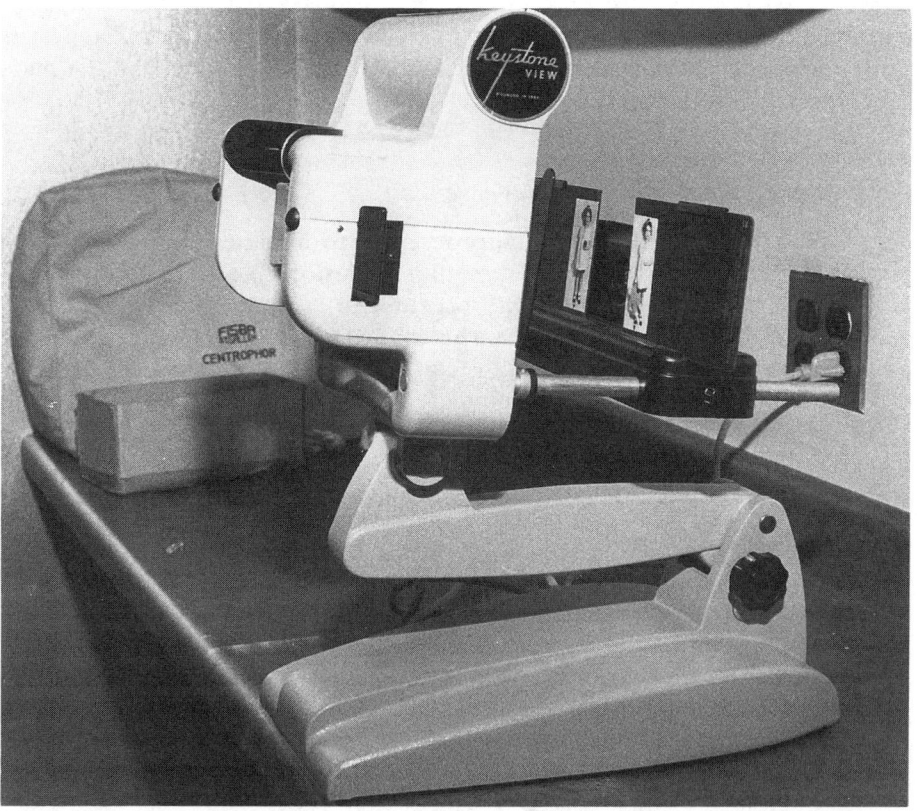

Figure 15.18 Stepping Stones to Fusion split cards in the Keystone Telebinocular.

Cheiroscopic Tracing

In cheiroscopic tracing, the patient views a target placed before one eye in either the Correct-Eye-Scope (Mast/Keystone) or the Bernell-O-Scope (Bernell Corp.). The patient holds a pencil before the other eye and begins to trace the picture seen by the fixing eye. Initially there is no fusion, since the target is seen by one eye only. Consequently, any oculomotor imbalance or instability tends to manifest, producing esophoric or exophoric posture as the patient traces. The visual-motor mismatch intrinsic to the Brewster stereoscope tends to induce proximal convergence, and esophoric posture is common (see Figure 12.10). Many patients show a progressive esophoric shift as the tracing is performed (see Figure 3.2) (Birnbaum 1985b).

The task demand is to maintain simultaneous perception of the target and the pencil, without suppression; to maintain approximate orthophoric posture; and to maintain postural stability as the tracing is performed. This is highly demanding, since there is no fusion lock when the tracing is begun and a strong tendency toward proximal convergence must be overcome. Shifts in position of the tracing as performance proceeds provide feedback regarding adequacy of performance. If the individual begins to overconverge, the tracing will appear to shift inward, and the patient must relax and attempt to look beyond the plane of regard to restore orthophoric posture.

Training Base-In Fusional Vergence

Base-in fusional vergence is more resistant to modification than base-out (Morgan 1944b), perhaps because attention and effort to fuse tend to generate overconvergence (Birnbaum 1984). Procedures to facilitate the development of base-in fusion include the use of transparent red-green life-savers cards, transparent eccentric circles, and Polaroid vectograms housed in hand-held transparent plastic holders, which allow the patient to more readily experience the feeling of looking through the target. The Quoits vectogram is particularly useful, since it provides little figure and is easy to look through.

The Plateau spiral (Figure 15.19), a black-and-white spiral affixed to a rotator, may be used to facilitate base-in vergence. Although the spiral is two-dimensional, a marked funnelling-away effect is produced when it is rotated clockwise. Watching the spiral funnel away helps to create a feeling of looking far, which may facilitate performance on subsequent base-in fusion tasks.

Forrest (1981) indicates that patients with persistent base-in difficulty frequently have poor visual imagery. Imagery ability aids in the development of base-in fusion. The ability to diverge beyond the plane of regard requires an ability to visualize, to imagine looking at something as if it were farther away than one knows it to be.

Imagery procedures in which the patient visualizes near or distant objects have been used to develop convergence and divergence, respectively (Cantonnet

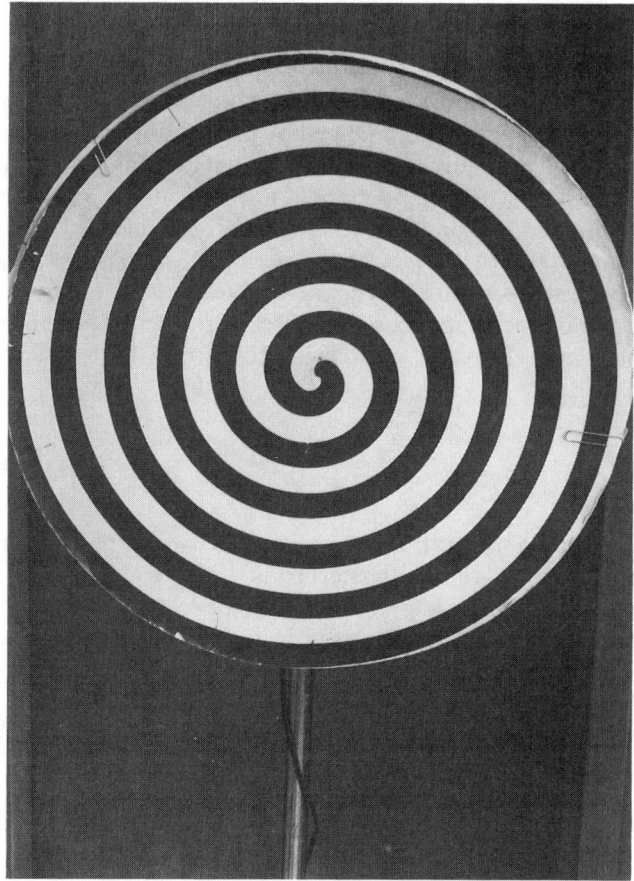

Figure 15.19 Plateau spiral.

and Filliozat 1934). Birnbaum (1978, 1990) describes an imagery/relaxation procedure to aid in expanding base-in vergence. The patient is seated in front of an instrument such as the Aperture Rule. The target is set at a base-in level just beyond that which he can achieve. The patient is asked to visualize a large wilderness lake, miles long, on a bright, sunny day; to see the ripples on the water and the sun glistening and reflecting off the ripples; to picture himself sitting in a clearing on one side of the lake; and to physically relax, feel the warmth of the sun on his body, and be aware of a wave of relaxation, beginning in the feet and moving up through the body, letting the feet, legs, body, shoulders, arms, hands, neck, jaw, and eyes relax; to look out across the lake at the mountains, trees, or sailboats miles away on the far side of the lake; and to keep the feeling of looking far away, miles across the lake, when he opens his eyes. Many patients achieve greater base-in vergence immediately upon opening the eyes. Visualization of a far away object facilitates the process of looking beyond the plane of regard, which is fundamental to base-in vergence.

When patients exert considerable effort to achieve during a vision therapy procedure, sympathetic activation induced by intense application may exacerbate overconvergence and interfere with ability to achieve base-in fusion (Birnbaum 1984; Forrest 1988). Instructing the patient to physically relax; to reduce tension in the shoulders, upper back, neck, and jaw; to breathe deeply; to smile; to "look easy"; and to maintain awareness of the periphery while performing the task; often aid the patient to localize vergence beyond the plane of regard. Practice with diaphragmatic breathing, progressive relaxation, and peripheral awareness procedures may aid relaxation and facilitate base-in performance (Birnbaum 1990).

Peripheral Awareness

During intense concentration, there is a narrowing of attention with constriction of peripheral awareness (Easterbrook 1959; Kahneman 1973). Heightened awareness of the periphery is characteristic of relaxed, passive concentration. Peripheral awareness procedures are used to foster a more relaxed attitude with less intense concentration, in order to reduce stress activation (Forrest 1976; Birnbaum 1978, 1990; Marrone 1991).

Peripheral awareness may be emphasized during any pursuit, saccadic, accommodative, or fusional vergence procedure. In performing thumb pursuits, for example, the patient is asked to maintain awareness of the surround as he moves his arm in a circle and fixates the thumb.

Specific additional peripheral awareness procedures include the following:

1. Binasal occlusion

    Binasal occluders are applied to Visitor's Specs, industrial safety fit-overs that can conveniently be taken on and off. The patient is asked to look easy and to maintain global awareness out of the corner of his eyes. He may stand still initially, and then walk about with the binasals on, guiding himself via peripheral visual input. The patient is asked to wear binasal occluders for a few minutes at a time, and to transfer this experience to daily seeing, attempting to maintain a relaxed, less intense, global, peripheral awareness as much as possible.

2. MacDonald Form Field Card

    The MacDonald Form Field card (MacDonald 1962) presents a central fixation dot surrounded by letters (Figure 15.20). The patient fixates the dot and attempts to relax, look passively, and maintain awareness of as many of the surrounding letters as possible. A variation, the Rothman card (Rothman 1985), contains each of the letters

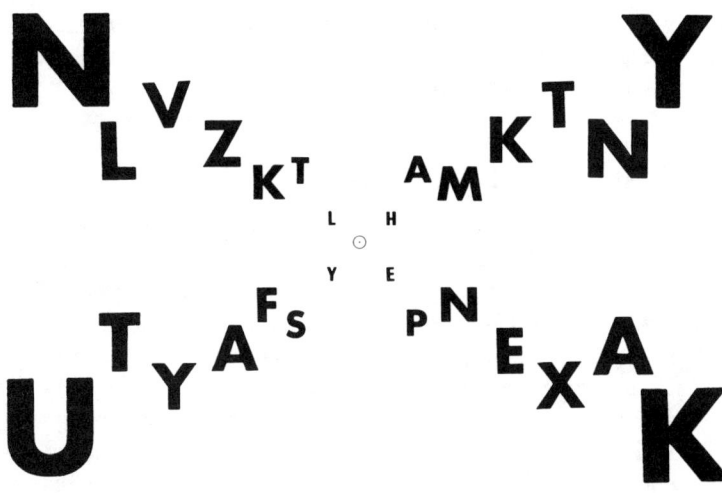

Figure 15.20   MacDonald Form Field Card.

of the alphabet; the patient maintains fixation on the central dot and attempts to find the alphabet in order using peripheral vision.

3. Hart Chart

A similar procedure is performed with a Hart chart (see Figure 11.5). The patient is asked to "look hard" at the central S on the chart, on a wall at arm's length, and then to relax and look easy at the S. Most patients see more of the surrounding letters when looking easy. This procedure is used to bring to conscious awareness the difference between looking intensely and a more passive, relaxed concentration. The patient is advised to maintain relaxed concentration with peripheral awareness as frequently as possible in everyday seeing.

Peripheral awareness is commonly incorporated when treating patients who are myopic or esophoric, who have difficulty with base-in vergence, or who are intense, focal, and detail-oriented in their approach to information-processing. The goal is not simply to see more out of the corners of the eyes, but to adopt a more relaxed, less intense concentration in daily seeing. To this end, patients are instructed to recreate in daily seeing, as often as possible, the feeling tones of the peripheral awareness procedures. Patients are told to "remind yourself many times each day to look easy, let your shoulders and body relax, smile internally, see as much of the surround as possible, and hold this feeling for 5 or 6 seconds." The value of the procedure lies in its frequent use, since relaxed, passive concentration may serve to reduce stress reactivity. Birnbaum (1978, 1990) suggests that peripheral awareness procedures that emphasize passive concentration may be used, like meditation, to elicit the relaxation response, a phys-iological counterstress response characterized by reduced activity of the sympathetic nervous system (Benson 1975).

VISUAL ACUITY TRAINING IN MYOPIA

Procedures to improve unaided visual acuity differ from the accommoda-tive relaxation procedures, described earlier in this chapter, that are used to reduce functional myopia. While myopia reduction seldom exceeds 0.50 to 0.75 D (Stoddard 1942; Woods 1946; Hildreth et al. 1947; Trachtman 1978; Tracht-man et al. 1981) significant improvement in unaided visual acuity is frequently obtained. Acuity improvement usually occurs not as sustained clarity in everyday vision, but rather in brief clear flashes. Acuity improvement during these flashes may be substantial, sometimes even extraordinary, and is often far out of pro-portion to any accompanying slight reduction in myopia. The capacity to achieve substantial improvement in unaided visual acuity is well-documented (Ewalt 1945; Woods 1946; Hildreth et al. 1947; Marg 1952; Epstein et al. 1978, 1981; Col-lins et al. 1981, 1982; Baillet et al. 1982; Gil and Collins 1983; Blount et al. 1984; Rosen et al. 1984; Berman et al. 1985). Consequently, training to improve unaided acuity is often successful in allowing myopic patients to qualify for jobs that require specific levels of unaided acuity, as with the police or fire depart-ments, from which they would otherwise be excluded.

Procedures to improve unaided visual acuity in myopic patients are de-scribed by Bates (1920), Kelley (1962), Rosannes-Berrett (1974), Epstein et al. (1978), Collins and Epstein (1979), Friedman (1981), and Gottlieb (1982). Ex-amples of such procedures include the following

1. Hart chart walkaway

    With corrective lenses removed, the patient views a Hart chart at the farthest distance at which the letters can be distinguished. The pa-tient stands with one foot well in front of the other, rocks forward so as to read the letters, and then attempts to distinguish the letters as he rocks back, trying to progressively increase the viewing distance over which the letters can be read. Advice to focus farther away, as if to look through or beyond the target, may aid performance. Viewing a Plateau spiral (see Figure 15.19) funneling into the distance; visual im-agery techniques in which the patient visualizes a faraway scene with eyes closed, then opens the eyes and attempts to keep the feeling of looking far away; and advice to maintain peripheral awareness, to breathe deeply and to physically relax, may significantly improve per-formance. Demand may be increased by performing the procedure through plus lens power rather than plano.

    A similar procedure using feedback and fading has been used by a group of research psychologists to improve myopic subjects' unaided acuity. Letters are presented in random order, and each correct response is reinforced by positive verbal comments (feedback). The viewing distance is increased by 20 cm (fading) when the patient correctly identifies 10 consecutive letters (Epstein et al. 1978; Collins and Epstein 1979). These principles have also been applied with a video computer (Gil and Collins 1983).

2. Deep fog

The patient, without refractive correction even if several diopters myopic, sits behind the refractor and views a distance Snellen chart through O.U. +2.00 D spheres. The chart is blurred and unreadable. As the patient views the chart, there are occasional brief flashes of clear vision. These clear flashes are not caused by squinting or refractive change. With practice, patients become more adept at creating flashes of clear vision. Acuity improvement is enhanced by the incorporation of visual imagery, peripheral awareness, and relaxation procedures.

3. PG 4

The Keystone PG 4 stereogram (Figure 15.21) contains a series of signposts which, when fused stereoscopically, appear to recede into the distance. The signposts present three-letter words with acuity demands that vary from 20/280 to 20/15, the letters becoming progressively smaller the more receded the signpost. The patient, with

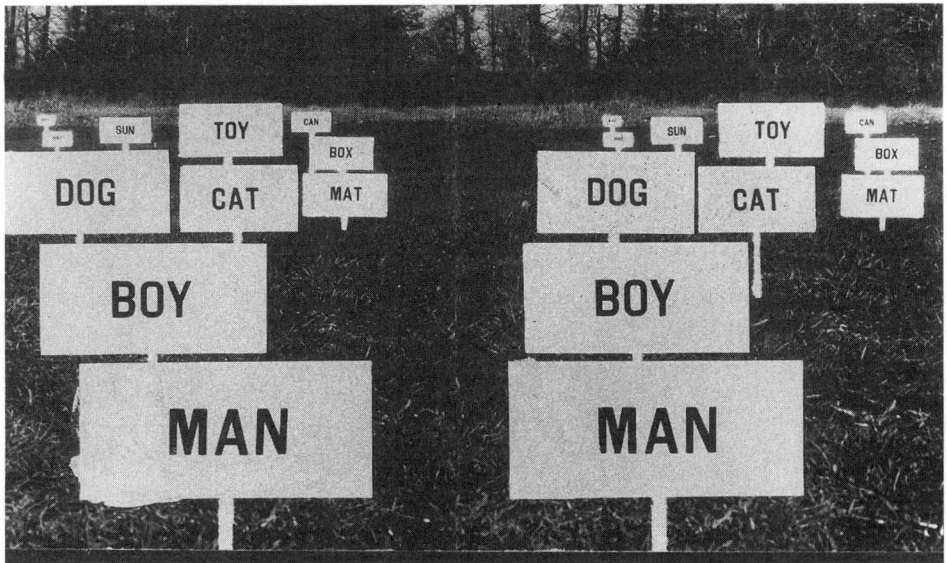

Figure 15.21 PG 4 stereogram.

refractive correction removed, views the target in a Keystone Telebino-cular or other Brewster stereoscope. As with the deep fog procedure, the patient uses visual imagery, peripheral awareness, and relaxation procedures to facilitate "looking away through the target" to generate flashes of clear vision. The technique is often performed with +2.0 D spheres to create additional fog.

4. Deep wink

The patient, with refractive correction removed, views an acuity chart at a distance just beyond that at which the letters are legible. The patient closes his eyes; physically relaxes while inhaling deeply; pauses for a second; and then simultaneously exhales forcibly through the nose while opening the eyes and physically tensing. The deep wink procedure frequently produces flashes of clear vision. As acuity improves, the patient performs the procedure at progressively increasing viewing distances. If the deep wink successfully produces flashes of clear vision, it may be used to aid performance with the Hart chart walkaway, deep fog, and PG 4 procedures.

5. Suggestion, relaxation, and visualization

Kelley (1962) describes a procedure that combines relaxation and visual imagery. The patient sits comfortably and imagines sitting in the sand at the beach, looking off toward the horizon. The thera-pist provides repeated suggestion for relaxation, and the patient at-tempts to maintain this feeling as he opens his eyes. Substantial improvement in unaided acuity is frequently obtained if the patient can maintain relaxation after the eyes are opened.

6. Auditory biofeedback

The Accommotrac Vision Trainer uses auditory biofeedback to train relaxation of accommodation to reduce functional myopia. Im-provement in unaided visual acuity has been reported by Trachtman (1978; Trachtman et al. 1981), Berman et al. (1985), and Gallaway et al. (1987), but no improvement was obtained by Koslowe et al. (1991).

7. Minimize use of refractive correction

The myope who wishes to improve unaided acuity should use re-fractive correction as little as possible. Although glasses are needed for driving and other high-acuity demand tasks, most myopes learn to function well without glasses for many everyday tasks. Practice in seeing without glasses in turn fosters acuity improvement. Low-plus fogging lenses may be used for noncritical tasks to exacerbate this ef-fect.

8. Bates method

The Bates system for myopia reduction and acuity improvement without glasses has anecdotal support, but lacks scientific documenta-tion (Bates 1920; Huxley 1942; Rosannes-Berrett 1974; Gottlieb 1982). Bates attributed refractive errors to muscular tension and mental strain induced by emotions, attitudes, and mental habits. He believed that effort and strain in seeing cause abnormal contraction of the extraocular muscles, which leads to distortion in the shape of the eyeball. Treatment procedures include the use of blinking, breathing, relaxation, and visualization exercises to foster learning to see effortlessly, without strain or tension. Patients are encouraged to remove glasses in nondemanding situations.

Bates indicated that, when attending to a task, especially when under tension and strain, individuals tend to stare and to blink less frequently and more tensely. Breathing becomes more shallow, and individuals tend to hold the breath for many seconds at a time. Attention narrows and patients tend to hold their eyes relatively steady for prolonged periods with reduced eye movements. To develop the ability to see without strain, patients are asked to blink more frequently and to breathe more deeply during everyday seeing, especially during tasks that require close attention. Patients are also encouraged to be more aware of the periphery, to look up frequently, and to move the eyes around and scan rather than stare.

Palming, swinging, and sunning are also used to foster relaxation. In *palming,* stimulation to the eyes is excluded as the patient, with eyes closed and elbows resting on the table, maintains relaxed awareness of breathing while covering the eyes with the palms of the hands. In *sunning,* the patient faces the sun or an artificial light with eyes closed, allows the warmth of the sun to penetrate the eyes, and maintains breathing while relaxedly turning the head from side to side. *Swinging* involves rotating the body from left to right and back so that eyes, head, and body all move together. The patient maintains awareness of movement, but does not fixate anything specific.

SUMMARY

Sequences and procedures are described for training pursuit, saccadic, accommodative, and fusional abilities. When performance is poor on any particular procedure, the therapist should seek to make the task less difficult, increase interest and motivation, increase feedback and kinesthetic involvement, and reduce distraction and concurrent demands. When the patient can perform a task, the therapist should attempt to shape further improvement by selecting progressively more difficult tasks and by developing the ability to maintain function as feedback and kinesthetic support are reduced, as less interesting procedures are selected, and as demands increase for concurrent physical and mental activity. Since the existence of adequate and equal monocular visual skills is important for optimal binocular function, monocular skills training of any particular function generally precedes binocular training. In training fusion ability in patients with nonstrabismic binocular vision disorder, the Flax-Brock sequence, beginning with large stereoscopic targets that serve as strong fusional stimuli, and developing the ability to maintain adequate binocular function with progressively weaker stimuli for fusion, is usually effective. Peripheral awareness procedures and training procedures to improve unaided visual acuity in myopia are also described.

SUGGESTED READING

Griffin JR (1982). *Binocular Anomalies: Procedures for Vision Therapy.* 2nd ed. Chicago: Professional Press.

REFERENCES

Allen MJ (1966). The Bartley phenomenon and visual rehabilitation in a home training technique. *Optom Weekly* July 28, 57:21–22.

Allen MJ (1988). Accommodative rock via computer. *J Am Optom Assoc* 59(8):610–613.

Balliet R, Clay A, Blood K (1982). The training of visual acuity in myopia. *J Am Optom Assoc* 53:719–724.

Bates WH (1920). *Perfect Sight Without Glasses.* New York: Central Fixation Publ.

Benson H (1975). *The Relaxation Response.* New York: William Morrow.

Berman PE, Levinger SI, Massath NA, et al. (1985). The effectiveness of biofeedback visual training as a viable method of treatment and reduction of myopia. *J Optom Vis Dev* 16:17–21.

Birnbaum MH (1977). The role of the trainer in visual training. *J Am Optom Assoc* 48(8):1035–1039.

Birnbaum MH (1978). Holistic aspects of visual style: A hemispheric model with implications for vision therapy. *J Am Optom Assoc* 49(10):1133–1141.

Birnbaum MH (1981). Perspectives on the contributions of Fredrick Brock. *Am J Optom Physiol Opt* 58(8):667–670.

Birnbaum MH (1984). Nearpoint visual stress: A physiological model. *J Am Optom Assoc* 55(11):825–835.

Birnbaum MH (1985a). Nearpoint visual stress: Clinical implications. *J Am Optom Assoc* 56(6):480–490.

Birnbaum MH (1985b). An esophoric shift associated with sustained fixation. *Am J Optom Physiol Opt* 62(11):732–735.

Birnbaum MH (1990). The use of stress reduction concepts and techniques in vision therapy. *J Behav Optom* 1(1):3–7.

Blount RL, Baer RA, Collins FL (1984). Improving visual acuity in a myopic child: Assessing compliance and effectiveness. *Behav Res Ther* 22:53–57.

Bogdanovich G, Roth N, Kohl P (1986). Properties of anaglyphic materials that affect the testing and training of binocular vision. *J Am Optom Assoc* 57(12):899–903.

Burian HM (1941). Fusional movements in permanent strabismus: A study of the central and peripheral regions in the act of monocular vision in squint. *Arch Ophthalmol* 26:626–652.

Burian HM (1947). The place of peripheral fusion in orthoptics. *Am J Ophthalmol* 30:1005–1010.

Cantonnet A, Filliozat J (1934). *Strabismus.* London: M. Wiseman, pp. 234–237.

Cohen AH (1981). Monocular fixation in a binocular field. *J Am Optom Assoc* 52(10):801–806.

Collins FL, Epstein LH (1979). Behavioral training for myopia. *Behav Med Adv* 2:3–5.

Collins FL, Epstein LH, Hannay HY (1981). A component analysis of an operant training program for improving visual acuity in myopic students. *Behav Ther* 12:692–701.

Collins FL, Ricci JA, Burkett PA (1982). Behavioral training for myopia: Long-term maintenance of improved acuity. *Behav Res Ther* 19:265–268.

Colorado Vision Consultants (1985). *Manual of Esotropia Therapy*. Boulder, CO: Colorado Vision Consultants (R. Bateman et al.).

Cooper J (1977). Intermittent exotropia of the divergence excess type. *J Am Optom Assoc* 48(10):1261–1273.

Cooper J (1988). Review of computerized orthoptics with specific regard to convergence insufficiency. *Am J Optom Physiol Opt* 65(6):455–463.

Crow G, Fuog HL (1937–39). *Basic Orthoptics and Reconditioning*. Optometric Extension Program Continuing Education Courses, Santa Ana, CA: Optometric Extension Program Foundation, Oct. 1937–Sept. 1939.

Daum KM (1983). A comparison of the results of tonic and phasic vergence training. *Am J Optom Physiol Opt* 60(9):769–775.

Daum KM, Rutstein RP, Eskridge JB (1987). Efficacy of computerized vergence therapy. *Am J Optom Physiol Opt* 64:83–89.

Easterbrook JA (1959). The effect of emotion on cue utilization and the organization of behavior. *Psychol Rev* 66(3):183–201.

Epstein LH, Collins FL, Hannay HJ (1978). Fading and feedback in the modification of visual acuity. *J Behav Med* 1:273–287.

Epstein LH, Greenwald DJ, Hennon D, et al. (1981). Monocular fading and feedback: Effects on vision changes in the trained and untrained eye. *Behav Modif* 5:171–186.

Eskridge JB (1989). Clinical objective assessment of the accommodative response. *J Am Optom Assoc* 60(4):272–275.

Ewalt HW (1945). The Baltimore myopia control project. *J Amer Optom Assoc* 17(5):167–185.

Flax N (1963a). Prism saccadic training. *Opt J Rev Optom* 100(9):31–33, May 1.

Flax N (1963b). The optometric treatment of intermittent divergent strabismus. *Eastern Seaboard Conference on Vision Training*, Washington, DC, transcript by Caryl Croisant, Morro Bay, CA.

Flax N (1968). *San Jose Vision Training Seminar*. San Jose, CA, transcript by Caryl Croisant, Santa Ana, CA.

Forrest EB (1976). Clinical manifestations of visual information processing. *J Am Optom Assoc* 47(1):73–80.

Forrest EB (1981). *Visual Imagery: An Optometric Approach*. Santa Ana, CA: Optometric Extension Program Foundation.

Forrest EB (1988). *Stress and Vision*. Santa Ana, CA: Optometric Extension Program Foundation.

Friedman E (1981). Vision training programs for myopia management. *Am J Optom Physiol Opt* 58:546–553.

Fujimoto DH, Christensen EA, Griffin JR (1985). An investigation in use of videocassette techniques for enhancement of saccadic eye movements. *J Am Optom Assoc* 56:304–308.

Gallaway M, Pearl SM, Winkelstein AM, et al. (1987). Biofeedback training of visual acuity and myopia: A pilot study. *Am J Optom Physiol Opt* 64(1):62–71.

Getman GN (1964). A new look at ocular motilities in visual development. Optometric Extension Program Continuing Education Courses, Santa Ana, CA: Optometric Extension Program Foundation, vol. 37, series 9, no. 1–3, Oct–Dec.

Gil KM, Collins FL (1983). Behavioral training for myopia: Generalization of effects. *Behav Res Ther* 21:269–273.

Gottlieb RL (1982). Neuropsychology of myopia. *J Optom Vis Dev* 13:3–27.

Griffin JR (1982). *Binocular Anomalies: Procedures for Vision Therapy.* 2nd ed. Chicago: Professional Press.

Grisham JD (1983). Treatment of binocular dysfunction. In: Schor CM, Ciuffreda KS (eds), *Vergence Eye Movements: Basic and Clinical Aspects.* Boston: Butterworth–Heinemann, pp. 605–646.

Hildreth HR, Mainberg WH, Milder B, et al. (1947). The effects of visual training on existing myopia. *Am J Ophthalmol* 30:1563–1576.

Hofstetter JW (1983). Graphical analysis. In: Schor CM, Ciuffreda KJ (eds), *Vergence Eye Movements: Basic and Clinical Aspects.* Boston: Butterworth–Heinemann, pp. 439–464.

Hugonnier R, Clayette-Hugonnier S (1969). *Strabismus, Heterophoria, Ocular Motor Paralysis: Clinical Ocular Muscle Imbalance.* Translated by S. Clayette-Hugonnier, St. Louis: C.V. Mosby.

Huxley A (1942). *The Art of Seeing.* New York: Harper and Bros.

Javal LE (1896). *Manuel Theorique et Pratique du Strabisme.* Paris: G. Masson.

Kahneman D (1973). *Attention and Effort.* Englewood Cliffs, NJ:Prentice-Hall.

Kelley CR (1962). Psychological factors in myopia. *J Am Optom Assoc* 33(11):833–837.

Kertesz AE (1981). Effect of stimulus size on fusion and vergence. *J Opt Soc Am* 71:289–293.

Kertesz AE (1982). The effectiveness of wide-angle fusional stimulation in the treatment of convergence insufficiency. *Invest Ophthalmol Vis Sci* 22:690–693.

Koslowe KC, Spierer A, Rosner M, et al. (1991). Evaluation of Accommotrac biofeedback training for myopia control. *Optom Vis Sci* 68(5):338–343.

Laxer M, Cohen J, Press LJ (1991). An expanded guide to the Keystone stereogram cards. *J Behav Optom* 2(3):59–66.

Lesser SK (1969). *Introduction to Modern Analytical Optometry.* rev. ed. Duncan, OK: Optometric Extension Program Foundation.

Macdonald L (1962). *Visual Training.* Optometric Extension Program Continuing Education Courses, Santa Ana, CA: Optometric Extension Program Foundation, vol. 35, series 1, no. 3 pp. 13–19, Dec.

MacDonald L (1965). *Lecture Transcripts.* Northwest Congress of Optometry, Portland, OR: The Report Co.

Marg E (1952). Flashes of clear vision and negative accommodation with reference to the Bates method of visual training. *Am J Optom Arch Am Acad Optom* 29(4):167–184.

Marrone MA (1991). Peripheral awareness. *J Behav Optom* 2(1):7–11.

Morgan MW (1944a). The clinical aspects of accommodation and convergence. *Am J Optom Arch Acad Optom* 21(8):301–313.

Morgan MW (1944b). Analysis of clinical data. *Am J Optom Arch Am Acad Optom* 21(12):477–491.

Peckham RM (1931). *Squint and Heterophoria.* Rochester, NY: C.G. Lymann.

Pierce JR, Greenspan SB (1971). Accommodative rock procedure in VT—A clinical guide. *Optom Weekly* Part I, 62(33):753–757, Aug. 19; Part II, 62(34):776–780, Aug. 26.

Press L (1987–88). *Computers and Vision Therapy Programs.* Optometric Extension Program Continuing Education Courses, Santa Ana, CA: Optometric Extension Program Foundation, vol. 60, Oct. 1987–Sept. 1988.

Punnett AF, Steinhauer GD (1984). Relationship between reinforcement and eye movements during ocular motor training with learning disabled children. *J Learn Disab* 17(1):16–19.

Rosannes-Berrett MB (1974). *Do You Really Need Eyeglasses?* New York: Hart Publ.

Rosen RC, Schiffman HR, Meyers H (1984). Behavioral treatment of myopia: Refractive error and acuity changes in relation to axial length and intraocular pressure. *Am J Optom Physiol Opt* 61:100–105.

Rosner J, Rosner J (1990). *Pediatric Optometry*. 2nd ed. Boston: Butterworth–Heinemann.

Rothman S (1985). Rothman field card—A modification of the MacDonald form recognition card. *30th Annual Invitational Skeffington Symposium on Vision*, Washington, DC, transcript by Caryl Croisant, Lebanon, OR, pp. 130–132.

Schor CM (1983). Analysis of tonic and accommodative vergence disorders of binocular vision. *Am J Optom Physiol Opt* 60(1):1–14.

Schroeder SR, Holland JG (1968). Operant control of eye movement. *J Appl Behav Anal* 1:161–168.

Schroeder SR, Holland JG (1969). Reinforcement of eye movements with concurrent schedules. *J Exp Anal Behav* 12:897–903.

Sethi BD, North RV (1987). Vergence adaptation changes with varying magnitudes of prism-induced disparities and fusional amplitudes. *Am J Optom Physiol Opt* 64(4):263–268.

Shankman AL (1988). *Vision Enhancement Training*. Santa Ana, CA: Optometric Extension Program Foundation.

Silbert JA, Alexander A (1987). Cyclotherapy in the treatment of symptomatic latent hyperopia. *J Am Optom Assoc* 58(19):40–46.

Somers WW, Hoppel AW, Phillips JV (1984). Use of a personal microcomputer for orthoptic therapy. *J Am Optom Assoc* 55:262–267.

Stoddard KB (1942). Physiological limitations on the functional production and elimination of ametropia. *Am J Optom Arch Am Acad Optom* 19(3):112–118.

Sutton A (1985). *Building a Visual Space World*. Optometric Extension Program Postgraduate Education Courses, Santa Ana, CA: Optometric Extension Program Foundation, vol. 57, series 1, no. 8, pp. 47–54 (May).

Trachtman J (1978). Biofeedback of accommodation to reduce functional myopia: A case report. *Am J Optom Physiol Opt* 55(6):400–406.

Trachtman J, Giambalvo V, Feldman J (1981). Biofeedback of accommodation to reduce functional myopia. *Biofeedback Self-Regul* 6(4):547–564.

Vaegan JL (1979). Convergence and divergence show large and sustained improvement after short isometric exercise. *Am J Optom Physiol Opt* 56:23–33.

Wick B (1985). Clinical factors in proximal vergence. *Am J Optom Physiol Opt* 62(1):1–18.

Wolff B (1970). *San Diego Behavioral Vision Seminar*. San Diego, CA, transcript by Caryl Croisant, Santa Ana, CA.

Woods A (1946). Report from the Wilmer Institute on the results obtained in the treatment of myopia by visual training. *Am J Optom Arch Am Acad Optom* 29(4):167–184.

Worth C (1903). *Squint: Its Causes, Pathology, and Treatment*. London: John Bale & Danielsson.

16

The Efficacy of Vision Therapy

Considerable evidence documents the effectiveness of vision therapy in the management of nonstrabismic (as well as strabismic) visual skills disorders. Research has demonstrated that inadequate accommodative, binocular, and ocular motility skills may be successfully treated, symptoms eliminated, and visual efficiency and performance improved through optometric vision therapy. This literature is reviewed by Greenspan (1971–72), Cooper and Duckman (1978), Suchoff and Petito (1986), Griffin (1987), Grisham (1988), and the 1986/87 Future of Visual Development/Performance Task Force (1988).

EYE MOVEMENTS

Busby (1985) reported improvement of pursuit eye movements in an enhancement program for special education students. The results of this controlled study showed statistically significant improvement, with persistence of therapeutic gains 3 months after discontinuation of the therapy.

In another controlled study, Heath et al. (1976) reported significant improvement in ocular pursuit ability (and reading scores) in a group of third and fourth grade students who initially scored poorly both on tests of reading ability and on tests of ocular pursuits.

Similar improvement in both eye movement ability and reading achievement following oculomotor training in a sample of reading disabled students was obtained in a controlled study conducted by Punnett and Steinhauer (1984). Eye movement training was most effective when feedback and reinforcement were provided. Similar results demonstrating that eye movements can be trained, and that such training is most effective when appropriate feedback is provided, were obtained by Schroeder and Holland (1968, 1969).

Wold et al. (1978) reported on 100 consecutive optometric vision therapy patients whose eye movement abilities were rated on the Heinsen-Schrock scale, a 10-point scale for observing and scoring pursuit and saccadic eye movement performance. Adequate performance was demonstrated by only 6% of the children prior to therapy, but was present in 96% on posttraining reevaluation. Cox and Hambly (1961) and Huelsman (1969) also reported improvement in pursuit and saccadic eye movement performance following vision therapy.

Fujimoto et al. (1985) demonstrated significant improvement in saccadic performance in a sample of children with poor saccadic eye movements. Similar gains were achieved with standard saccadic training procedures and with a newly developed saccadic training videocassette program.

Additional studies document that inefficient eye movement patterns during reading can be significantly improved through vision training. Eye movement recordings before and after training demonstrated a reduction in fixations and regressions and an increase in span of recognition and reading rate following vision training, confirming patients' subjective impressions of increased reading fluency (Solan 1967, 1985a, 1985b; Winter 1974; Young et al. 1982).

ACCOMMODATION

The ability to successfully train accommodative function has been documented objectively through the use of sophisticated optometers that permit continuous monitoring of accommodation. Randle (1970) used auditory biofeedback to demonstrate the trainability of accommodation. Cornsweet and Crane (1973) similarly demonstrated that subjects provided with auditory feedback of accommodation, with no feedback as to clarity or blur, could learn to voluntarily control accommodation to change pitch of a tone in a desired direction. Once learned, control of accommodation could be transferred to other tasks. Subjects also learned to control accommodation voluntarily in response to visual stimuli, changing the accommodative response so as to vary the position of a line on an oscilloscope to match a reference line.

Provine and Enoch (1975) demonstrated that subjects could be trained to voluntarily accommodate as much as 9.0 D. Once voluntary accommodation was learned, it could be elicited on command, even in total darkness.

Hung et al. (1986) reported changes in several parameters in symptomatic patients with accommodative and vergence disorders following orthoptic therapy. TA, slope of the fixation disparity curve, slope of the accommodative response/stimulus curve, the CA/C ratio, and the $+2.0/-2.0$-D monocular accommodative flipper rate all showed changes toward the mean demonstrated by asymptomatic patients. These physiologic changes were accompanied by significant reduction in symptoms.

Liu et al. (1979) objectively demonstrated improvement of accommodative function through vision training in young adults with accommodative insufficiency. Subjects showed changes in the dynamics of accommodation, including reduced time constants and latencies. These objectively monitored physiologic changes correlated well with rate of clearing accommodative flippers and elimination of subjective symptoms.

Lovasik and Wiggins (1984) used an objective testing procedure, the visually evoked response (VER), to verify reduced accommodative ability and to demonstrate increase in amplitude of accommodation as a result of accommodative rock training.

Bobier and Sivak (1983) provided additional objective evidence of the efficacy of orthoptics in the treatment of patients with slow accommodative response (accommodative infacility). Using dynamic photorefraction to document accommodative response, they reported that speed of both accommodation and accommodative relaxation improved and latency reduced following training. Further, improved accommodative flexibility was retained after cessation of training.

Haynes and McWilliams (1979) reported that the time required to make response shifts from far to near and back reduces with training.

FUSIONAL VERGENCE

In the 1930s and 1940s, Fry (1937, 1938, 1943), Hofstetter (1945), and Morgan (1944) investigated the relationship between accommodation and convergence and developed the concept of graphical analysis of the zone of binocular vision. Hofstetter (1945) reported that the width of the zone of clear, single binocular vision can be increased by training. He found that the range of relative convergence could be increased, particularly on the positive side. Further, when the width of the zone is increased at one fixation distance, a corresponding increase is found at all other fixation distances. Fry (1943) and Flom (1954) obtained similar results, reporting that the width of the zone is readily varied by training. Flom indicates that the near point of convergence and the positive side of the zone appear to be the most trainable.

Morgan (1944) compared phorometric changes in a sample of 50 vision training patients and 50 controls to determine which findings were amenable to alteration through training. He found that the positive convergence blur and break findings at near point were the easiest findings to change through training.

Morgan (1944) ranked the various findings in order of ease of modification through training:

A. Findings easiest to alter
   1. positive fusional convergence at near (#16B)
   2. positive relative convergence at near (#16A)
   3. base-out at distance (#10)
   4. negative fusional reserve at near (#17B)
   5. positive relative accommodation (#20)
   6. negative relative convergence at near (#17A)
   7. abduction (#11)
B. Findings alterable to a limited degree
   1. negative relative accommodation (#21)
   2. nearpoint phoria (#13B)
   3. farpoint phoria (#8)

    4. amplitude of accommodation (#19)

    5. monocular and binocular cross-cylinder findings (#14A, #14B)

  C. Findings not significantly alterable

    1. gradient AC/A

In a series of studies, Daum (1982, 1983a, 1986a, 1986b; Daum et al. 1987, 1988) confirmed the ability to alter vergence measures through vision training. Daum (1982) administered vergence training procedures over a 3-week period to asymptomatic young adults with normal binocular function. Subjects showed marked gains in base-out vergence, which were largely retained, with some decrement, following 5 months without vision training. Gains in negative fusional vergence were less pronounced, but actually showed a slight further increase 5 months after termination of treatment.

In double-blind controlled studies of the efficacy of fusional vergence training, Daum (1986a, Daum et al. 1988) demonstrated significant improvement in positive vergence at distance and near. Training over short, frequent intervals was most effective. Improvement in positive fusional vergence through training has also been demonstrated in studies by Norn (1966), Kertesz (1982), and Pantano (1982), as well as in studies of computerized vergence therapy by Cooper and Feldman (1980), Sommers et al. (1984), Daum et al. (1987), and Cooper (1988a). Griffin et al. (1982) documented an increase in base-out fusional vergence at distance through training.

  . Cooper and Feldman (1980) used random dot stereograms and operant conditioning, and reported significant improvement in convergence ranges in children with binocular dysfunction who had previously been unsuccessful with conventional stereograms without formal operant conditioning; patients were then able to transfer improved convergence ability to vergence tasks using vectograms and prisms.

Daum (1986b) demonstrated that negative vergence can also be improved substantially through training, although gains are more difficult to achieve and are usually smaller in magnitude than those obtained with positive vergence. Increased negative fusional vergence with training has also been documented by Jampolsky (1970) and Vaegan (1979).

Vaegan (1979) reported significant increases in both base-in and base-out prism vergence following brief but sustained exposure to base-in and base-out prism vergence demands. Significant improvement in the direction trained occurred after only 5 minutes of training, and lasted after training had ceased. Vaegan emphasized the importance of sustained effort in the desired training direction as a key requirement for improvement, especially for divergence. Vaegan also demonstrated that push-up exercises produced a significant, long-lasting increase in convergence ability.

Infrared eye position recordings have been used to objectively document changes in vergence dynamics with orthoptics. Vergence tracking rate, a measure of the ability to make rapid and appropriate vergence change to track a step-vergence staircase stimulus, improves as a result of training in patients with mild binocular dysfunction. This improvement correlates with an increase in clinically measured vergence ranges (Chan and Grisham 1975; Grisham 1983; Grisham et al. 1991). Vaegan and McMonnies (1979) also used an objective recording device to document sustained improvement in convergence with training.

Orthoptic training has been demonstrated to increase the rate and amplitude of prism adaptation, and to cause a flattening (reduced slope) of the forced vergence fixation disparity curve (Arner et al. 1956; Sheedy and Saladin 1977; Vaegan 1979; Sheedy 1980; North and Henson 1982).

Manny (1980) demonstrated that vergence can be trained even in the absence of retinal disparity information. Subjects given feedback of eye position learned to produce both adduction and abduction in response to prism, even though one eye was occluded. The clinical significance of this study lies in the demonstration of the importance of appropriate feedback. Vergence ranges can be trained even under adverse conditions (absence of fusion and disparity information), as long as appropriate feedback is provided,

Although vertical vergence is less amenable to training than is lateral vergence, several reports suggest that vertical vergence can be increased in some cases. Although such increase is usually quite small, very large increases in vertical vergence have been obtained in some cases, particularly when intermittent or noncomitant hypertropia is present (Crone 1973; Duke-Elder and Wybar 1973; Robertson and Kuhn 1984, 1985; Metz 1986; Rutstein et al. 1988). Rutstein et al. (1988) indicate a tendency for vertical vergence training to flatten the slope of the vertical fixation disparity curve and improve the ability to adapt to vertical prism.

Cooper (1988b) reported little improvement in vertical fusional vergence through training, but found that fusion ability in hyperphoria is significantly improved by training horizontal vergence. In four patients with vertical deviation, only one showed improvement in vertical vergence, and this improvement was minimal. However, Cooper reported that the need for full-time vertical prism correction was eliminated in all four patients by prescribing the minimum prism necessary to eliminate diplopia; using vision therapy to expand horizontal fusional ranges; reducing the vertical prism by 2^Δ; repeating horizontal fusion range extension; and repeating the process until reaching a plateau. Since vertical vergence range improved in only one case, he suggests that the ability to reduce vertical prism correction results from improvement in the slow-fusional vergence adaptation system.

The biofeedback literature indicates that even functions once thought untrainable can be brought under voluntary control when appropriate feedback is provided (Brown 1974). Perhaps the most extraordinary demonstration of plasticity in the vergence system is the demonstration of a capacity to train voluntary torsion movements. Balliet and Nakayama (1978) trained conjugate cyclorotary eye movements as great as 30 degrees using a visual feedback technique. The implication is that even functions which are resistant to training may be modified with the development of procedures and techniques which provide adequate feedback.

CLINICAL STUDIES: EFFICACY OF TREATMENT OF ACCOMMODATIVE AND VERGENCE DISORDERS

The preceding studies document the capacity to improve accommodative and vergence function. Numerous clinical studies report the efficacy of vision therapy in the treatment of nonstrabismic visual skills disorders. These studies document improved function, with elimination or reduction of both clinical disorder and subjective asthenopic symptoms in a high percentage of cases.

As early as 1944, Duthie (1944) reported an 88% cure rate following orthoptic treatment for convergence insufficiency. Mayou (1945) reported achieving cures in 72% of 364 patients with convergence deficiency treated between 1938 and 1944. Campbell and Mein (1944) reported successful treatment of 85% of exophores and 85% of esophores who completed therapy; completion generally required 10 to 15 visits.

Bryer (1961) investigated the long-term effects of treatment of heterophoria. Of 89 patients whose initial symptoms were completely relieved during orthoptic treatment, 81% remained symptom-free on follow-up 6 to 10 years after discharge. Only 4% experienced recurrence of symptoms severe enough to require further treatment.

Cooper and Duckman (1978) summarized the results of orthoptic treatment of convergence insufficiency as reported in 13 studies. They report that most authorities indicate that convergence insufficiency responds well to vision therapy. In the 13 studies they summarize, 94% of the patients treated showed relief from initial symptoms. Cure rates of 75% or better were reported in nine of the 13 studies.

Grisham (1988) similarly reviewed 15 studies of vision therapy for convergence insufficiency over a 47-year period. These studies survey nearly 2,000 patients and report an overall cure rate of 72%, with improvement in an additional 19% and failure in only 9% of cases.

Cooper et al. (1983) treated seven convergence insufficiency patients with automated fusional convergence training using random dot stereograms. All showed significant increase in base-out vergence, significant reduction in asthenopia, and flattening of the base-out portion of the fixation disparity curve. Following the gains obtained via automated fusional convergence training with random dot stereograms, the introduction of traditional accommodative and vergence training procedures produced further increase in base-out fusion range and reduction in asthenopia. It appears that the use of varied methods of vergence stimulation helps to generalize function and maximize improvement.

Daum (1984) reported on treatment of 110 patients with convergence insufficiency, treated on a home basis for an average of 4.3 weeks. Treatment consisted mainly of exercises to strengthen the positive vergence system. Total success was achieved in 41% and partial success in 56%. Daum documented improvement in a number of functions: (1) nearpoint exophoria decreased; (2)

stimulus AC/A ratio increased; (3) base-in vergence measures increased despite the fact that base-in training was not performed; (4) positive fusional vergence measures showed substantial improvement; (5) convergence near point improved; and (6) amplitude of accommodation improved.

Dalziel (1981) reported the results of vision training in 100 patients with convergence insufficiency who failed to meet Sheard's criterion at near (that is, positive fusional convergence was less than twice the nearpoint exophoria). Training stressed stimulation of positive fusional vergence, was primarily home-centered, and lasted an average of 6 weeks. Eighty-four percent of the patients successfully met Sheard's criterion after therapy.

Daum (1983b) reported on the treatment of 96 patients with accommodative insufficiency. He found improvement in amplitude and facility of accommodation, stereopsis, and fusional vergence following brief orthoptic treatment. Fifty-three percent of the patients achieved total success, with normalization of accommodative function and elimination of subjective symptoms, and 43% improved but did not achieve total success. Only 4% failed to improve.

Cooper et al. (1987), in a controlled study, demonstrated marked improvement in accommodative amplitude and facility following automated monocular accommodative facility training. Improvement was accompanied by a reduction in asthenopia in all five subjects.

Hoffman et al. (1973) reported an overall success rate of 90% in the treatment of nonstrabismic visual skills disorders. Their criterion for success was the normalization of phorometric findings as per Morgan's expecteds. Their sample included 129 patients with accommodative dysfunction, convergence insufficiency, and general skills disorders. Accommodative cases constituted the majority of the sample. Patients were seen for an average of 25 treatment visits.

Wold et al. (1978) reported improvement in ocular pursuits. saccadic fixations, accommodative amplitude and flexibility, and binocular visual function following vision training in a sample of 100 patients with nonstrabismic binocular vision disorder, all of whom also exhibited learning dysfunction.

Studies by Weisz (1979), Hoffman (1982), and Atzmon (1985) document not only that deficient vergence and accommodative function can be remediated, but that such improvement transfers to other functions. Among children diagnosed as having accommodative dysfunction, Weisz (1979) found greater improvement in accuracy of performance on a nearpoint paper-and-pencil task in children receiving accommodative training than in a control group that received perceptual-motor training unrelated to accommodation. Hoffman (1982) reported that, in a sample of 5- to 8-year-old children with accommodative disorder, treatment of accommodative deficiency was accompanied by concomitant improvement in visual perceptual skills related to visual discrimination, attention, and visual-motor integration. In a sample of children with reading disability and deficient fusional vergence, Atzmon (1985) reported that orthoptic improvement in fusional vergence was accompanied by improvement in reading and other aspects of school performance in 85% of the subjects. These studies suggest that vergence and accommodative disorders interfere with efficient visual information-processing, and that remediation of such dysfunction transfers to improved visual efficiency and task performance.

Improvement in stereopsis has been documented to result both from specific therapy to increase sensitivity to retinal disparity (Wittenberg et al. 1969), and nonspecific therapy designed to alleviate underlying disorders of fixation, vergence and accommodation (Dalziel 1981; Saladin and Rick 1982; Daum 1983b).

Remediation of clinical deficits is commonly accompanied by elimination of asthenopic symptoms, increased visual efficiency, heightened ability to process visual information, and improved classroom performance and reading ability. Improved reading and academic function following remediation of functional vision disorder is documented in several studies (Ludlam et al. 1973; Heath et al. 1976; Getz 1980; Haddad et al. 1984; Punnett and Steinhauer 1984; Atzmon 1985; Mazow et al. 1989). In addition, Dowis (1977) reports a substantial reduction in rate of recidivism among juvenile delinquents receiving vision therapy to remediate functional vision disorder, presumably as a result of increased capacity for achievement.

Although vision therapy is often associated with children and young adults, presbyopic and geriatric patients may benefit as well. As presbyopia progresses, exophoria frequently increases as accommodation and accommodative convergence diminish (Eames 1933; Morgan and Peters 1951; Hokoda et al. 1991). Many patients with vergence dysfunction develop convergence insufficiency. Wick (1977) and Cohen and Soden (1984) report good success in treating older adults with convergence insufficiency.

Wick (1977) reported on the efficacy of vision training in 161 presbyopes with visual skills disorders. Convergence insufficiency was the most common problem (83%). Success was achieved in 92%, using objective and subjective criteria; 97% of the patients reported elimination of subjective complaints.

Similarly, Cohen and Soden (1984) reported on the treatment of 28 geriatric (over age 60) patients with convergence insufficiency. All but one patient achieved both subjective and objective criteria for success. Long-term retention of gains was demonstrated in 83% of patients reevaluated 9 months after treatment.

Vision therapy is often helpful even in cases in which vision disorder is of organic rather than functional origin. Improvement has been reported in cases of accommodative, convergence, and fusional disorders arising from head injury (Candler 1944; Cohen and Soden 1981; Krasnow and Griffin 1982). Duckman (1980, 1984) has demonstrated that accommodative dysfunction is prevalent in persons with cerebral palsy and can be remediated with vision training.

SUMMARY

Numerous research reports document that vision therapy is effective in remediating deficient pursuit and saccadic eye movements, inefficient eye movements while reading, inadequate accommodative function, and restricted base-out and base-in fusional vergence ranges. Vision therapy has been reported to increase both the rate and amplitude of vergence adaptation. Several studies provide incontrovertible evidence, in the form of objective recordings, of the ability to improve ocular function.

Clinical studies indicate that vision therapy is successful in remediating oculomotor, accommodative, and binocular vision disorders with elimination or reduction of symptoms in most cases. Treatment for convergence insufficiency has been reported to be effective in presbyopic and geriatric patients, as well as in younger populations. Remediation of vergence and accommodative disorder has been reported to be accompanied by improved nearpoint task performance, visual perceptual skills, stereopsis, and reading and other academic abilities.

SUGGESTED READING

1986/87 Future of Visual Development/Performance Task Force (1988). The efficacy of optometric vision therapy. *J Am Optom Assoc* 59(2):95–105.

Cooper J, Duckman R (1978). Convergence insufficiency: Incidence, diagnosis and treatment. *J Am Optom Assoc* 49(6):673–680.

Greenspan SB (1971–72). Research studies of visual and perceptual-motor training. Optometric Extension Program Continuing Education Courses, Santa Ana, CA: Optometric Extension Program Foundation, vol. 44, Oct. 1971–Sept. 1972.

Griffin JR (1987). Efficacy of vision therapy for nonstrabismic vergence anomalies. *Am J Optom Physiol Opt* 64(6):411–414.

Grisham JD (1988). Visual therapy results for convergence insufficiency: A literature review. *Am J Optom Physiol Opt* 65(6):448–454.

Suchoff IB, Petito GT (1986). The efficacy of visual therapy: Accommodative disorders and non-strabismic anomalies of binocular vision. *J Am Optom Assoc* 57(2):119–125.

REFERENCES

1986/87 Future of Visual Development/Performance Task Force (1988). The efficacy of optometric vision therapy. *J Am Optom Assoc* 59(2):95–105.

Arner RS, Berger SI, Braverman G, et al. (1956). The clinical significance of the effect of vergence on fixation disparity—A preliminary investigation. *Am J Optom Arch Am Acad Optom* 33:399–409.

Atzmon D (1985). Positive effect of improving relative fusional vergence on reading and learning disabilities. *Binoc Vis* 1(1):39–43.

Balliet R, Nakayama K (1978). Training of voluntary torsion. *Invest Ophthalmol Vis Sci* 17(4):303–314.

Bobier WR, Sivak JG (1983). Orthoptic treatment of subjects showing slow accommodative responses. *Am J Optom Physiol Opt* 60:678–687.

Brown BB (1974). *New Mind, New Body. Biofeedback: New Directions for the Mind*. New York: Harper and Row.

Bryer ZJ (1961). Assessment of the results of orthoptic treatment in heterophoria. *Br Orthopt J* 18:87–89.

Busby RA (1985). Vision development in the classroom. *J Learn Disab* 18:266–272.

Campbell DA, Mein J (1944). Civilian heterophoria. A record of cases treated at the Coventry and Warwickshire Hospital. *Br Orthopt J* 2:42–49.

Candler R (1944). Some observations on orthoptic treatment following head injury. *Br Orthoptic J* 2: 56–62.

Chan CL, Grisham JD (1975). Objective verification of fusional vergence orthoptics. O.D. thesis. School of Optometry, University of California, Berkeley.

Cohen AH, Soden R (1981). An optometric approach to the rehabilitation of the stroke patient. *J Am Optom Assoc* 52(9):795–800.

Cohen AH, Soden R (1984). Effectiveness of visual therapy for convergence insufficiencies for an adult population. *J Am Optom Assoc* 55(7):491–494.

Cooper J (1988a). Review of computerized orthoptics with specific regard to convergence insufficiency. *Am J Optom Physiol Opt* 65(6):455–463.

Cooper J (1988b). Orthoptic treatment of vertical deviations. *J Am Optom Assoc* 59(6):463–468.

Cooper J, Duckman R (1978). Convergence insufficiency: Incidence, diagnosis and treatment. *J Am Optom Assoc* 49(6):673–680.

Cooper J, Feldman J (1980). Operant conditioning of fusional convergence ranges using random dot stereograms. *Am J Optom Physiol Opt* 57:205–213.

Cooper J, Selenow A, Ciuffreda KJ, et al. (1983). Reduction of asthenopia in patients with convergence insufficiency after fusional vergence training. *Am J Optom Physiol Opt* 60(12):982–989.

Cooper J, Feldman J, Selenow A, et al. (1987). Reduction of asthenopia after accommodative facility training. *Am J Optom Physiol Opt* 64(6):430–436.

Cornsweet TN, Crane HD (1973). Training the visual accommodation system. *Vis Res* 13(3):713–715.

Cox BJ, Hambly LR (1961). Guided development of perceptual skill of visual space as a factor in the achievement of primary grade children. *Am J Optom Arch Am Acad Optom* 38(8):433–444.

Crone RA (1973). *Diplopia*. New York: American Elsevier, p. 80.

Dalziel CC (1981). Effect of vision training on patients who fail Sheard's criterion. *Am J Optom Physiol Opt* 58:21–23.

Daum KM (1982). The course and effect of visual training on the vergence system. *Am J Optom Physiol Opt* 59(3):223–227.

Daum KM (1983a). A comparison of the results of tonic and phasic vergence training. *Am J Optom Physiol Opt* 60(9):769–775.

Daum KM (1983b). Accommodative insufficiency. *Am J Optom Physiol Opt* 60 (5):352–359.

Daum KM (1984). Convergence insufficiency. *Am J Optom Physiol Opt* 61:16–22.

Daum KM (1986a). Double-blind placebo-controlled examination of timing effects in the training of positive vergences. *Am J Optom Physiol Opt* 63(10):807–812.

Daum KM (1986b). Negative vergence training in humans. *Am J Optom Physiol Opt* 63(7):487–496.

Daum KM, Rutstein RP, Eskridge JB (1987). Efficacy of computerized vergence therapy. *Am J Optom Physiol Opt* 64:83–89.

Daum KM, Rutstein, RP, Cho M, et al. (1988). Horizontal and vertical vergence training and its effect on vergences and fixation disparity curves: I. Horizontal data. *Am J Optom Physiol Opt* 65(1):1–7.

Dowis RT (1977). The effect of a visual training program on juvenile delinquency. *J Am Optom Assoc* 48(9):1173–1176.

Duckman RH (1980). Effectiveness of visual training on a population of cerebral palsied children. *J Am Optom Assoc* 51:607–614.

Duckman RH (1984). Accommodation in cerebral palsy: Function and remediation. *J Am Optom Assoc* 55:281–283.

Duke-Elder WS, Wybar K (1973). *Ocular motility and strabismus*. In: Duke-Elder WS (ed), *System of Ophthalmology* Vol. VI. St. Louis: C.V. Mosby, pp. 730–731.

Duthie OM (1944). Convergence deficiency. *Br Orthopt J* 2:38–41.

Eames TH (1933). Physiological exophoria in relation to age. *Arch Ophthalmol* 9:104–105.

Flom MC (1954). The use of accommodative convergence relationship in prescribing orthoptics. *Penn Optometrist*, 14:3–8, 17–18.

Fry GA (1937). An experimental analysis of the accommodation-convergence relation. *Am J Optom Arch Am Acad Optom* 14:402–414.

Fry GA (1938). Further experiments on the accommodation-convergence relationship. *Trans Am Acad Optom* 12:65–74.

Fry GA (1943). Fundamental variables in the relationship between accommodation and convergence. *Optom Weekly* 34:153–155, 183–185.

Fujimoto DH, Christensen EA, Griffin JR (1985). An investigation in use of videocassette techniques for enhancement of saccadic eye movements. *J Am Optom Assoc* 56:304–308.

Getz DJ (1980). Learning enhancement through visual training. *Academic Ther* 15(4):457–466.

Greenspan SB (1971–72). Research studies of visual and perceptual-motor training. Optometric Extension Program Continuing Education Courses, Santa Ana, CA: Optometric Extension Program Foundation. vol. 44, Oct. 1971–Sept. 1972.

Griffin JR (1987). Efficacy of vision therapy for nonstrabismic vergence anomalies. *Am J Optom Physiol Opt* 64(6):411–414.

Griffin JR, Hattan MA, Hertneky RL (1982). Vision therapy with stereoscopic motion pictures: A comparative evaluation. *Am J Optom Physiol Opt* 59:890–893.

Grisham JD (1983). Treatment of binocular dysfunction. In: Schor CM, Ciuffreda KJ (eds), *Vergence Eye Movements: Basic and Clinical Aspects*. Boston: Butterworth–Heinemann, pp. 605–646.

Grisham JD (1988). Visual therapy results for convergence insufficiency: A literature review. *Am J Optom Physiol Opt* 65(6):448–454.

Grisham JD, Bowman MC, Owyang LA, et al. (1991). Vergence orthoptics: Validity and persistence of the training effect. *Optom Vis Sci* 68(6):441–451.

Haddad HM, Isaacs NS, Onghena K, et al. (1984). The use of orthoptics in dyslexia. *J Learn Disab* 17(3):142–144.

Haynes HM, McWilliams LG (1979). Effects of training on near-far response time as measured by the distance rock test. *J Am Optom Assoc* 50:715–718.

Heath EJ, Cook P, O'Dell N (1976). Eye exercises and reading efficiency. *Academic Ther* 11(4):435–445.

Hoffman L (1982). The effect of accommodative deficiencies on the development level of perceptual skills. *Am J Optom Physiol Opt* 59:254–262.

Hoffman L, Cohen AH, Feuer G (1973). Effectiveness of non-strabismic optometric vision training in a private practice. *Am J Optom Arch Am Acad Optom* 50(10):813–816.

Hofstetter H (1945). The zone of clear single binocular vision. *Am J Optom Arch Am Acad Optom* 22(7):301–333; 22(8):361–384.

Hokoda SC, Rosenfield M, Ciuffreda KJ (1991). Proximal vergence and age. *Optom Vis Sci* 68(3):168–172.

Huelsman CB (1969). *The Influence of Vision Training Upon the Subsequent Reading Achievement of Fourth Grade Children*. U.S. Office of Education, project no. RF 1603, contract no. OE3-10-089.

Hung GK, Ciuffreda KJ, Semmlow JI (1986). Static vergence and accommodation: Population norms and orthoptic effects. *Doc Ophthalmol* 62:165–179.

Jampolsky A (1970). Ocular divergence mechanisms. *Trans Am Ophthalmol Soc* 68:730–822.

Kertesz AE (1982). The effectiveness of wide-angle fusional stimulation in the treatment of convergence insufficiency. *Invest Ophthalmol Vis Sci* 22:690–693.

Krasnow DJ, Griffin JR (1982). Fusional convergence loss following head trauma: A case report. *Optom Monthly* 73(1):18–19.

Liu JS, Lee M, Jang J, et al. (1979). Objective assessment of accommodation orthoptics. I. Dynamic insufficiency. *Am J Optom Physiol Opt* 56(5):285–294.

Lovasik JV, Wiggins R (1984). Cortical indices of impaired ocular accommodation and associated convergence mechanisms. *Am J Optom Physiol Opt* 61:150–159.

Ludlam WM, Twarowski C, Ludlam DP (1973). Optometric visual training for learning disability—A case report. *Am J Optom Arch Am Acad Optom* 50(1):58–66.

Manny RE (1980). Monocular vergence movements produced by external visual feedback. *Am J Optom Physiol Opt* 57(4):236–244.

Mayou S (1945). The treatment of convergence deficiency. *Br Orthopt J* 3:72–82.

Mazow ML, France TD, Finkleman S, et al. (1989). Acute accommodative and convergence insufficiency. *Trans Am Ophthalmol Soc* 87:158–173.

Metz HS (1986). Think superior oblique palsy. *J Pediatr Ophthalmol Strab* 23:166–169.

Morgan MW (1944). Analysis of clinical data. *Am J Optom Arch Am Acad Optom* 21(12):477–491.

Morgan MW, Peters HB (1951). Accommodative-convergence in presbyopia. *Am J Optom Arch Am Acad Optom* 28:3–10.

Norn MS (1966). Convergence insufficiency incidence in ophthalmic practice. Results of orthoptic treatment. *Acta Ophthalmol* 44:132–138.

North RV, Henson DB (1982). Effect of orthoptics upon the ability of patients to adapt to prism-induced heterophoria. *Am J Optom Physiol Opt* 59(12):983–986.

Pantano FM (1982). Orthoptic treatment of convergence insufficiency: A two year follow-up report. *Am Orthopt J* 32:73–80.

Provine R, Enoch J (1975). On voluntary ocular accommodation. *Percept Psychophys* 17:209–212.

Punnett AF, Steinhauer GD (1984). Relationship between reinforcement and eye movements during ocular motor training with learning disabled children. *J Learn Disab* 17(1):16–19.

Randle R (1970). Volitional control of visual accommodation. In: *Conference Proceedings, Advisory Group for Aerospace Research and Development.* vol. 82, pp. 15–17.

Robertson KM, Kuhn LD (1984). Successful vision training for alternating sursumduction. *J Am Optom Assoc* 55:911–914.

Robertson KM, Kuhn LD (1985). Effect of visual training on the vertical vergence amplitude. *Am J Optom Physiol Opt* 62:659–668.

Rutstein RP, Daum KM, Cho M (1988). Horizontal and vertical vergence training and its effect on vergences, fixation disparity curves, and prism adaptation: II. Vertical data. *Am J Optom Physiol Opt* 65(1):8–13.

Saladin JJ, Rick JO (1982). Effect of orthoptic procedures on stereoscopic acuities. *Am J Optom Physiol Opt* 59:718–725.

Schroeder SR. Holland JG (1968). Operant control of eye movements. J Appl Behav Anal 1:161–168.

Schroeder SR, Holland JG (1969). Reinforcement of eye movement with concurrent schedules. *J Exp Anal Behav* 12:897–903.

Sheedy JE (1980). Fixation disparity analysis of oculo-motor imbalance. *Am J Optom Physiol Opt* 57:632–639.

Sheedy JE, Saladin JJ (1977). Phoria, vergence, and fixation disparity in oculomotor problems. *Am J Optom Physiol Opt* 54:474–478.

Solan HA (1967). The improvement of reading efficiency: A study of sixty-three achieving high school students. *J Read Spec* 7(1):8–13.

Solan HA (1985a). Deficient eye-movement patterns in achieving high school students: Three case histories. *J Learn Disab* 18(2):66–70.

Solan HA (1985b). Eye movement problems in achieving readers: An update. *Am J Optom Physiol Opt* 61(12):812–819.

Somers WW, Happel AW, Phillips JD (1984). Use of a personal microcomputer for orthoptic therapy. *J Am Optom Assoc* 55:262–267.

Suchoff IB, Petito GT (1986). The efficacy of visual therapy: Accommodative disorders and non-strabismic anomalies of binocular vision. *J Am Optom Assoc* 57(2):119–125.

Vaegan JL (1979). Convergence and divergence show large and sustained improvement after short isometric exercise. *Am J Optom Physiol Opt* 56:23–33.

Vaegan JL, McMonnies C (1979). Clinical vergence training. *Aust J Optom* 62:28–36.

Weisz CL (1979). Clinical therapy for accommodative responses: Transfer effects upon performance. *J Am Optom Assoc* 50:209–221.

Wick B (1977). Vision training for presbyopic nonstrabismic patients. *Am J Optom Physiol Opt* 54(4):244–247.

Winter JF (1974). Clinical oculography. *J Am Optom Assoc* 45(11):1308–1313.

Wittenberg S, Brock FW, Folsom WC (1969). Effect of training on stereoscopic acuity. *Am J Optom Arch Amer Acad Optom* 46:645–653.

Wold RM, Pierce JR, Keddington J (1978). Effectiveness of optometric vision therapy. *J Am Optom Assoc* 49:1047–1059.

Young BS, Pollard T, Paynter S, et al. (1982). Effect of eye exercises in improving control of eye movements during reading. *J Optom Vis Dev* 13(2):4–7.

Recommended Texts and Manuals of Vision Therapy Procedures

Colorado Vision Consultants. *Manual of Esotropia Therapy.* R. Bateman et al., Boulder, CO: Colorado Vision Consultants, 1985.

Francke AW. *Introduction to Optometric Visual Training.* Santa Ana, CA: Optometric Extension Program Foundation, Oct. 1974–Sept. 1975.

Functional Vision Associates. *Vision Therapy Manual.* Dallas, OR: Functional Vision Associates, c/o G.D. Kappel, O.D.

Getz DJ. *Strabismus and Amblyopia.* Santa Ana, CA: Optometric Extension Program Foundation, series 1 and 2, Oct. 1973–Sept. 1975.

Hoffman G. *Vision Therapy Manual.* Fullerton, CA: Southern California College of Optometry, 1984.

Kraskin R. *Visual Training in Action.* Santa Ana, CA: Optometric Extension Program Foundation, series I–III, Oct. 1965–Sept. 1968.

MacDonald LW. *Visual Training.* Santa Ana, CA: Optometric Extension Program Foundation, series I–III, Oct. 1962–Sept. 1965.

Richman JE, Cron MT. *Guide to Vision Therapy.* South Bend, IN: Bernell Corp., 1988.

Rosner J, Rosner J (1988). *Vision Therapy in a Primary-Care Practice. Procedures Manual.* New York: Professional Press.

Schrock RE. *Introduction to Vision Training.* Santa Ana, CA: Optometric Extension Program Foundation, series I and II, Oct. 1965–Sept. 1967.

Schrock R, Heinsen A. *The Schur-Mark Out-of-Office Vision Training System.* 3rd ed. Davenport, IA: Keystone View Co., 1966 (out of print).

Swartwout JB. *Manual of Techniques and Record Forms for In-Office and Out-of-Office Optometric Vision Training Programs.* Published by VisionExtension, Inc. 2912 S. Daimler, Santa Ana, CA 92705, 1991.

Wold R, Getz DJ, McGraw L. *In-Office Vision Therapy Manual.* Books 1 and 2. Los Angeles, CA: A-V Scientific Aids, 1974.

Directory of Vision Therapy Equipment Distributors

Academic Therapy Publications
20 Commercial Blvd.
Novato, CA 94947

American Optical Company
14 Mechanic St.
Southbridge, MA 01550

American Vision Training, Inc.
1558 E Port Ct.
P.O. Box 197
Cicero, IN 46034

Bernell Corporation
750 Lincolnway East
P.O. 4637
South Bend, IN 46634-4637

Biofeedtrac, Inc.
57 Hicks St.
Brooklyn, NY 11201

Clement Clark, Ltd.
3128 D E. 17 Ave.
Columbus, OH 43219

Creative Therapeutics
155 County Rd.
Cresskill, NJ 07626

Educational Developmental Laboratories
P.O. Box 210726
Columbia, SC 29221

GTVT
18807 10th Place W
Lynnwood, WA 98036

Instructional/Communications Technology, Inc.
10 Stepar Pl.
Huntington Station, NY 11746

J.W. Engineering
8 Dike Dr.
Wesley Hills, NY 10952

Learning Frontiers, Inc.
190 Admiral Cochran Dr.
Annapolis, MD 21401

Manico/Bloomington
418 E. 17th St.
Bloomington, IN 47408

Mast/Keystone
4673 Aircenter Circle
Reno, NV 89502

Optometric Extension Program Foundation
2912 S. Daimler St.
Santa Ana, CA 92705

Pacific Prisms
P.O. Box 700
Rexburg, ID 83440

Dr. Jack Pierce
School of Optometry/Medical Center
University of Alabama at Birmingham
University Station
Birmingham, AL 35294

Alfred J. Poll, Inc.
40 W. 55 St.
New York, NY 10019

R.C. Instruments, Inc.
1558 E. Port Ct.
P.O. Box 109
Cicero, IN 46034

Stereo Optical Co.
3539 N. Kenton Ave.
Chicago, IL 60641

Synthetic Optics Corp.
1600 Parker Ave.
Fort Lee, NJ 07024

Titmus Optical Co.
P.O. Box 191
Petersburg, VA 23804

Michael Tyner, O.D.
555 Brookwood Village
Birmingham, AL 35209

VTC Enterprises
3408 Acadia Ct.
Bloomington, IN 47401

Wayne Engineering
1825 Willow Rd.
Northfield, IL 60093

Dr. Michael Wesson
University of Alabama at Birmingham
Sparks Center for Developmental and Learning Disorders
1720 Seventh Ave. S.
Birmingham, AL 35233

Index